HSM 510

ETHICAL CONSIDERATIONS IN HEALTH CARE DELIVERY

CALIFORNIA COLLEGE FOR HEALTH SCIENCES
222 West 24th Street
National City, CA 91950

Published by:

California College for Health Sciences
222 West 24th Street
National City, CA 91950

ISBN 0-933195-23-0

FROM THE AUTHOR

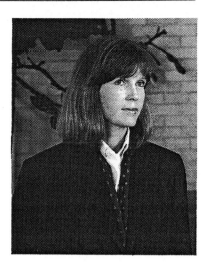

I've read and thought and written about ethics in the
care of patients. I'm a nurse and I know the reality that
good patient care is the basis of ethics. I'm a lawyer
and I know the reality that ethics is the basis of law.
Most important, I am a cynical person from the "show
me" state. I wrote this course-text to teach people to be
skeptical of ethical authority and to make ethical
decisions for themselves.

Jacqulyn Hall, RN, JD

Table of Contents

INTRODUCTION

SEX AND GENDER

You will see the word gender confused with the word "sex." Squeamish as you may be about saying it, the correct term for the difference between males and females, men and women, is their SEX. Gender is the word for the pronouns used in speech or writing, as in "Susie had her hair cut." Use of the pronoun "her" is the gender. Susie's femaleness is not her gender, it's her sex. As for gender in this course, we will use "him" and "her" and "his" and "hers" and "he" and "she" whenever it occurs to us, without pattern.

USING THE WORD: "PATIENT"

We will use the word "patient," not "client." First, everyone knows what the word means. Second, to use another word is a futile attempt to change the relationship. If we are to change the relationship with, or to, patients, we must do that, CHANGE THE RELATIONSHIP—not merely change the name.

Maybe use the word "client?" The word "client" signifies a person who is a dependent, on a higher-up patron. I don't believe that is the relationship you have with people you take care of, so we won't use "client."

The root of the word "patient" comes from a word for suffer, endure in latin. The words "compassion" and "compatible" are from the same root. They mean to suffer with, to feel with. The patient suffers—endures; and we suffer and endure with her.

Recently I have heard practitioners use the word "customer." We devoutly hope that our nurse feels differently about us than the sales clerk at the store does. The word "customer" comes originally from a customs-gatherer, toll-gatherer, tax collector. None of those words describe the relationship we have with patients.

This course will focus a lot on the words we use. Words are the only way we can communicate meanings to each other.

It's Illness Care

In this course we will not (except when we forget) use the term "health care." Most of us care for people who are <u>ill</u>. People who are healthy can take care of themselves. Some practitioners work at preventing illness. They may care for well babies and mothers, people who are healthy now. But healthy people get care only because they are in some way at risk of becoming ill.

Examples Are Going To Be Simple

Some of the examples will seem easy. The answers will be obvious. I could use harder examples, where the answer is not so easy, where the arguments come out even on both sides. But I think you need to be able to do simple stuff before you can handle more complex situations. You don't start teaching blood gases with a case where the blood gases are mixed acidosis and alkalosis.

Most ethics cases <u>are</u> easy. Most of the time, things pretty much go right. You can figure out the right thing to do. It goes without any big conflict or hassle. It is the hard cases, the edges of what is right, which attract the writing and thinking and abstract pondering of ethicists.

Thanks

I owe a lot to the RT's I've known and consulted with, and the nurses, and lab techs, and pt's and doctors and administrators and secretaries, too, who work in the care of patients. Incredible, wonderful people, like you, who are in it for a lot more than the money. And that "more than the money," <u>plus</u> the money, is what ethics is about. Thanks to you all.

HSM 510

ETHICAL CONSIDERATIONS IN HEALTH CARE DELIVERY

COURSE POLICIES

COURSE/TEXT OBJECTIVES

Upon successful completion of this course, you will be able to:

Discuss philosophical views reflecting views of the world as ideal, and real.

Distinguish between law and ethics.

Define terms and concepts often encountered in the ethics of patient care.

Recognize the values underlying all ethical issues.

Discuss current ethical issues in illness care in four areas:

1) A Time to Be Born
2) Professionals and Employees
3) Share of Care
4) A Time to Die

Express feelings clearly and articulate informed opinions about ethical conflicts.

Recognize and describe the effect of your personal feelings on thoughts and actions.

ABOUT THE COURSE

Who needs this course? Why are you taking it? Of course, for the credit, for the eventual degree, for the piece of paper that will qualify for the job. That's great. But the degree, and hopefully this course in bioethics in particular, will do more. It will be an unintended consequence.

Your intended consequence is that you'll have a piece of paper and a better job and more money and all that. The unintended consequence is that you'll be better educated. It isn't that you will act all that differently. You may even <u>do</u>, act, or behave, generally the same as if you didn't have this extra education. But now you will know why you act. You'll be more comfortable, content, happier with yourself. That's worth a lot, with or without a job that requires the piece of paper.

Having an education, a bachelor's degree, means more than a piece of paper; it sets up an expectation from other people that you have certain knowledge, that you have certain attributes, that you're a certain kind of person.

COURSE GOAL

What this course will do is teach you what the people who are talking about "ethics" are saying. It will teach you how to interpret the words they are using into plain English. It will teach you how the things they are talking about relate to practitioners.

Our hope is that you will be better prepared to think about these things, make up your own mind, and act on your own values. You may not act differently than if you hadn't had the course. But you will know why you acted and on what values, and you will be happier with your action.

By the act of taking this course and reading these words you demonstrate that you are someone out of the ordinary, so we assume that you'll make a difference in illness care. Right now, working to help people as you do makes a big difference every day in some life. We assume that you may make even more of a difference in the future.

Taking this course, eventually getting this degree, will have intended consequences for you. What you don't know about are the unintended consequences. After the degree, you will limit yourself more. You'll be more specialized. For example, having the degree may cause you to limit your work to administration. Then there will be fewer kinds of jobs you'll take. You'll be less limited in some ways. You will be eligible for those kinds of jobs in many more different agencies and locations. The unintended consequences may be enormous.

PROCEDURES

Each unit will have objectives and study questions listed at the beginning of the unit to give you some idea of what's coming. Be thinking about the questions and answering them as you complete the unit. After completion, compare your answers with possible answers given at the end of the unit.

Remember that in ethics, there is usually no wrong or right answer. Be able to defend your answer. Write out what you would say if someone asked why you wrote what you did. Put down why you think your answer is the right answer.

TESTING AND STUDENT EVALUATION

UNIT EXAMS

This course has five (5) "open-book" Unit Exams and a proctored "closed-book" Final Exam. The Unit Exams are located at the end of each module of this course. Mark your answers to the Unit Exam items on the enclosed Scantron forms and submit them to CCHS. We will send the results to you in a timely manner.

When completing the Unit Exams, you may use your textbooks and other available reference materials for assistance. It is important that you put forth your best effort when you take the Unit Exams because **the score you receive will be used in calculating your course grade.** *You will not be given an opportunity to improve your grade by retaking the exam.* Since these exams are open-book and untimed, you have an opportunity to check and double-check your answers. You should NOT send in the Scantron forms until you are confident you have answered all test items correctly.

You will not be able to schedule your Final Exam until you have *successfully completed* all of the Unit Exams. Successful completion means that you have submitted a Scantron form with at least 90% of the items answered correctly. In the event that you do not correctly answer at least 90% of the items when the exam is submitted initially, you will need to correct your errors and resubmit the answers to all items on a new Scantron form. The purpose of this requirement is to help you succeed on the Final Exam. Because the Final Exam is closed-book and proctored, we feel that the effort you exert in correcting your errors will increase your likelihood of success on the Final Exam.

NOTE: Keep in mind that the purpose for correcting your errors on the Unit Exams is to ensure your understanding of the course material before you take the Final Exam and that the corrections will not affect your Unit Exam scores. Therefore, we strongly encourage you to make certain that your original answers are correct in order to help you earn a good grade and to avoid the necessity of resubmitting your test answers prior to scheduling your Final Exam.

FINAL EXAM

The Final Exam is a 100-item multiple choice test that will be administered by an approved proctor. The proctor is to verify that you have completed the exam without the aid of study materials or outside assistance of any kind. You have the responsibility for identifying someone who is willing to proctor your exam and for gaining approval of the person identified. (See "Selection of a Proctor" below for further details.)

GRADING

Your grade for the course will be determined by your performance on the Unit and Final Exams. The exams will be weighted as follows:

Unit Exams (10% each)   = 50%
Final Exam   = 50%
Total   = 100%

Letter grades will be assigned only at the end of the course. Successful completion of the course requires an overall score of 75% or better. The following scale will be used to determine your course grade:

A	=	94-100
B	=	88-93
C	=	81-87
D	=	75-80

CREDITS

Upon successful completion of this course, you will receive three (3) semester units of college credit.

SELECTION OF A PROCTOR

At least one month before you expect to take your Final Exam, you should identify someone to serve as a proctor. The proctor should be a responsible individual who has no direct involvement with you, either personally or professionally. The following individuals qualify as CCHS proctors: hospital administrators, Director of personnel/human resources, Director of education, librarians, counselors, or school officials. Once you have identified someone, complete the enclosed Final Exam Scheduling Card and send it to CCHS. You and your proctor will need to schedule the exam at a time that is convenient for both of you. The exam will be sent directly to your proctor who then administers the exam and submits your responses to CCHS for scoring.

DO THESE EXERCISES FOR EACH UNIT

Exercise: Write a case of your own describing an ethical conflict you have observed from your experience or have read about in the newspaper, or have seen on television. Analyze it by the STOP, LOOK, LISTEN, AND STOP method given in Unit 3. Present the case and your analysis to a group at work or to some individual you respect.

Exercise: Write a letter to the editor of a newspaper, a professional journal, or to your legislator (state or federal). Analyze a problem in the Unit of the course that you are currently working on. Propose a solution for the problem. Hold the letter until after you finish this course. See if you've changed your idea, and how. Revise it if needed, and MAIL IT.

REFERENCES

Throughout the course I will not footnote, but you will be able to find information on the topic discussed in the References. In formal writing, all facts or quotes obtained from a source must be put in a reference in a footnote or endnote. There will also be Resources listed. In formal writing, these are sources you can use to learn more about a subject generally. They haven't been specifically referred to in the text.

A lot of the references and resources in this course are from medical journals. These journals discuss the same issues as the bioethics journals. Many are written by the same writers as the journals on medical ethics and bioethics. The advantage to you is that you may be able to find them in your agency or hospital library if it's large enough. If not, your local branch librarian can usually hook up with a medical school library in your state to get you the article free. Or you can contact the medical school librarian yourself. Librarians are another helping occupation. Like lawyers.

ABBREVIATIONS USED IN REFERENCES:

JAMA: Journal of the American Medical Association
AIM: Archives of Internal Medicine
NEJM: New England Journal of Medicine

Here are some places you can write directly if you're interested in more information. Remember, every piece of information you get in ethics has a built-in bias. Ethics is an art, not a science.

National Reference Center for Bioethics Literature
Kennedy Institute of Ethics
Georgetown University
Washington, D.C. 20057
1-800-MED-ETHX
1-202-687-3885
FAX: 1-202-687-6770
(established 1971)

A bibliographic BIOETHICS database produced here is available on-line through the National Library of Medicine's MEDLARS system. The Center produced and has available Scope Notes on several specific bioethical issues, such as Maternal-Fetal Conflict.

The International Directory of Bioethics Organizations, available from the above center, lists one or more organizations for bioethics in 25 states in the U.S. and 25 countries.

Midwest Bioethics Center
410 Archibald, Suite 200
Kansas City, MO 64111

Institute of Society, Ethics and the Life Sciences
The Hastings Center
360 Broadway
Hastings-on-Hudson, New York 10706
(established 1969)

Scholl Institute of Bioethics
2606 1/2 West 8th Street
Los Angeles, CA 90057-3810
(213) 382-2156

ADDITIONAL REFERENCES:

American College of Physicians. *Ethics Manual*, available from *Annals of Internal Medicine*, Subscriber Service Division, American College of Physicians, 4200 Pine Street, Philadelphia, PA 19104. And printed in *Annals Int. Med.*, 1984; 101:129-37, and 101:263-74.

Anderson, Gary R., Glesnes-Anderson, Valerie A. *Health Care Ethics.* Aspen, Rockville, MD, 1987.

Beauchamp, Tom L., Walters, Leroy, Eds. *Contemporary Issues in Bioethics.* Wadsworth, Belmont, CA, 1995.

Cassell, Eric J. *The Place of the Humanities in Medicine.* The Hastings Center, Hastings-on-Hudson, NY, 1984.

Guidelines on the Termination of Life-Sustaining Treatment and the Care of the Dying. The Hastings Center, Hastings-on-Hudson, NY, 1984.

Halverson, William H. *A Concise Introduction to Philosophy.* Random House, New York, 1981.

Halverson, William H. *Concise Readings in Philosophy.* Random House, New York, 1981.

Hayek, F. A. *New Studies in Philosophy, Politics, Economics and the History of Ideas.* University of Chicago Press, 1985, Chicago.

Monagle, John F., Thomasma, David C. *Medical Ethics.* Aspen, Rockville, MD, 1988.

Ross, Judith Wilson. *Handbook for Ethics Committees.* American Hospital Association, Chicago, 1986.

Waymack, Mark H., Taler, George A. *Medical Ethics and the Elderly.* Pluribus Press, Chicago, 1988.

REQUESTING HELP

If you have any questions about how to proceed through the course, or regarding any CCHS policy or procedure, the easiest way to get help is to use one of the Request for Help Forms included at the end of the course material.

DISCUSSION OF TERMS AND DEFINITIONS

BIAS, SELF-INTEREST, AND SELFISHNESS

Bias

A lot of people write in the field of ethics. All of them, your teacher, too, have personal biases, particular views of the world, certain sets of assumptions. And our writing reflects that bias, world view, assumption. You should be able to detect the biases in this course. You can detect the biases of others, also. For example:

> *"A morally good community is one whose common commitments are grounded in something other than self-interest and meet criteria of moral validity." Pellegrino, Edmund D., "The Medical Profession as a Moral Community," Bulletin of the New York Academy of Medicine, Vol. 66, No. 3, May–June 1990, pp. 24-35.*

Dr. Pellegrino has written more on the place of the humanities in medicine than perhaps any other contemporary thinker. And you can see that he's written from the view of the world that self-interest is not a good, moral position. He writes with the assumption that self-interest is not the highest good. He assumes that moral validity demands something more than self-interest. He has a bias about self-interest. He might never say it was a bias; he believes he is speaking truth.

Self-Interest

I have a bias in favor of self-interest. I, like Dr. Pellegrino, believe that my bias is the truth. Enlightened self-interest serves us best. Self-interest enlightened means self-interest that is fully informed about the consequences of choices to be made.

Self-interest is the only real motivation for human beings. Whenever it appears that we act in other than our own interest we are expressing self-interest in a different way. Donating a kidney to one's sister? Self-interest in preserving the family, the good opinion of others, the good opinion of one's SELF. Self-interest in expressing love of the sister, the wish to have her around.

Self-interest is not the same as the bad connotations of selfishness. We often put other's interests ahead of our own, but we do so for a reason that will ultimately benefit us, even if no more directly than we will have a better world to live in. This is why cooperation, not competition, is the theme of human history. Working together, people have always accomplished more than working alone or against one another—to the good, the self-interest, of each and all.

People's self-interest is not just about economics, unless you expand the meaning of economics to include all human action and desires. It's a part of self-interest to want to live in a peaceful world, a world with enough for all, a world in which all can achieve some measure of success, however they define that.

So I disagree with Dr. Pellegrino on the above statement. A morally good community (that's a load of value terms) cannot exist outside the self-interest of each, of all. The strongest effort for good (defining good quickly as peace and plenty) can be had when each is acting in his self-interest. That self-interest is to benefit all so that each gains. That is how humans work.

We choose to obey laws, volunteer our time, our money, work longer hours, charge less for our services, put our patients before ourselves, take care of other people the way we would want to be cared for. Because somewhere not so far down in our consciousness we know that we are not so tough, so big, so strong. We could have been born like someone else, or we could lose our job or get sick.

We act as though this world is a place where the weak are safe. We work to make the world like that. Then when, or if, we become weak, we'll be safe, too.

Selfishness Is Good for Everyone?

There is also a theory, first written down by Dr. Bernard Mandeville in the early 1700's, that actual selfishness, not just enlightened self-interest, is good for everyone. It goes like this: People who act in their own self-interest, however selfish it seems, are in one way or another indirectly or directly benefitting all others.

For example, say you "selfishly" buy a uniform for a cheap price, made by a poor person working in a factory. Some people say this is exploitation of the workers, and urge you not to buy such things.

But say you ignore this advice and buy the uniform. If enough people do so, the worker will get paid to make more. He'll be paid more money for each uniform, too, as they are more desired by you and your selfish friends. The "unselfish" person does not get the uniform at a low price. If she is successful in her efforts to keep you from buying the uniforms, the worker will not be hired to make any more. There will be no more demand for the uniforms. The "unselfish" person will bask (unselfishly?) in the glow of her goodness.

References: Mandeville, Bernard. *The Fable of the Bees*. Oxford University Press, 1924.

Hayek, F. A. *New Studies in Philosophy, Politics, Economics and the History of Ideas*. University of Chicago, 1985.

LIMITS TO ETHICS AND LAW

Humans are wonderful creatures. We can arrange our lives nearly any way we want—NEARLY.

There are some limits on our behavior toward each other and ourselves. We don't know them in advance, only when they start to get us into trouble. For example, we can walk anywhere we want, theoretically. But when we walk out onto the lake or ocean we discover the physical limits of our ability. So too, there seem to be limits to the ways that we can arrange our relationships with other people.

We can call this religion, or Natural Law, or Natural Rights, or moral imperatives. There are a few things that are constant in all those systems. They all say that it is wrong to kill, to steal, to lie, to hurt other people. The bioethical issues we discuss in this course all come back to these "shalt nots" and how we apply them to our work with people who need our help.

FREEDOM TO MAKE MISTAKES

There are limits, but we have to discover them for ourselves. We seem to do the best when all of us have the freedom to get ourselves into trouble. Of course we would like to protect ourselves and others from ever getting into trouble. And we do to some extent. For example, we pass laws to make everyone wear seat belts.

We would rather protect people from the bad consequences of their actions. Unfortunately the control necessary to keep them out of trouble causes more trouble than the bad consequences of their freely chosen actions would.

If we could and did protect people from all the consequences of their actions, they would never learn what reality is, what humans can and cannot do. The central planning of the economy in the Sovlet Union is a good example. When the factories made poor shoes, they never "learned" that there were consequences to making poor shoes. They went on making bad shoes and the shoes never got any better.

Protecting people from their mistakes is a natural tendency for parents, and practitioners who take care of other people. It's not an evil thing, but it just doesn't work. People learn about reality from making mistakes. People have to learn about reality to survive. You have to learn that you cannot walk on the water, or you'll drown.

INTENDED CONSEQUENCES

We act rationally to achieve intended consequences. We can usually see pretty well what the intended consequences will be. For example, Massachusetts lawmakers intended that the elderly people in their state should get cheaper medical care. They required all the physicians in the state to accept Medicare patients for a minimum payment. To keep their licenses, the doctors could not bill the patient more than Medicare would pay.

UNINTENDED CONSEQUENCES

The problems come with the unintended consequences of our actions. We can never know with certainty what these will be. In Massachusetts, the Medicare-covered people got cheaper care, as intended. But the unintended consequence of the law was that many physicians left the state. Instead of cheaper care, some of the people received no care.

See the section in Unit 5, Professionals and Employees, for a discussion of this example.

LEARNING FROM OTHERS' MISTAKES

We can estimate what some of the unintended consequences of our actions will be by using our own and other people's experiences. That is why we study history. We can see how other people acted and what the unintended consequences of their actions were.

It helps to know what the outcome of the Massachusetts law was, so that we don't make the same kind of mistake in other states. By examining others' experiences, we can make better estimates of the unintended consequences of our actions. We can make those consequences better, or not so bad.

We can extend what we learn from others. Learning from Massachusetts: If all states would require practitioners to accept minimum payments for Medicare, there would be no advantage to leaving for another state. We'd have them. Or would we? We know what the practitioners did in that situation. And we can imagine that if the requirement were burdensome enough, at some point an unintended consequence of our scheme would be that many would leave the occupation. They might go to law school! We can't force them to stay in practice—the 13th Amendment of the Constitution prohibits involuntary servitude. We can think of the unintended consequences, to some extent, when we use experience that others have already gained.

Reference: Von Mises, Ludwig. *Human Action*. Yale University Press, New Haven, 1949.

UNIT ONE

Chapter One
Why Bioethics?

Objectives

Upon successful completion of this chapter, you will be able to:

1. List two consequences of taking this course.

2. Describe what the course will do for you.

3. Give one reason practitioners study ethics.

4. Define "bioethics."

5. Define "ethics" in terms of a concept or construct.

6. Restate, in your own terms, how words come to represent real things and actions.

7. Identify the limits of the course.

8. Describe what is not the goal of the course, and what is the goal of the course.

Study Questions

This is not a test. Read the study questions before you begin the chapter. Answer them as you go along or after you finish the chapter. Then look at the suggested answers at the end of the chapter to see if you agree with the answers.

1. What are two consequences of taking this course?

2. What will the course do for you?

3. What is one reason practitioners study ethics?

4. What is bioethics?

5. What is ethics? Is it a "real" thing?

6. How do words come to represent real things and actions?

7. What are the limits of the course?

8. What is <u>not</u> the goal of the course, and what <u>is</u> the goal of the course?

WHY STUDY BIOETHICS?

Why study bioethics? Isn't it enough that you're technically good at your job? Why not just do what you're told? You may not be able to change decisions in some cases no matter what your own ethics. It seems many people get along fine without a course in ethics. What is this going to do for you?

Ethics is part of the "liberal arts" like philosophy, literature, art, history. The reason to study ethics is the reason you study any of them. Dr. Edmund Pellegrino, influential writer on the subject of humanities in medicine, gives you a reason:

> *"The liberal arts are attitudes of mind, not disciplines or bodies of knowledge. They have since classical times been those intellectual skills needed to be a free man—not only in the political sense, but more critically in the sense of being free of the tyranny of other men's thinking and opinions, free to make up one's own mind and take one's own position. The liberal arts comprise those skills most commonly associated with being human—the capability to think clearly and critically, to read and understand language, to write and speak clearly, **to make moral judgments**, to recognize the beautiful, and to possess a sense of the continuity between man's present and inherited past."*

Pellegrino, Edmund, in Cassell, Eric J. *The Place of the Humanities in Medicine.* The Hastings Center, Hastings-on-Hudson, NY, 1984, p. 30.

ILLNESS PRACTITIONERS USE ETHICS MORE

Practitioners who care for sick people, face more difficult and immediate conflicts than people in other jobs. The people we care for are weak and unable to fend for themselves. They have less information or knowledge than when they need other services.

If you take your car to the mechanic, you're usually walking upright and not dependent on him to save your life. The lawyer you hire can usually explain your legal situation pretty quickly in lay language. But a patient may not even be conscious, and may be totally dependent on your action. And his care and condition may be so complex that he has to rely on you to take actions he could never understand.

Most of you are at both undergraduate and professional study levels. You should have the opportunity for a systematic exposure to ethics, equivalent to at least one semester. That's what the experts say. The ideal is a separate course in ethics, and that's what you've got here. Nearly every medical and nursing school in the U.S. teaches ethics in one form or another.

Lawyers typically study ethics for at least a semester. They do not study ethics as a subject. They study the particular and specific provisions of their code of ethics, the rules of professional responsibility. These rules are not ideals to be adopted voluntarily. They are rules that lawyers must follow or risk discipline and possible loss of their licenses. You will learn more on codes of ethics in Chapter Five, Professional Employee.

ETHICS IS A CONSTRUCT

Bioethics is simply ethics applied to biology. Ethics, like law, philosophy, sociology, religion, history, or science, is a construct, or a concept. These examples are all artificial divisions to help us think about things. We make up, conceptualize, or construct these divisions to help us organize and classify the things we think about and act upon.

Ethics is a concept, like any other idea that is not something that can be touched or seen. Concepts exist only in our minds. They mean only what we mean when we think of them.

For example, "health" is a construct. What really exists are people that we agree to label "healthy" or buildings with the word "health center" on them, and people with name tags that have the word "health care worker" on them. But "health" is just a word. The word origin is "whole, hale, hearty." And "health" (like ethics and bioethics) is just a concept, not a touchable, seeable thing—neither are ethics nor bioethics.

Health is at least the absence of illness. Many writers and the World Health Organization (WHO) say it is more than that. They say health means a wholeness, using the origin of the word, a more positive image.

The World Health Organization definition states: "Health is a state of complete physical mental, social well being and not merely absence of disease or infirmity." That is an ideal state. No real person ever has been or is likely to be healthy under that definition. It is an example of Plato's Ideal Type (see Chapter Two, View A, Imagine the Ideal). No individual could be more than a shadow of health, a poor image of the ideal.

Reference: WHO's Basic Document: Preamble to the Constitution of WHO in Gillon, Raanan, "On Sickness or Health," *British Medical Journal*, 1986; 292:318, 319.

Diseases or conditions are treated as if they are real entities, when in fact they are conceptualizations. But, you say, surely we can measure blood sugar and diagnose diabetes. You lab techs should know that in the old days they tasted the urine for sugar.

Is high blood sugar the same as diabetes? What is diabetes? It's a concept again, a way to organize our thinking about something. It's a collection of symptoms and signs, of certain treatments, certain outcomes we have decided on. There are continual changes; we invent new diseases all the time. See discussion of Persistent Vegetative State in Chapter Six, "A Time to Die."

Psychosomatic illnesses all existed. "Psycho" means mind; "soma" means body. Which illness that we treat now do you think will be classed as psychosomatic in the future—as not "real?" These usually are real to the individual. They are not faked. As an example, hysteria has been a real disease since the middle ages. Now it's in such disrepute that even the name (hysterical) suggests a malady based only on emotion. *Hysteria* is the Greek word for uterus. Women were "sick" because they had uteruses.

Hysteria disappeared about the time of psychoanalysis. The theory is that when doctors referred these patients to psychiatrists, the validity (value) of their disease disappeared. If it isn't in the body, it isn't "real." That's still a prevalent attitude among practitioners.

Are hypoglycemia and total allergy disease psychosomatic? Perhaps a certain percentage of people are susceptible genetically to psychosomatic diseases. Perhaps they have something real after all. They have "psychosomatic disease syndrome."

Reference: Shorter, Edward. *From Paralysis to Fatigue: History of Psychosomatic Illness in the Modern Era*, The Free Press, 1991.

Mental "health" is a particularly slippery diagnosis. Note the inappropriate use of the word "health" again. We are not talking about mental health, but mental illness. Often there are no measurable things to diagnose from, as there are in physical medicine. Psychiatry is on the edge of medical science, between science and the social sciences or philosophy.

The potential for abuse is great. For example, in the old Soviet system, if you didn't like communism, you were crazy and sent to a Soviet mental hospital. Now, if you like communism, you are crazy and sent to a Russian mental hospital. What if you don't like to wear clothes, and you want to live on the street? You're crazy and you go to an American mental hospital. What if you don't want surgery that might save your life? You're declared "incompetent" and might be forced to have it.

Reference: Szasz, Thomas, "The Myth of Mental Illness," in *Contemporary Issues in Bioethics*, Tom Beauchamp and LeRoy Walters, Eds., Dickenson Publishing Company, Belmont, CA, 1989, pp. 110-14.

"ETHICS" IS ONLY A WORD

"Ethics" is a word, and words mean only what we all agree that they mean. By using it in different ways, we change the meaning of a word constantly, a little, until it may mean something entirely different than before.

One of the animals said to Alice (in the Wonderland), "I can make a word mean anything I want. The question is, who's to be the master? The word, or me?"

That's an independent attitude. If you use words as something other than what people think they mean you'll be constantly explaining in other words what your "special" word means. We are doing some of that in this course, with "illness care," and with "share of the care" (see Chapter Four, Share the Care). There is a limit to how we can change the words we use and still communicate, which is the function of language.

Words have no meaning in themselves. They have meaning only as long as they refer to things that we can then construct in our minds. For example, when we read or hear the word "tree," we "see" in our minds a woody thing with leaves. That is, we see it if we have been taught that connection as children or in language class.

People who speak only Spanish merely hear a strange sound when you say "tree." What do you think when you hear the word "arbol?" You may have learned that's Spanish for tree, so you think of a woody thing with leaves. People in the Midwest just hear a funny word, "arBOLL." They don't think of anything, except that you've said a strange word.

People who speak English, have agreed that the word "tree" refers to the thing (woody with leaves).

THINGS TO THOUGHTS TO WORDS

Even if we change the words we use for something, if the thing we speak about is the same, the meaning to us will be the same. If we use the word "terminate" instead of "kill" we may be confused or distracted temporarily, since we are not familiar with the word. And we may then think the word refers to something different.

But when we realize that in both "terminate" and "kill," the patient dies, the meaning to us will be the same. The picture in our minds will be the same whether we hear the word "terminate" or the word "kill."

Eventually we find out that when we changed the word we did not change the thing. From "graveyard" to "cemetery" to "memorial park," we changed the words. We did not change the thing—a place where dead people are buried. Using "baby" instead of "fetus," changing "unsound mind" to "incompetent" to now "incapacitated;" none of those changes of words has changed the reality of the people described.

Reference: Crookshank, F. G., M.D., F.R.C.P., "The Importance of a Theory of Signs and a Critique of Language in the Study of Medicine," in *The Meaning of Meaning*, Ogden, C. K., Richards, I. A., Eds., Harcourt, Brace & World, New York: 1959, pp. 337-55.

AMERICAN BIOETHICS

American Bioethics for practitioners is the subject of this course. Ethics is the concept of "doing the right thing." We assume Spike Lee doesn't own that phrase. We further limit our subject by defining bioethics as doing the right thing relating to biology. Further limiting our subject is doing the right thing by practitioners of illness care. The practitioner limit means we'll discuss things that are relate to people who work in caring for people with present or potential illnesses.

By limiting the subject to American bioethics, we can focus on issues most important to us in this country. There is much we could learn from other cultures, other religions, other countries. We have a limit on time and space. We leave you, the student, to explore those for yourself if you're interested.

This course was created especially for California College for Health Sciences, instead of requiring a book that was written by someone else. No single textbook on bioethics or medical ethics that we examined spoke as clearly as necessary. What follows is a distillation of what the major thinkers and authors in bioethics have to say, with explanation and some analysis.

THE GOAL OF THE COURSE IS NOT

The goal of this course is not to make you a "moral" practitioner. That can be defined only by you.

The goal of a lot of ethics courses is to increase morality. The morality is defined by the instructor. If the goal of this course were "to increase morality," it would be the teacher's kind of morality that we'd want to increase, not yours.

We're not "moral" enough to foresee all the different situations that you are going to encounter, or to anticipate how you should act in each one. You are already as ethical as you are able to be.

An "ethical" person is a human being like us who wants the best for self, without hurting anyone else. What really does teach "ethics," or right behavior, is experience. With experience we can see the intended consequences and some of the unintended consequences of our acts. Your experiences are more valuable in teaching you about right behavior than any course in ethics can be. What you gain with experience is greater ability to anticipate the consequences of your actions, the intended and un-intended consequences. Allowing abortion on demand will produce one desirable intended consequence, freedom. Freedom, autonomy, is one of the highest values we have for patients and ourselves. Abortion on demand allows the freedom of women to bear children or not. But the unintended consequence may be that people will abort more female (girl) babies, or homosexual or handicapped babies. See Chapter Three, A

Time to Be Born, for discussion of the issue. That unintended consequence, of fewer females born, fewer homosexuals, fewer handicapped, may not be what we wanted.

THE GOAL OF THE COURSE IS

The goal of this course is to give you some information about bioethics. You can use that information, with what you already know, to work on problems in illness care. You know better than anyone how difficult the problems are. Let's get you informed, and working on the problems!

References: *The Teaching of Ethics in Higher Education*, A Report by the Hastings Center, Hastings-on-Hudson, New York, 1980.

The Place of the Humanities in Medicine, Eric J. Cassell, M.D., The Hastings Center, New York, 1984 quoting Pellegrino from "The Humanities in Medical Education, *Mobius* 2:133-41, 1982.

Teaching Ethics in the Health Care Setting, Coutts, Mary Carrington, Kennedy Institute of Ethics, Washington, D.C., September 1991.

STUDY QUESTIONS WITH ANSWERS

These are suggested answers. If you have something like these answers in your own words, consider yourself successful. If you have more (quality, not quantity) than these answers, consider yourself excellent.

1. What are two consequences of taking this course?

   • You will have more credits toward your degree.
   • You will better understand your actions.

2. What will the course do for you?

   The course will help me understand my actions better. In adding credits toward my degree, the course will help me realize some of the intended and unintended consequences in getting the degree.

3. What is one reason practitioners study ethics?

    The people who practitioners care for are more dependent on the goodness, the rightness, the ethical behavior of practitioners than in other fields.

4. What is "bioethics?"

    "Bioethics" is biology applied to ethics.

5. What is "ethics?" Is it a "real" thing?

    "Ethics" is doing the right thing. It is a construct or a concept, something in our minds.

6. How do words come to represent real things and actions?

    People use words, and the things are pictured in their minds. People to some extent agree that the words represent the things.

7. What are the limits of the course?

    The course is limited to ethics for practitioners of illness care in America.

8. What is _not_ the goal of the course, and what _is_ the goal?

    The goal of the course is _not_ to make the practitioner a more ethical or moral person. The goal of the course _is_ to give the practitioner information she can use to make her own ethical decisions.

SELF-TEST

This is NOT a unit exam, and it is NOT to be sent to CCHS for scoring. This is a practice test to prepare you for the unit exams that will follow each of the remaining chapters of this course. However, in order to get the most out of this practice test, you should take it without looking at the text materials. The answers can be found at the end of the test, and if you missed any questions you should review the course material to see why you were wrong.

1. One consequence of having taken this course in ethics is:

    a. You will be more ethical.
    b. You will have fewer credits toward your degree.
    c. You will better understand your actions.
    d. You will be an ethicist.

2. What is one reason practitioners study ethics?

    a. They are more ethical.
    b. The people they care for are more vulnerable.
    c. They want to be more ethical.
    d. Ethics is a required subject.

3. Define bioethics.

    a. The ethics of mineral things.
    b. The ethics of plant things.
    c. Biophysical meta-ethics.
    d. Biology applied to ethics.

4. Define ethics.

    a. A concept; doing the right thing.
    b. A measurable concept; doing the right thing.
    c. A science of meta-ethics.
    d. A physical entity; doing the right thing.

5. Choose the correct statement about how words come to represent things and concepts:

    a. People agree the word "means" the thing pictured in their minds.
    b. People make up words and convince others the word means something different.
    c. Committees decide which words mean what things.
    d. People can change actual things by changing the words that represent the things.

6. The goal of this course is:

    a. To make you an ethical practitioner.
    b. To make you a more ethical practitioner.
    c. To help you practice more ethically.
    d. To give you information about ethics.

NOTES

Answers:

1. C; 2. B; 3. D; 4. A; 5. A; 6. D

CHAPTER TWO
WHICH BIOETHICS?

OBJECTIVES

Upon successful completion of this chapter, you will be able to:

1. Describe three issues in recent American bioethics that are still issues.

2. Imagine and describe a bioethical conflict that predates written history.

3. List three professions important in the development of bioethics in America.

4. Realize that bioethical problems arise from, or result in, conflict between people.

5. Describe your personal feelings about contemporary ethical conflicts.

6. Define "metaphysical" as not physical.

7. Know that ethics is part of the metaphysical, not physical, world.

8. Define "ethics" as custom.

9. Describe the current German attitude toward bioethics and state the reason for the attitude.

10. Identify two views of the world as 1) ideal, and 2) real.

11. List five philosophers who more nearly represent the view of the world as "Ideal."

12. Quote Descartes' words by which he believed he proved his existence by thought alone.

13. Identify five philosophies related to the view of the world as "Ideal."

14. List two philosophers identified with the view of the world as "Real."

15. Identify five philosophies related to the view of the world as "Real."

16. Describe in your own words that no person has a philosophy or view of the world that is totally either "ideal" or "real."

17. Identify the local library as a resource for information on philosophy.

18. Understand that there are only seven values in bioethics.

19. Define "beneficence" in bioethical terms.

20. Identify a self-interest that practitioners have in being beneficent to patients.

21. Describe an example of paternalism in patient care.

22. Identify one reason that practitioners seem less paternalistic at present.

23. Identify the phrase "first, do no harm," as <u>primum non nocere</u>.

24. List one self-interest that practitioners have in being nonmaleficent.

25. Describe in your own words that the values of beneficence and nonmaleficence cause professional codes of ethics to suggest continuing competence and continuing education.

26. Identify malpractice as the legal remedy available to the patient who is harmed by a practitioner who fails to be beneficent, or who is maleficent.

27. Define "patient autonomy."

28. Describe an example of relative, not absolute, autonomy.

29. Identify conflict between provider and patient as the situation in which discussion of patient autonomy is likely to occur.

30. Identify the practitioner's self-interest in valuing autonomy.

31. Describe the relationship between autonomy and individualism.

32. Identify what is represented by the scales that a statue of Justice holds in her hand.

33. Identify the controversial concept associated with the word "justice."

34. Give an example of the concept of "equality" under distributive or social justice.

35. Describe what can happen if social justice is applied to illness care.

36. Define Rawls' Original Position.

37. Describe the principle that Rawls believes would result from the Original Position.

38. Define the Knowledgeable Position.

39. Identify one self-interest practitioners have in the value justice.

40. Identify the self-interest practitioners have in distributive or social justice.

41. Identify at least one value in the list of values that is protected by the U.S. Constitution.

42. Describe the benefit to the individual and to the system from the value of veracity.

43. State in your own words why the word "consent" does not need the word "informed" in front of it.

44. Describe what you think is the purpose of veracity.

45. Imagine a conflict that you as a practitioner might experience with veracity relative to a patient.

46. Describe the practitioner's interest in the value of veracity.

47. Identify one of the basic human relationships that underlie the value of fidelity.

48. Describe the relationship of the fidelity value to the idea of confidentiality.

49. Identify the self-interest inherent in fidelity.

50. Speculate on what might be the result as we deal more with strangers in our lives.

51. State your view on whether you think the value of life is absolute or relative, and why.

52. Identify the self-interest in the value of life.

53. Quote the Nazi phrase used to justify killing people.

54. Distinguish how withdrawing treatment from terminally ill or PUP's is different from what the Nazis did.

55. Define the conditions under which we consider a patient's quality of life.

56. Define "quality of life."

57. Describe how the Quality Adjusted Life Years measurement works.

58. Identify the value usually hidden, but always present, in bioethical conflicts.

59. Identify the economic system in which work is exchanged for work.

60. Identify the medium used to exchange work more easily, more freely, with more people with more and different goods and services.

61. List some of the common ideas from the text that are identified with work/money.

62. Identify the self-interest of the practitioner in the value of work, aside from your own money and work.

63. Define "law."

64. Distinguish ethics from law.

65. Describe why we must use caution when told something is ethical, or has ethics.

66. Discuss the distinction some people make between ethics, morals, and values.

67. Differentiate between what some authorities call "moral reasoning" and "ethical practice."

68. Describe Kohlberg's theory of moral development.

69. Indicate why feminists dispute Kohlberg's theory.

70. Describe concerns about theories and tests of morals or ethics.

71. State the occupations of the members of the ethics committee in your agency.

72. Describe how members are selected for your ethics committee.

73. Describe how ethics committees relate to courts of law.

74. Answer whether your ethics committee does the following:
    - Sets policy
    - Provides education
    - Initiates case investigation
    - Receives requests from any person for consultation
    - Does case consultation
    - Has patients or family present for discussion
    - Has an ethicist on staff
    - Has a physician consultant
    - Decides DNR orders over family disagreement

75. Describe how the Danforth Amendment affects ethics committees.

76. State whether your agency has an Institutional Review Board and an AIDS committee to review the work situation of practitioners who are HIV positive.

77. Disagree or agree with the following statement and explain your position: "An ethicist is an ethical person who has a Ph.D in ethics and who has no bias."

78. Identify the highest value in the two methods of bioethical conflict resolution given.

79. List the steps in the conflict resolution process described in this section and explain each step.

80. Describe the purpose of the courts.

STUDY QUESTIONS

This is not a test. Read the study questions before you begin the chapter. Answer them as you go along or after you finish the chapter. Then look at the suggested answers at the end of the chapter to see if you agree with the answers.

1. What are three issues that were issues in recent American bioethics that are not issues now?

2. What is an example of a bioethical conflict that predates written history? Imagine and describe.

3. Which are three professions that have been important in the development of bioethics in America?

4. What is an example of a bioethical problem that did not arise from, or result in, conflict between people?

5. What are your personal feelings about the Nancy Cruzan case (feeding tube removed from young woman diagnosed as being in a Persistent Vegetative State); or the Clarence Thomas—Anita Hill hearing (Supreme Court Justice Candidate accused of sexual harassment by Law Professor)?

6. What is the meaning of "metaphysical," using two words?

7. Is ethics part of the physical or metaphysical world?

8. What is the definition of "ethics," in one word?

9. What is the current German attitude toward bioethics? What is the reason given for it?

HISTORY

The Egyptian living 2000 years before Christ examined the stump of his leg. "That damn doctor is a quack. If I'd had good treatment I wouldn't have lost my leg. There should be some system to compensate me for my loss. The government ought to do something." The government did. It had a schedule of payments to compensate patients injured by physicians, a cross between malpractice insurance and workers' compensation.

Every generation believes that the world began when it was born. We are no different. Reading the current literature, it would seem that bioethics was discovered in the last 40 or 20 or 10 or 2 years, depending on the writer's age.

RECENT HISTORY

The last few years of bioethics history is instructive. We have changed what we worry about. And we will change again. We still worry.

We used to worry about who would receive kidney dialysis. When the taxpayers started paying for everyone who needed it, presto, no more ethical problem. What if we stop paying again? (See the British limits and the Diagnostic Related Group problems in Chapter Four, Share the Care.)

Organ transplantation across species was at one time a big topic. Remember Baby Fae, the baby who "experimentally" received a baboon's heart? With the use of bone marrow from primates and organs from pigs, the issue arises again.

Not many years ago, many people were domiciled in mental hospitals. We debated the ethics of calling them "dangerous" and forcing them into the institution. Now they are on the streets. No more ethical problem? No, now the question is whether it is ethical to force them to accept housing. Some states have laws against "abuse" which include definitions of "neglect." Yes, you can "neglect" yourself and be forced into an institution for care.

They get less publicity, but forced institutionalization and treatment for self-neglect or dangerousness are still ethical issues. Some people, such as severe manic depressives, who are prone to mental conditions that will be subject them to forced hospitalization.

Serious suggestions have been made that these people should write a "living will." This living will, which is different than the one explained in Chapter Six, A Time to Die, indicates while they are "sane", what they would wish to happen when they are "insane" again.

Reference:　　Chodoff, Paul. "Involuntary Hospitalization of Mentally Ill as a Moral Issue," *American Journal of Psychiatry*, 1984; 141:3, pp. 384-89.

Another ethical issue that has come back is the definition of death. "Brain death" was accepted as the answer some years ago. Now a new definition, "persistent vegetative state," is being advocated. See the issue in Chapter Six, A Time to Die.

The ethical issue of whether the patient could be denied the treatment she wanted, because it was not "good" for her, came up years ago. People with cancer wanted to have therapy with laetrile, an extract of apricot pits. The federal government sought to protect them from what was considered useless and possibly harmful therapy. Then several states passed laws allowing their citizens to use laetrile. End of ethical issue?

No, the issue of the patient's ability to have the treatment she wants, regardless of harm, continues with silicone breast implants. If the evidence is that the implants cause side-effects in a minority, should the majority be denied the implants—even if they know and accept the risk? Another controversial drug involving ethical issues is RU486, the French abortifacient. (See Chapter Three, A Time to Be Born, for discussion.)

LONGER HISTORY

Looking at history, we can see that conflict about doing the right thing with sick people has been going on since records have been made and doubtless before recorded history, if we can speculate from the behavior of aboriginal people. We can easily imagine a scenario in a tribe of hunters. A sick individual is either to be carried and cared for, or left to die. We can imagine the discussion between two carriers—and the carried.

We have records of early peoples who feared children born that looked different from the tribe, or children born as twins. They were killed at birth. The degree of "difference" of individual babies must have been debated. The mother of the baby may have had something to say. The Greek philosopher Plato recommended that children born handicapped or inferior in some way be left to die. That is not so far from the issue of fearing a Downs syndrome baby, and aborting before birth.

We can contrast that with evidence from prehistorial America. Some archeological studies show that aboriginal peoples in America held certain values, certain ethics. Skeletal remains have been found of a child born with spina bifida, with the spinal cord exposed; these children are very difficult to care for even now with our high technology. The remains show that the child lived to be a teenager, indicating a high degree of care for a "different" child.

These ethical problems are not new. The conflicts now are not different in principle, only in detail. The technology is better. We can do more for people than ever before, and sometimes we do more than they want. The issues of who lives, who dies, who is considered a human being with rights and protections . . . these are not new. We have talked about them since we have been able to talk.

We have written about them, too. Realize that this is an enormous topic, with an immense body of literature written about it. A lot of the writing has been done recently, within the last 10-20 years. There are many experts. They build on others' thoughts, adding their own. They don't have all the answers. In a subject that is a concept, one that is not measurable, no one has the answers for anyone else.

We can learn from each other. We learn from the experiences we have had and from other's experiences. That is the value of reading the literature. That is the value to you of taking this course—to know other people's ideas about ethics.

BIOETHICS IN AMERICA

Bioethics in America is a development of law, religion, and medicine. We didn't always have practitioners of those occupations in this country. In 1728, William Byrd, a prominent official and landowner in Colonial Virginia, said:

> *The New Proprietor (of New Jersey) inveigled many over by this tempting account of the Country: That it was a Place free from those 3 great scourges of mankind, Priests, Lawyers and Physicians. Nor did they tell a word of Lye, for the people were too poor to maintain these Learned Gentlemen.*

We've come a long way, baby?

Reference: Ebert, Robert H., "The Medical School," Scientific American, *September 1973, p. 139.*

ETHICS IS ABOUT CONFLICT

You will usually hear the word "ethics," in connection with conflict between people. If we all agree on what the right thing is to do, no conflict exists. There will be no discussion of ethics. We don't discuss whether it is ethical to treat a 40-year-old (otherwise healthy) man for his first heart attack. We all agree that it is the right thing to do.

We do talk about "ethics" when we discuss whether we should treat vigorously a 90-year-old demented man for long-standing congestive heart failure. In that case, we do not agree on what is the custom, the right thing to do.

You might hear that "values are in conflict here." Values are not in conflict with other values. People with values are in conflict with other people, who have different values.

People do not have much internal ethical conflict. They quickly prioritize their conflicting interests, and have one interest as a priority.

People act in accord with their interests. That's how you tell what their interests are—by what they do. You can tell what a person's values are by her actions. Not by what she says she believes, but by what she does. If she says she values her profession, but she's never joined the professional association or read about it or been to a meeting, then you know she really doesn't value what she said.

In any conflict situation, and especially if it is labeled an ethics conflict, look to see who the people involved are, and look to see what their interests are. If the government has an interest in some ethical problem, think further. The government is a shorthand way of saying "the people in a group."

The government is a construct, too, not a "real" thing. Notice that the government does not put you in jail for tax evasion; the Sheriff, a real person, does. In the Missouri Supreme Court's Cruzan decision, the justices said the state had an interest in keeping Nancy alive. The state's interest could have been in her as a taxpayer (she wasn't) or a soldier (she couldn't). Finally, they said the state (we) had an interest in protecting the life of a person who couldn't protect herself. An increasing interest of the government (us) and the people who work for us, is to reduce cost. Look for that interest every time in an ethical conflict.

Other people with interests are always in the ethical conflict. The patient most of all has an interest, or her "surrogate decision maker" does if she's incompetent. Her family will have interests. Her practitioners have interests. The hospital has interests. Her priest or "ethicist" has an interest too; don't assume that this person has no personal interest, that he or she is a neutral person.

Religion was the basis of ethics in the past. Much of what we call "ethical" behavior still is reflected in religions. Religions are deontological systems, prescribing rules for conduct. (See the discussion, "View A people," below.) This religious base of ethics and association with ethics is so strong that some newspapers who before had pages for "Religious News," now say "Religion and Ethics" (such as the St. Louis Post-Dispatch).

"ETHICS" IS PERSONAL

Some people say they don't feel emotion about things ethical. They can think purely and abstractly about what is the right thing to do. Some say that this is a "higher" or better way to be, without emotion. These are Type or View A people.

Others (Type Bs) believe ethics is personal. We decide how we feel about an issue—what should be done—by how we react personally. When the Nancy Cruzan case was being decided, people reacted according to how they projected themselves into the case.

You may have said, "I wouldn't want to live like that." You may have been in favor of whatever action would allow her to be relieved of her existence. Or you said, "I wouldn't want them to kill my sister." In that case, you were for whatever principle would protect her life.

Either way, you identified, or felt at one with, someone in the situation. You felt with Nancy, or her parents, or her nurses, or yourself, imagining you were one of the people in the situation. In effect, you projected yourself personally into the situation.

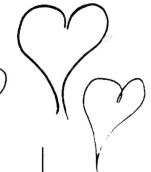

The same happened in the Clarence Thomas—Anita Hill hearings. Either you identified with Thomas, as a victimized Supreme Court nominee who felt wronged by a vindictive woman opposing you for your beliefs. Or you identified with Hill as a victimized employee who felt compelled to come forward with the truth at a critical moment. The depth of feeling in these cases can come because people feel personally involved.

People who demonstrate in favor of abortion rights, or in opposition at abortion clinics, feel personally about the issue. They are not issues of calm distant reason. They affect us personally. We believe we have been or could be in the same kind of situation, or we empathize with people who are.

It is good to be logical and not more emotional than necessary. It would be nice to think logically. We don't have to get lost in the emotion. But it helps to realize that the emotion, the bias, is there and that it motivates us in one direction or another. Once we recognize what our emotion is, we can think reasonably about the issue. We can see if what we feel is a good idea, for us as individuals or for us in the large group.

I may be emotional about reporting what I see as a violation of patient autonomy. Once I realize that it's emotion and think about the consequences to the patient and myself and the agency, I may or may not decide to report the incident.

You may emotionally feel that we should allow abortion or euthanasia. After thinking about the consequences, you may realize some limit on those activities is good. Or, you may emotionally feel that abortion and euthanasia should be forbidden. After thinking about the consequences, you may realize that some allowance for those activities is good.

Either way, you have to feel first, then recognize and acknowledge your feeling. My analysis of the Cruzan case started out as personal feeling. I heard all the logical arguments for and against removing her feeding tube. I realized I didn't want Nancy killed because I had taken care of so many like her. To say her life was without value was, to me, to say that my work for all those people was without value, too. Now I recognize that was emotion, and I still feel it, but I also realize why I am more likely to listen to and agree with arguments against euthanasia.

ETHICS IS PHILOSOPHY AND CUSTOM

Philosophy is a word for love of learning; "phil" means love, and "sophy" means learning. Philosophy for a long time, until after the middle ages, included all of knowledge. Science was part of philosophy, too. Only in the 1400s was "natural philosophy," or science, separated from "moral philosophy," which is all the rest of knowledge.

The humanities (history, art, literature) were included in philosophy, as was ethics, law, and religion. The early divisions of psychology and the social sciences were part of philosophical studies too. That was before their practitioners decided it was more prestigious to be included with medicine in the "hard sciences" such as physics.

All of knowledge that rests on belief and can't be measured is called "metaphysics." Aristotle called it in Greek, meta ta phusika, meaning "after or beyond, the physical things which are Nature." Anything that is not physical is metaphysical.

Reference: Partridge, Eric. *Origins: A Short Etymological Dictionary of Modern English*, Greenwich House, New York, 1983.

The origin of the word "ethics" comes from the Greek ethike tekne, the moral art. In Latin the word becomes "ethos," or "character." Adopted into English, it means "character and spirit of a people, or custom."

Our ethics are our customs. When we say something is not ethical, we mean it is outside our custom. The United States is a plural society; we have people with many different customs here. Because of that it is sometimes hard to say with certainty exactly what our custom, our ethic is in a situation. We may have to tolerate the idea that there is not one "right" behavior for all situations.

GERMAN ETHICS?

But we may find that some actions are outside what we want to be the "American custom." We can decide what that should be. Some actions are outside all human customs. The German National Socialist custom or ethic seems to have been to kill Jews and priests and labor leaders and gypsies and Poles.

But because individuals or groups have killed, stolen, oppressed, does not mean that is their custom. The Nazis did not really have a "custom" or ethic of genocide, or they would have done it openly, proudly, as a value of the German people.

The Nazi years still affect what happens in Germany now. There's a lesson for us here. Bioethical discussion reminds the Germans now of the Nazi slippery slope of human life values. Germany has an anti-bioethics movement. They will not hear discussion about euthanasia or withholding treatment from handicapped children.

They vow never again to question anyone's right to life. This is the view of both right- and left-wing groups. The society has developed a deeply rooted taboo against evaluating the worth of human life, because of what happened there 50 years ago.

They have prevented speeches by a writer on ethics, Peter Singer. He supports "preference utilitarianism," which is actively ending the life of severely disabled newborns if the parents request it. German opponents argue that Singer's position is murder. They call it "deadly ethics," and say that there is no right to free speech for a murderer's talk. Such speech is not within desired academic freedom either; they oppose rational discussion about life. They believe if one can rationally analyze life, it is possible that one can come to the same conclusions the Nazis did.

Reference: Schone-Seifert, Bettina, and Rippe, Klaus- Peter. "Silencing the Singer: Anti-Bioethics in Germany," *Hastings Center Report*, November-December 1991, pp. 20-26.

STUDY QUESTIONS

1. What are the names of the two views of the world, to be described in the text?

2. Who are five of the philosophers who represent the View A "Ideal" world?

3. What are the words of Descartes, by which he believed he proved his existence by thought alone?

4. What are five of the "isms" or philosophies related to the View A "Ideal" world?

5. Who are two of the philosophers mentioned in the View B "Real" world? (Realists don't get their names on philosophies as much as idealists.)

6. Which are five of the "isms" or philosophies related to the View B "Real" world?

7. What is your view of the world? Is it totally either "ideal" or "real?"

8. Where can you go to get more information on a certain philosophy (should you want it)?

TWO VIEWS OF THE WORLD

Again, ethics is a subdivision of philosophy. Your ethics, your belief in what is the right thing to do, **comes from** your own personal philosophy. That is your idea of what life is all about. You need to understand some philosophy to know where ideas come from. These same philosophies or ideas are the basis of action for other people, whose actions affect your life, including your life at work as a practitioner, and your life as a citizen of this country.

What follows is a very short and simplified framework of major ideas and philosophers in Western history—that is, the Western world as distinct from the Eastern philosophies, not Western as in cowboys and abo-Americans. This will be just enough to get you by when a discussion or article on ethics mentions of one of these people or concepts.

These ideas are all discussed as they relate to bioethics in America in the late 1990s and early 21st Century. If you encounter other terms (and you will), and if you are interested, you can look them up. The major encyclopedias in your branch library will be of help, and especially good if you find it is the *Dictionary of the History of Ideas*, Scribners, New York, 1973.

I'm going to describe two ways of looking at the world. One view is "Imagine the Ideal." The other is "Describe the Real." We will tie all the major philosophies and philosophers into one or the other. All ideas which are not listed are variations of one view or the other. There are no new ideas in the world, and there probably won't be until new kinds of humans are made.

If you're a student of philosophy you will know I've taken great liberty with specifics here. If you're a student of philosophy you probably didn't need this course. People taking this course need a short sweet augenblick, which is German for a little glance. If you are someone interested in the specifics of philosophies and philosophers through history, excellent books await you in the library. But this short view will get you through most ethical discussions.

See if you're more of a type A or a type B.

VIEW A: "IMAGINE THE IDEAL"

This view of the world is best represented by **Plato**, the Greek philosopher who lived about 200 B.C. In this view, people are perfectible, or at least society is. In a structured, ordered system, **a utopia**, people are educated for their use to society. Things get ranked and put into a hierarchy. Some things, values, or people are better than others.

Thinking is better than feeling, reasoning better than emotion. Be a Rationalist, not a Emotionalist. People who think are superior to people who do. Don't deal with cases (particulars) go for the big picture -- the generalization (the ideal). Use **deduction**, the process of taking the big idea and applying it, or deducing to the particular example or case involving your patient. Start with a big theory and then think down to the application of the idea in the real world.

Everything evolves. **Evolution** means things get better; stuff progresses inevitably from stage to stage. Darwin didn't invent this, he just applied it to species differences. And **Marx** then applied it to governments, that capitalism evolves to socialism to communism, the planned utopia. He would be confused to see Eastern Europe now.

We find this in technology; we tend to believe that every new machine is better than the old, though sometimes machines merely have more bells and whistles. Later in this chapter, you will also see this idea of hierarchy, of evolving and bettering and getting higher, in the idea that morality develops.

You have probably studied the progression in psychology of **Maslow's** hierarchy of needs, from physical to safety to love to "self-actualization." You recognize in it his use of the idea that some "needs" are higher than others, that as the needs evolve, basic ones are met and people get "better."

Another totalitarian and collective system, **fascism,** also envisioned an ideal, utopian world. The German National Socialist constructed an ideal world occupied by a pure, superior, Aryan <u>volk</u> (people) and worked toward that. When we discuss genetics and abortion for genetic reasons, we have to consider whether an ideal like this is at work.

Hobbes, an English philosopher of the 1600s, developed the ideal government along the idea of a body analogy. The workers were the legs, the government was the brain (the <u>government</u>?). Some bureaucrats and legislators believed that they were appointed and elected because they were somehow smarter, knew better what to do than the people who put them in office. For example, the insurance clerk who knows better than the practitioner whether a patient's treatment was necessary.

To focus on the ideal is to be indifferent to the physical world—like the **Stoics** in ancient Greece. Their idea was to live only for virtue (good) and to avoid vice (evil). Be tough, be a man, be a queen. Keep a stiff upper lip. If you can't change the world, bear the pain with grace. Focus on higher values. A practitioner who puts his ideal view of his work above his need for a coffee break fits this description.

Rene **Descartes** (pronounced day-<u>cart</u>), a Frenchman of the 1400s, was also of view B. He said the mind and body are dual, separate, "I think, therefore I am." The mind exists independent of the body. The mind, not the body, is the person. A physician on a panel discussing Nancy Cruzan (brain damaged, body not) testified for Descartes when he said "She's not a person."

Idealists would say that you can know something by just figuring it out in your mind, without seeing or touching it or by any other sense experience. **A priori** (ah preeORY) is Latin for knowing something prior to, before any experiment or knowledge of the senses, just by reason. See <u>a posteriori</u> (ah postEERYory) in View B for the opposite. Religious people, philosophers, and some ethicists are big on <u>a priori</u> thinking. Scientists use mostly the opposite, in View B.

When <u>a priori</u> reasoning is applied to bioethics, it means you can know what is right by reasoning about it, by thinking about it a lot. That is, without finding out any facts or doing any research. You could think about it and figure out whether people wanted to be resuscitated.

Emmanuel **Kant** was a philosopher who believed that it was possible to do this. His name is associated with the "Categorical Imperative", which states that you should judge every act you do by whether you would choose the same behavior for everyone in the world. His later followers were Hegel, Engels, and eventually Marx. His philosophy flowed from stoicism, the idea of living for virtue. When you are tempted to skip the breathing treatment for the uncooperative patient, and chart it anyway, Kant would have you consider the categorical imperative.

Kant's categorical imperative has loaned its power in philosophical circles to a new term or two. You'll hear "moral imperative" and "ethical imperative." The word **"imperative"** means something that has to be done, about which there is no choice, no debate, no differing point of view. When someone tells you something is a moral or ethical imperative they mean you don't get to argue about it—they're right and that's that.

The word "imperative" is predictably from the word "imperial," as in Emperor, Imperial. The moral imperative would have us all moving toward a dream of fulfilled human potential to attain a supportive community of peace, justice, and freedom in a sustaining natural environment, a utopian ideal. Advocates believe humans need an ideal, something more than the material world to live and strive in. The problem comes when the ideal is imposed, creating an imperative for people who do not share it.

The Categorical Imperative sounds somewhat like the Christian "Do unto others as you would have them do unto you." Christian thought is View A, valuing the ideal over the real. Christianity advises turning the other cheek, living for the reward of virtue or afterlife. Material things are unimportant or less important than spiritual ones.

Deontology means using rules instead of experience to decide what is right. (Of course the rules may have been developed from much experience.) It means adhering to a set of rules or ideal values. We do a thing because it's the rule, God said so. You might refuse to pull the plug on a patient because the ten commandments say Do Not Kill. (See the opposite, Teleology, in View B.)

Jacques **Rousseau**, a Frenchman of the 1700s, believed the ideal was the "natural" state of some unspoiled time. The noble savage was the ideal human. Rousseau wrote that under an ideal social contract, we all make a deal with each other to live together harmoniously. Romanticism, the idealization of emotion and an ideal world of nature, is closely related.

Natural rights or natural law is a principle of justice that some philosophers say can be known just by logic, **a priori**. That means you can discern the law just by thinking about what it should be, without considering experience. This philosophical principle developed as the influence of religion declined in Europe (called "the enlightenment"—see Humanism under View B).

Natural law replaces and in many instances mirrors the tenets of Christianity. It purports, however, to be human law instead of God's law.

Since it is not written down, it may be determined only by reference to what one believes is "natural." This principle was fully developed by the time of the Revolutionary War. The United States Declaration of Independence states: "We hold these truths to be self-evident; that all <u>men</u> are created equal and endowed by the Creator with certain <u>inalienable rights</u>, among them life, liberty and the pursuit of happiness." (Emphasis added.)

The courts have used the concept of natural law when no written law was available to use, to mandate the result they desired or felt necessary. In years past, "liberal" justices of the U.S. Supreme Court used natural law; lately a "conservative" justice endorsed the concept (Justice Clarence Thomas, nominated by President Bush and confirmed in 1991).

"Liberal" is a word whose meaning has changed from that of its use 100 years ago. As it was used then, the word would describe the opposite of what a "liberal" is considered now. The terms "liberal" and "conservative" and "right-" and "left-wing," are not very helpful. An individual with one label may hold a number of opinions that vary from that label.

You will hear "natural law" and "natural rights" invoked when any group or person wishes to bolster its desire for some action with an appeal to law. This is especially so when there is no written law mandating the action these people want, and the group wants some law to be written.

For example, the pro-choice side in the abortion debate insists that the right to choose to abort a fetus is a natural right of women, even if not written specifically in the Constitution. Thus we must not pass laws that prohibit abortion. On the other side, the pro-life side insists that a child before birth has a natural right to life, even if that isn't written specifically in the Constitution. Thus we must pass laws to prohibit abortion.

If the Devil can quote Scripture from the Bible for his purpose he can quote natural law as well. Which side, if either, is the Devil in this issue? (More about abortion later in Chapter Three, Around Birth.)

VIEW B: "DESCRIBE THE REALITY"

Aristotle, the Greek (what else) philosopher who lived before Christ, best represents View B's emphasis on the real world instead of an ideal in the mind. He was a student of Plato's, but had quite a different philosophy. He strove for the middle, the "golden mean" (or average). He sought to avoid extremes, and advocated moderation.

The virtues (values) he advocated were temperance, prudence, and wisdom. All those values involved controlling your physical side (your appetite and passion) with your mind. Mind over matter. From these ideas come Freud's "id," the appetite; his "ego," human reason; and his "superego," spirit or passion. View B is big on reasoned behavior as is View A, but reason as applied to the real, not an ideal, world.

In this century, medicine relies more on Aristotle's philosophy. Scientists are more likely to describe the real world than to invent an ideal one. The social scientists, like, the sociologists and psychologists, are likely to construct worlds more like Plato's abstract ideal in View A.

Reference: Edelstein, Ludwig. "Platonism or Aristotelianism,"*Bulletin of the History of Medicine*, 1933; vol. 7, no. 6, pp. 757-69.

Existentialism is a philosophy more in harmony with view B. Camus (pronounced ka-moo) is a name you will hear associated with it. This idea is that human existence is the basis for all ideas, that humans and their individual existence come first and are the only reality. Building on Descartes' words, this view is more like, "I am, therefore I think." If you think your patient is, exists, as only what you can see and touch, you're more like an existentialist.

Immediately, you can see that also in View B are the philosophies of humanism and individualism. Humanism says that humans are the paramount creatures in the world, as opposed to God. This idea of humanism has been rediscovered several times, from the Renaissance (rebirth) in Italy in the 1400s, to the enlightenment -- the dramatic times around the American and French revolutions of the 1700s.

The idea of **individualism** means that the individual is more important than the collective, the society. Anything with society or socialism related to it is more likely related to View A above, the ideal. That's because ideas are in the abstract, while people are real. Individualism has been an important philosophy in the United States. If you value the autonomy of your patient above all other values (see below), that is part of the philosophy of individualism.

The philosophy of **Utilitarianism** comes under view B. It's based on the idea that actions are not good or bad in themselves, only as judged against their outcomes (their utility). Good actions are those that gain the greatest good for the greatest number of people. In some sense it is the opposite of individualism (see below). Advocates would argue that the probability is that any one individual will be better off if this were the philosophy of the society.

When planners, government analysts, or epidemiologists consider the effect of any given act on the whole population, they are considering its social utility; its usefulness to the whole society.

Do the interests of the individual and the society conflict? They may if planners forget that the society is a construct (a concept) for a group of individuals. The society is individuals. There is no "society" in the sky, only a group of people here on earth.

As an example of utilitarianism: Oregon by adopting its Medicaid revision, spends the taxpayers' money for immunizing many children, rather than for bone marrow transplants for a few. Oregon hopes that many children will grow up healthier than they would have otherwise, while a few will die for lack of treatment. By prioritizing the care, they put a higher value on a longer life for a healthy child than any life for a sick child. (More about Oregon in Chapter Four, Share the Care.)

The greatest good for the greatest number is the thought underlying all cost-benefit analysis; when for example, screening a whole population for detection of cancer is proposed. The names most often heard in connection with utilitarianism are Jeremy Bentham, an English philosopher who lived in the late 1700's, and John Stuart Mill, also English, born in the 1800s.

Teleology is the opposite of deontology, which was described in View A of doing something because it is right. Teleology is the idea that we should do something because then things will come out the way we want them to, not necessarily because it's the right thing to do in the first place. Sometimes this attitude is criticized as "situation ethics."

Going from cases to bigger principles is called **casuistry**. The base of the word is "cases." It's the opposite of **absolutism**. The term also refers to the system of judge-made law in England and English-founded countries including Canada, Australia, India, Jamaica, and the U.S., in which a system of decisions in individual cases together comprise a body of principles or laws.

The term is used in a negative way suggest excusing people from the effect of a law you don't want to apply, on a case-by-case basis -- As in the pejorative use of "situation ethics." Critics of casuistry as a method of finding principles say that principles can't be gotten this way, because people change their principles depending on the cases.

This criticism implies that people wake up in a new world for each case. It assumes that they don't apply prior experience or learning from prior cases. A study of nurses showed that nurses with experience, not fresh out of school, were "better" at making ethical decisions. Experience was given as the 3rd most used source of 13 factors, for ethical decisions by RN students in a BSN program. Generic (non-RN) students in the same kind of program predictably put their reliance on experience in ethical decisions in 8th place. Since these students are likely to be younger than the RN's, their ranking of experience as a resource probably will rise.

Reference: Cassells, Judith M., and Redman, Barbara K. "Preparing Students to Be Moral Agents," *Nursing Clinics of North America*, 1989; 24:463-73.

Materialism falls under View B. It is the idea that what exists is not the ideal but the material, and that the highest value is not ideas but material things. A practitioner who values his car, his house, his income more than his ideals is adhering to the philosophy of materialism. Also under View B would come **Emotivism** and "Intuitivism". Emotivists use words to express real emotions, not to represent things abstractly or objectively. Intuitivists believe that your first "gut" reaction is a valid indication of the rightness or wrongness of an action.

"Determinism" is related under View B, and represents the idea that things are predetermined, that they will happen a certain way no matter what the circumstances. Some religions believe this. Look for this when issues of genetics and behavior come up. (See the discussion in Chapter Three, Around Birth, and Chapter Five, Professionals and Employee.)

Under View B would come research to find out what people think of Advance Directives, versus knowing what your patient thinks without asking him. That's the **empirical**, not the **theoretical**, view. An advocate of such research in bioethics is David Thomasma.

Reference: Thomasma, David C. "Empirical Methodology in Medical Ethics," *Journal of American Geriatrics Society*, vol. 33: 1985; 313-14.

This approach suffers the dilemma of all social science "research." It's done by questionnaire, asking people to give answers. People sometimes lie, or tell what they think the tester wants to hear. Often they can't anticipate what they'd do, or remember what they did, or care.

No matter what they say they'd do, studies constantly show that people change their behavior when confronted with a real situation. This is particularly true when people make "Advance Directives." (See the discussion on that topic in Chapter Six, Around Death.)

Induction was mentioned in View A as the opposite of Deduction. Induction is going from the case to figure out some big principles. In reality, we don't think specifically in one way or the other, but a combination. We always start with a case, with a problem, so then we induce to the principle above.

But probably we have heard or read of some principles; perhaps we've heard them in church or your mother said it or they are just in human's heads as part of the collective unconscious. If you've studied psychology you'll remember that was Jung's theme; he discussed the dreams that express the collective unconscious.

The theory of law most related to View B is **Positivism**, which states that we can only know about things that exist; that we can imagine only what is here and now. Applied to law, this means that the law is just what is written and nothing else -- not what it should be or could be.

After seeing the two views, you know that none of us is a total realist or a total idealist. The philosophies and philosophers included in one view or the other are there for convenience, arbitrarily grouped by the author. They more nearly represent ideas or reality values. We use the two views only to organize our thinking. You can see that your own personal philosophy, your view of what the world and life are all about, would be neither all View A nor all View B.

What Does That Word Mean?

You may hear or read about many terms in bioethics conversation that are not defined here. If the meaning is not obvious, it may not be very important. Experts usually know their subject well enough to explain it in pretty simple terms. They write so that nonexperts can understand their writing.

Some ethical terms are made up by the writer or speaker. You need to listen to them or read closely to find out what they mean by their words. Some of the terms may be in an ordinary dictionary. Some may have particular use just about ethics. You would have to go to a dictionary of philosophy or ethics.

Look it up

All these books have indexes, in alphabetical order. You know the ABC's! Some of the books have glossaries with definitions, too.

Use the library

The libraries are paid for with tax money—yours. Get some of your money's worth. Librarians are in a helping profession (like illness practitioners). Ask them for help.

Study Questions

1. Do you agree with the statement that there are only seven values in bioethics?

2. What is the definition of "beneficence" in taking care of patients?

3. What is one self-interest that practitioners have in being beneficent to patients?

4. What is an example of paternalism in patient care?

5. What is one reason that practitioners seem less paternalistic at present?

6. What is the old medical Latin phrase that means "first, do no harm?"

7. What is one self-interest that practitioners have in being nonmaleficent?

8.   What, in your own words, do the beneficence and nonmaleficence values cause professional codes of ethics to suggest?

9.   What is the legal remedy that the patient who is harmed has against a practitioner who fails to be beneficent, or who is maleficent?

10.   What is the definition of "autonomy" from the patient's view?

11.   Who, for example, is relatively, but not absolutely, autonomous?

12.   In what situation is a discussion of patient autonomy likely to occur?

13.   What is the practitioner's self-interest in valuing autonomy?

14.   How are autonomy and individualism related?

15.   What do the scales represent that a statue of Justice holds in her hand?

16.   What is the controversial concept associated with the word "justice?"

17.   Give an example of the concept of "equality" under distributive or social justice.

18.   What can happen if social justice is applied to illness care?

19.   What is the definition of Rawls' Original Position?

20.   What is the principle that Rawls believes would result from the Original Position?

21.   What is the definition of the Knowledgeable Position?

22.   What is one self-interest practitioners have in the value justice?

23.   What is the self-interest practitioners have in distributive or social justice?

24.   What is one value in this list that is protected by the U.S. Constitution?

25.   What is the benefit to the individual and to the system from the value of veracity?

26.   Why does the word "consent" not need the word "informed" in front of it?

27.   What is the purpose of veracity or free speech?

28.   What kind of conflict might you as a practitioner experience with veracity relative to a patient?

29. What is the practitioner's interest in the value of veracity?

30. What is one of the basic human relationships that underlie the value of fidelity?

31. What is the relationship of the fidelity value to the idea of confidentiality?

32. What is the self-interest inherent in fidelity?

33. What might be the result as we deal more with strangers in our lives?

34. What is your view on whether you think the value of life is absolute or relative, and why?

35. What is the self-interest in the value of life?

36. What is the National Socialist phrase used to justify killing people?

37. How is withdrawing treatment from terminally ill or PUP's different from what the National Socialists did?

38. What are the conditions under which we consider a patient's quality of life?

39. What is the definition of "quality of life?"

40. How does the Quality Adjusted Life Years measurement work?

41. Which is the value usually hidden, but always present, in bioethical conflicts?

42. Which is the economic system in which work is exchanged for work?

43. Which is the medium used to exchange work more easily, more freely, with more people with more and different goods and services?

44. What are some of the common ideas from the text that are identified with work/money?

45. What is the self-interest of the practitioner in the value of work, aside from your own money and work?

VALUES: SEVEN OR SO

There is an old myth that there are seven people in the world and you keep running into them, disguised and with other names. After you read ethics for a while, it will seem that there are only seven ideas in the history of the world, and that you keep encountering them. They go out, then come back into fashion.

The values that we define are like that. We will define seven of the most prevalent in bioethics for American practitioners now: autonomy, life, beneficence, nonmaleficence, justice, and fidelity. And one more may be silent but it is always there: work (money).

These are called principles, too, but they look more like things we value or want for ourselves applied to us. Inherent in all the values is our primary self-interest, discussed in Chapter One.

1. BENEFICENCE

The word comes from Latin; bene means "good," ficence means "to do or make." This is the idea that we act for the good (the benefit, the health) of another, our patient. This is in our self interest, too. As we do good for others we feel good about ourselves; we value ourselves. We believe we are seen as good people.

Practitioners adopt a system that places this value above all others in "professional" behavior. We also believe that helping people increases the odds that we may get help when we need it—"what goes around comes around," and all those related sayings.

With Beneficence comes paternalism. Pater means father in Latin. Paternalism connotes acting in a father-like or mother-like way toward our patients. The temptation is that because we are acting for the good, beneficence, of our patient, we know what is best for her. The patient's wishes come second.

Total paternalism ignores the patient's autonomy or freedom to choose her own action. The assumption is that to do good for our patients, we do what is best for them no matter what they want, because we know more about what they need than they do. We have the information; they don't, is the reasoning.

Practitioners are more careful about paternalism now; patients are refusing to trust practitioners to make decisions for them. That's different from the time when we all knew each other better. And, in another time people trusted and obeyed authority more. They did not insist so on their autonomy/freedom.

Also, practitioners are increasingly unwilling to take responsibility for another's choices. They see themselves not as trusted father or mother figures. They are technicians or advisors whose patients make their own decisions. This means the patient, not the practitioner, has responsibility for the decision.

2. NONMALEFICENCE

From Latin, non means "not," mal means "bad," and ficence means "to do or make." The value is to not harm the patient. If we can't help people, then at least we can avoid making them worse. This can be a real problem sometimes with the amazing things we can do to people.

There's a real risk in just coming to the hospital at all, considering the iatrogenic (provider-caused) illness possible. The old Latin medical saying is "Primum non nocere" (first, do no harm). Pronounce that "preemum non no-cherry" and nobody will laugh—unless they don't know how to pronounce classical Latin!

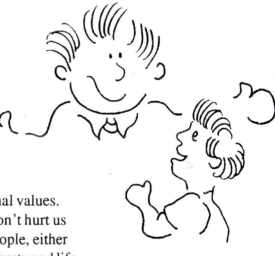

The self-interest here is the same as for beneficence. We'll feel good, be seen as good, adhere to our professional values. In particular, we hope that if we don't hurt others, they won't hurt us either. There are laws to punish people who hurt other people, either intentionally or negligently. Criminal prosecution costs liberty and life, and civil lawsuits cost psychic pain and money.

From beneficence and nonmaleficence come the mandates for the practitioner to provide competent care. Professionals are supposed to continue their education to keep their skills and to practice competently. These ideas come from the values of doing good for your patient and causing him no harm. As you will see in Codes of Ethics in Chapter Five, Professionals and Employees, most codes for professionals encourage continuing education and competent practice.

Also note that in theory the malpractice suit is a result of these two values, beneficence and nonmaleficence. The people through law wish to compensate the patient if the practitioner fails to do good. They may also wish, through malpractice suits, to punish the practitioner who harms.

3. AUTONOMY

Some writers rank this value first; they believe it is the most important of all. There is probably no absolute rank of these values in any given case, but we value freedom. Autonomy is the freedom to choose and act in your own life. Autonomy is the expression of freedom in the real world, the autonomy to decide and do what you want short of restrictions of the law and restrictions you have voluntarily assumed.

Autonomy is always relative, just as all values are. We don't allow people to do just anything they want to us or to other people. If that happened there would be anarchy, where only the temporarily strongest are safe.

Autonomy is not absolute. While you are a child, when you are declared incompetent, when a prisoner, in the military, in school, on the job, you do not have absolute freedom.

Autonomy is the value recognized in cases where the patient wants something different from what the practitioner wants. Otherwise there'd be no conflict, no reason to talk about autonomy. We rarely notice autonomy problems when at the grocery. We do notice them in the hospital.

There is self-interest here, too. You value such freedom, autonomy, control, power (synonymous with autonomy) for yourself, too. In a civilization (the opposite of anarchy) the only way you can have autonomy is to grant it to others.

As you saw in the View B philosophies, freedom or autonomy is the essence of individualism. The opposite of individualism is collectivism, which considers people only as members of a group (e.g., Communists and Fascists). Then the freedom and autonomy "belongs" to the group, not the individual. The philosophy of collectivism assumes that society (or the group) is a real thing that exists, not merely a construct of our minds.

4. JUSTICE

People should be treated fairly under the law. That is justice. The same process should be applied to everyone, without bias. The statute of justice has a blindfold, and she is holding a scale that can't be unfairly weighted. She treats all people the same; everyone gets a fair deal. The outcome does not have to be equal, but under justice, no one should be treated with bias, for or against her.

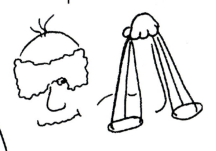

That meaning of justice is not the one is used in most discussions of bioethics. Equality of people in the legal process is not usually an ethical problem; at least we agree that it is to be valued. What is in controversy, is another use of the word "justice."

"Distributive justice" or "social justice" are concepts that have been around as long as socialism (and before that in the idea of a utopia). The equality of the outcome is the point in these concepts. In the area of race, for instance, equality of outcome is attained when there are blacks in school in numbers proportional to the people in the community who are black. If the proportion of women working for the company, is "equal" to the proportion of women in the town, that's social justice.

Basketball teams don't count.

Social justice is not completely compatible with autonomy/freedom. For instance, if all people have a socially just share of illness care, all will have equal shares. As it is now, there's an inequality. All people have access to care, but some cannot buy as much as others.
The answer from social distributive justice in that case is to redistribute. The only solution for keeping things equal is to limit access to care for people who can afford more. It would be necessary to prevent others with more money from buying more illness care. Their autonomy, their freedom, would have to be curtailed to that extent.

To achieve distributive social justice in health care, we would have to give everyone a share of the care. If distributive social justice is to be had, no person can have more care than any other person. Otherwise there will be more than one level of care, and that would be socially unjust. The concept is controversial.

John Rawls, a writer on the subject of social justice, suggests that we can imagine what the laws of society should be by taking what he calls the Original Position. Imagine that you are making laws for the society.

You are hidden behind an imaginary "veil of ignorance." You don't know what your "place" or rank in the society will be, so you make laws that benefit everyone in case you are in the lower "rank."

We see immediately that Rawls assumes there is a class or hierarchical system. Marx postulated such a "class struggle" a hundred years earlier. Rawls suggests that the morally correct laws made by one in such an Original Position would look like this: No one could work to get more than another, unless his actions would at the same time benefit the lowest member of society.

Remember the idea from Chapter Two that absolute selfishness also may benefit all other people. Rawls believes that he is truly objective in his development of this Original Position, as Kant also believed he was in proposing the Categorical Imperative.

Reference: Rawls, John. *A Theory of Justice.* Harvard University Press, Cambridge, 1971.

Practitioners take more of what I call a Knowledgeable Position every day. They know that someday they will be patients. They work to benefit their patients, knowing that if the system works, someone later will work to benefit them.

Our self-interest in Justice is that it keeps down the fighting. When people are not treated fairly they will eventually take to the streets. Each of us wants to be treated justly. The surest way to get that justice is to support and participate in a system that provides justice for all. That way you get treated justly, too.

The self-interest in social distributive justice is in an ideal—that no person will have less or more than another.

5. FIDELITY

Fide means "loyalty" in Latin. This value is about keeping promises, telling truth (veracity), and keeping secrets (confidentialism). Loyalty is important every time we have a professional/employer conflict. What should we do for a patient if he has a conflict with us or our agency?

The basis of fidelity:

We value our selves, family, our friends, our agency, our profession. By extension we value our patients more than "strangers." These are all "us," and "we," extensions of "me." Therefore they're more familiar, more valued. Our town, our school, our hospital, are all exhibitions of loyalty. Can techs do care as well as nurses? "Ah, but they're not **nurses** and we are." The whole union movement and related activity is built on this. Loyalty to the union, to the cause, to the sisterhood. Don't betray (what a word!) your sisters. This loyalty can conflict with loyalty to your patient, or employer, or the law. Even the words used in loyalty conflicts are loaded with emotion; as in tattle, rat, whistle-blow (See this part in Chapter Five, Professionals and Employees).

Truthfulness is another subdivision of Fidelity

Another word for this is veracity. Vera means "truth" in Latin. This part of fidelity is somewhat less often mentioned; it's hardly a controversy any more that patients should be told the truth. It's a "good" thing. Your mother told you to do it. The First Amendment protects it under freedom of speech.

When people tell the truth about things we get information about reality, about the world. We need that information to make decisions about our actions. What if the map maker is lying and we end up in the wrong town? What if the government official lies and we end up paying more taxes when we budgeted for less? "Read my lips."

When we get told the truth we benefit. What if the lab lied when we asked for blood chemistries? What if the RT doesn't do the blood gases, just draws and makes them up? The system breaks down if we can't rely on others to give us information. If we had to get all information for ourselves, we would accomplish much less.

Another piece of veracity in the patient business is consent. The term is sometimes modified with the word "informed." But consent is not valid, it's not consent, unless the person is informed about what he is consenting to. "Lack of consent" implies battery (unconsented - to physical contact) we are concerned here with "lack of informed consent." The law now requires that we not be paternalistic for our patient. We must tell her of the dangers her consent will subject her to. We not only should tell the truth, ethically; we are mandated to do so, or we risk legal liability.

More truth gives better information and a better outcome. The outcome is at least more likely to be based on reality. But more truth carries some risk. You have to be prepared to deal with the information you are seeking. For example, don't culture all the obstetrics department personnel for staph unless you know what you'll do with the information you seek. Know what you'll do if your staff has staph, or don't seek the information.

This better outcomes from better information is the purpose of promoting free speech. The First Amendment guarantee of freedom of speech is not just a vague ideal, meaningless by itself.

Truth-telling is a relative value (like all others). Some writers believe the protection of speech must be subject to furtherance of the goals of the society. Law Professor and English Department Chair at Duke, Stanley Fish, is a proponent of subordinating speech to the good of society. Problems: what is good, and to whose society? Which goals should the speech serve? This approach legitimizes propaganda. It gives free speech only to whichever group controls society.

Fish defends enforcement of Politically Correct speech. He believes that now conservatives control society so only their speech is free. Charged that P.C. rules chill speech, Fish replies that such speech as "nigger," "cunt," "kike," and "faggot" should be chilled.

Reference: Zubler, Todd. "Fish Tackles 'Free Speech,' Denounces Hatred," *Student Life*, Washington University, St. Louis, Missouri, September 13, 1991, pp. 1, 3.

The free speech issue concerns practitioners. Practitioners have had their licenses endangered for exercising free speech in telling patients of therapy that their physicians don't want them to hear. (See issues in Chapter Three, A Time to Be Born, and Rust v. Sullivan and Licensure in Chapter Five, Professionals and Employees.)

The criminal also law punishes lying, especially when lying is done to gain something from another. It's called fraud; that is, lying for gain. The law also imposes civil liability (and monetary remedies) for lying: In libel, slander, and civil fraud causes of action.

Those penalties alone make us have a self-interest in telling the truth. We benefit in other ways when we tell the truth. Others then see us as people to rely on for information that can help them. They turn to us, value us, and we are better off for that directly. We also participate in that bigger system of veracity that benefits us as well as all others.

Keeping confidentiality secrets is sometimes listed as a separate value, but it's related to fidelity. Confidentiality is hiding a truth; not telling a truth that could hurt. You know that truth, because the patient saw you as faithful (loyal) to him. He trusted you, trusted in a whole system to be faithful and loyal to him and to be "on his side."

The self-interest in fidelity must be evident. We take care of our own, they take care of us. For a long time in human history and prehistory, strangers were the unusual. They were dangerous.

Our world has changed. We must deal with strangers daily. We have to care for them without fear or hate. We cope with a society that is open, plural. We work not to hate or distrust the strangers.

Must we at the same time not be so loyal to our group? Can we stay loyal to "us," and still love the stranger? The German Nationalsozialismus, the "National Socialists" gave us the Nazis. Is patriotism, or love of country, something we will have to give up to live in a small world in peace?

6. LIFE

This value is also called sanctity of life; some religions teach that life is sanctified, or blessed by God. We are talking about human life here, not animal or plant. (See the research section in Professionals and Employees for that.) Many people adhere to an absolute value of life, of all life, whatever the condition or quality. Others think that life should not be valued or preserved at all costs. That makes the valuation of life relative.

Then life's value depends on quality or conditions. Quality of life is always subjective, meaning the individual herself has to decide what the "quality" of her life is. She personally has to decide how valuable her life is to her. When is life not valuable to a person? The same question: When is a person better off dead? People try to make the quality of life a number, like the weather forecast. The Quality Adjusted Life Years Scale is an attempt to make another person's quality of life objective, numerical, and impersonal.
In such discussion about life, we recognize instinctively that life is valuable, ours and other people's. If we don't value others' lives, our existence would be the temporarily strong dominating all others; war against all by all.

A group of people for whom life was not "sacred," most valued of all values, were the Germans who were National Socialists. The value of life for other than their own volk (folk or people) was relative. The Nazis had a term for other than their own people's lives; Lebensunwertes Leben, Leben (life) unwertes (unworthy) of Leben (living). Those were the people judged, according to a cost-benefit analysis, as costing more than they were worth.

Under Nazi programs, thousands of children diagnosed with congenital handicaps, mental retardation, and as mentally deficient were marked for "treatment." That was the Nazi word for killing. Next to go were the "incurables" with schizophrenia, epilepsy, syphilis, encephalitis, and Huntington's disease. Then the handicapped adults, "asocial" persons, Jews, Gypsies, Poles, Slavs, Catholic and Protestant "troublemakers," and on and on. Estimates are that 6,000,000 Jews and 4,000,000 "others" were killed.

ARE WE NAZIS?

Is withdrawing or withholding treatment from the terminally ill or Persistent Unconscious Patients (PUP's) the same as Nazi "treatment?" No, some say, because our motives are different. We are not doing it for cost saving, or because we don't value their lives. We are doing it to help the patients; acting in their best interest.

The Chief Medical officer of the National Socialists was Dr. Karl Brandt, whose feeling for hopelessly ill patients made him want to find for them "a peaceful end." He defended, until his death by hanging after the War, his compassion in giving painless deaths to such people. He designed gas chambers that could kill thousands "painlessly."

We can forget the Nazi experience if we believe that unlike us, Germans were particularly unethical, vicious, or stupid people. Or if we believe that Hitler was a madman superman, able to carry all that out entirely alone. None of that is true.

Could it happen here, in this country, now? No. But only because we continue to remember what happened there, and we measure our motives and actions by that experience. The French memorial at Dachau outside Munich says "Jamais rien"—Never again.

Reference: "Contested Terrain: The Nazi Analogy in Bioethics," *Hastings Center Report* 1988, August-September, pp. 29-33. By Hentoff, Callahan, Crum, and Cohen.

QUALITY OF LIFE

Note that quality of life is discussed only when we have an incompetent patient who cannot express his wishes. When people can express their wishes they can decide for themselves. Some decide to live and fight for life in situations that amaze us. We project that we would have long ago given up in the same situation.

Their life and its quality is their decision. We recognize that. But when they are not able to decide, we may decide for them. How do we assess the quality of life for someone else? How do we decide if or when their life is more burden than benefit to them?

The term "quality of life" has no generally accepted meaning. Three possible definitions are proposed:

1. An individual's subjective satisfaction with his own life. That's the philosophy of individualism. Since we only consider the quality of life when the individual cannot decide his own subjective quality of life, this is not a helpful definition.

2. An outsider's estimate of another's life, either as a reasonable person, as used in law, or by a person in similar situation of age and illness. This is a substituted judgment test described in Chapter Six, A Time to Die. It, too, reflects the philosophy of individualism, the priority of the individual.

3. The degree of achievement of success valued in our society. This would take into account the social status and wealth of the individual, and his use to society. The philosophies you can see here are utilitarianism and materialism.

A major study was done in which physicians made decisions in a hypothetical situation whether to intubate or not to intubate a patient. Among the doctors who decided not to intubate, 87% said their decision was supported by quality of life factors given for the patient. Of the doctors who decided to intubate the patient (same hypothetical), 83% said their decision was supported by quality of life factors, too!

These doctors saw the patient's quality of life differently; some decided to intubate based on that perceived quality, and some decided not to intubate based on the same information. There is no generally agreed upon or accepted criterion for quality of life. The doctors used their own values. It is important that you know and be able to identify when your own values are involved and at work.

Reference: Pearlman, Robert, and Jonsen, Albert. "The Use of Quality-of-Life Considerations in Medical Decision Making," *Journal of American Geriatrics Society,* 1985; vol. 33, no. 5, pp. 344-52.

The Quality Adjusted Life Year is the attempt to reduce the quality of life to a number. To explain generally, the patient is assessed by taking his age, computing the <u>average</u> life expectancy he has left, and factoring in a number for how sick he is. That means that people who have more life left (younger), and who are less ill (healthier), have higher QALY's. They will get better or more treatment under any system that prioritizes care by the numbers.

Experts admit that the concept is difficult to grasp. They disagree as to how to compute it. They lack reliable data to calculate it. They actually admit they may be attempting the impossible—to reduce the quality of life to a number. Over 50 years ago, investigators said that such an approach led to a serious <u>loss</u>, not gain, of information. PRESENT day experts still insist, it's better than nothing.

References: Stoutman, K. and Falk, I. S. "Health Indexes: A Study of Objectives Indexes of Health in Relation to Environment and Sanitation," *Bulletin of Health Organizations*, League of Nations, 1936; 5:901-96.

Cubbon, John. "The Principle of QALY Maximisation as the Basis for Allocating Health Care Resources," *Journal of Medical Ethics*, 1991; 17:181-84.

Harris, John. "Unprincipled QALYs: A Response to Cubbon," *Journal of Medical Ethics*, 1991; 17:185-88.

Editorial. "Which Medical Condition Shall We Treat First," *The Lancet*, Nov. 29, 1988, pp. 1175-76.

AND MORE

7. MONEY—WORK

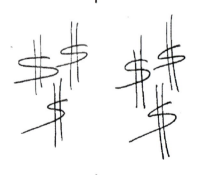

You won't see this listed as one of the "values" in usual illness care texts. Yet it's always there in ethical conflicts; it must be. Conflicts do not exist just in people's minds. They exist in the real world, too. In the real world, someone must pay the bill. Someone must do the care. Someone actually must pull the plug. Someone must watch the patient die, and pull the tubes and wash the dead body. There is <u>work</u> to be done. This subject is not as much fun as the "clean" values like beneficence, but it must be considered when ethical conflicts arise.

Translate the word money to the word <u>work</u>, in the following way: In simple exchanges between people, I can exchange my work for yours. I will work and grow some potatoes, you will work and raise some chickens. We will get together and trade. Both of us can eat chickens and potatoes. We can exchange services; I will clean your house every week, and you can give my mother her insulin injection every day.

These are simple exchanges of work for work, known in economics as barter. It's a great system. It goes on all the time, even now. But it's limited to situations where I want something you have, and you want something I have. That doesn't always happen.

Money is a way to exchange work, more easily. I exchange my work for something (call it "money"). Then I exchange the money for your work. You take the money I gave you, and exchange it for someone else's work. That's all there is to money; it's a substitute for work.

Schematic of Work for Money for Work

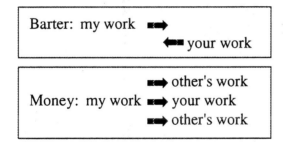

Reference: Rothbard, Murray. *Man, Economy, and State*, Menlo Park: Institute for Humane Studies, 1970.

Several ideas come up in ethical discussions around work (money). One is the idea of not wasting. This is pure Aristotle. Find the middle, not the extreme. Use only so much to do a job, enough to do a good job, but not too much. Moderation in all things, the "golden mean." We've all heard "Waste not, want not." Ever hear, "Use it up, wear it out, make it do, or do without?" We may hear it again.

These ideas are the essence of environmentalism (of conservation). You say nobody cares if it's not their personal work (money) being used, wasted in illness care? Ah, but it <u>is</u> their money, either in taxes for Medicare, or insurance money that will result in higher premiums.

That's the self-interest in valuing work. Even though it might seem that you personally benefit when you get paid for work that is not going to be useful, if it drives up costs for all in the long run it will cost you, too. That's the indirect self-interest everyone has in using illness care dollars (work) wisely. They cost everyone in the long run when wasted. The tricky part is to tell the difference between need and waste.

OTHER VALUES

"Is that all there is?" Are those all the possible values there are?

These are the most socially accepted ones now. We also value power, leisure, status, prestige, college, cars, houses, clothes, especially money. We've put that in above, but on a more general scale, not a personal one. All these other values are personal self-interests. We value self above all else, and we express that in all these "values." Self is the highest value of all, and is implied in all the others.

STUDY QUESTIONS

1. What is the definition of law?

2. How can you distinguish ethics from law?

3. Why must we use caution when told something is ethical?

4. What difference do some people make between ethics, morals, and values?

5. What is the difference between what some authorities call moral reasoning, and ethical practice?

6. What is Kohlberg's theory of moral development?

7. Why do feminists dispute Kohlberg's theory?

8. What are some concerns about theories and tests of morals or ethics?

ETHICS IS LAW AND IT IS NOT LAW

Law is a minimum ethics written down and enforced. Law is mandated behavior that is the minimum of <u>some</u> one's ethic.. There are crimes that will be punished, but that are not considered by <u>most</u> people to be ethically wrong, such as speeding at 57 miles per hour (some people consider breaking any law to be "unethical"). However, speeding at 100 miles per hour through a playground would be considered unethical by most people. The more severe the penalty for breaking the law, the more likely the law is an ethic of the majority of the people, being enforced.

Ethics and law are guides for human behavior (for human action). Ethics resembles but differs from law. We can separate law out from ethics. Law is behavior that we have agreed should be mandatory—or prohibited.

Ethics and law are on a continuum of human behavior. The continuum concept is very helpful to think of a number of things, from acidosis to ethics. You can arbitrarily draw a line and say "here at this number starts acidosis," and you can do the same thing with law—arbitrarily draw a line and say "here starts law" and mandated behavior. Do remember that it's an arbitrary, human-made, constructed line.

Ethics

draw the line

Law

Both law and ethics are a part of our efforts to live together. We hurt each other as little as possible. We help each other as much as we can in a given situation. Law is way down on the bottom of the continuum. It's behavior that we either mandate (prescribe) as what must be done, or behavior that we prohibit (proscribe) as what must not be done.

Law usually is about extremes of behavior. We have together in our system of government decided that certain actions must be done. You must care for your child. We have decided that certain actions will not be tolerated. You must not abuse your child.

Together, we elect or authorize other people to enforce the law. The word is important. Force is implied in law. That's not just persuasion, as we try to do with ethics. As we mentioned in the Justice part of Values above, in statues and paintings of Justice, she (!) is blind so she's impartial. She holds a scale to weigh the case in one hand. That symbolizes her judgment.

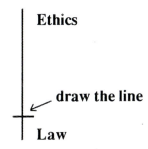

Do you remember what she has in the other hand? Find a statue of Justice at the courthouse and check it out. She has a sword in her other hand, which symbolizes force. Enforcement. Without force, we have no law. If we're all going to live together, we can't allow force to be used by anyone but people with authority of law.

Still on the continuum of human action, ethics is higher, in the area of behavior we desire. We wish people would act ethically but we're not going to make them. If we force and not persuade, that's law and not just ethics.

Law and ethics are guides for human action. Law has force, ethics does not. In law we use the words "must," and "shall." Ethics words are usually like "should" and "may."

A further difference: Laws have to be written down, by people with authority to write them. Remember the course you had in junior high? There are three branches of government, and they are the three sources of law. The Legislature makes statutes, the judiciary decides cases, and the executive writes rules or regulations.

Conceptual Framework of Law and Ethics in Human ActionEthics

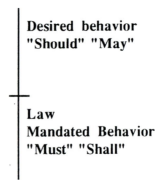

Desired behavior
"Should" "May"

Law
Mandated Behavior
"Must" "Shall"

Credit is due to Dr. Harold Werner for the original idea for this schematic.

Can a law be unethical? Can obeying a law be unethical? Sure, because the law is the lowest standard of behavior. The law is not the highest ethic; if something is merely legal, by definition it is not fully ethical (a higher behavior). The immediate example comes from Nazi law, in which judges, lawyers, doctors, nurses and all kinds of other people obeyed laws that were legal but certainly unethical by our standards. It's easy; if something is legal, then some merely say "It's the law; I don't have any ethical choice to make." This was done every day in those Nazi years.

Say your patient has designated his niece to be his surrogate decision maker. The law says the decision maker has authority to withhold treatment. You know the niece has ordered you to stop the breathing treatments because the patient will die without them, and she wants her inheritance. Must you stop any ethical analysis and just obey the law?

Ethics can be "unethical" too. You may decide that some "ethics" and standards written by someone else are really unethical according to your standards. It's legal to perform abortions, to help in executions, and in one state (Oregon) perhaps will be legal to assist suicide. Is it ethical for an illness care practitioner to do so?

But Who Makes The Ethics?

We have to be careful about ethics. Ethics is a guide for human behavior. It can be used to guide human behavior in different directions. Law is used this way, too.

But we can control the way law guides us. We have some control over the law makers. The laws must be made by people with authority. In our system we must give them the authority. Laws must written down, and we can see them.

People who "make" ethics or "write" ethics, or purport to establish standards of ethical behavior, are not controlled at all. Some people will use ethics to get other people to do what they want. Remember, ethics makers have not been elected or appointed to guide behavior. They don't have authority, unless you believe them.

Sometimes people want you to do something or believe something that they believe. They will put this in ethical terms, in terms of "you should." Or they might say that what they want is a moral imperative.

Morals=Values=Ethics?

"Morals," "values," "ethics" are words that are used interchangeably. Some authorities regard morals and values as concepts that pertain to what **is**, now. They mean that morals and values are the guides that exist now in our behavior. And they define ethics as what **ought** to be—the ideal, the goal.

By that definition we can never actually be ethical. We could be moral. Ethics would be always out of reach. We'd have to strive continually to be better, to be more than we are. This idea is quite familiar; it's common in religions in which the individual is somehow unclean, or inferior, or sinful. The individual strives for salvation or nirvana. The end, perfection, is always out of reach.

This attitude assumes that people are not okay as they are. But it does keep people always working to improve.

NOTES

MORALITY DEVELOPS?

Some writers distinguish moral reasoning from ethical practice. They say that moral reasoning, also known as moral judgment, or moral development, is thinking. Ethical practice, they say, is the action of ethics. (Since we can't see the thinking, all we have to go by to determine ethics is the acting).

Some writers say this can be separated with tests; for example, you can ask, "What do you think the practitioner should do for the patient in this situation?" That would measure the thinking, the moral reasoning. Then you could ask, "What do you think the practitioner will do for the patient in this situation?" That way they will tell you about the ethical practice (the action).

Reference: "Ethics, Part I: Issues in Nursing," *Nursing Clinics of North America*, June 1989, 24; 2:463–579.

Theories are proposed and accepted by some that people "develop" morally as they get older, more experienced, better educated. We learn, from growing up, from living, from better studying. Ideally, as we learn we use that knowledge to act "better" or more efficiently and cooperatively to get what we want. We cooperate, see the value to ourselves in assisting others, have more knowledge of how we affect the world and how it affects us.

A little baby just wants. Teenagers want and go for their wants pretty directly. Older people want and go for what they want more cooperatively, with more knowledge of the world (or maybe not, depending on what they learned or believe).

Kohlberg echoes the pervasive idea that people "evolve" from babyhood. This is the same idea shared by Darwin, Piaget, Maslow, and all the Platonists. Kohlberg thought he could "measure" stages of ethical behavior from "lowest" ethical behavior to "highest." Here again is the View A idea of hierarchy, ranking, elitism.

Kohlberg believes people develop ethically in stages that are invariable in sequence: They move from simple thought to complex moral reasoning. At higher stages, they use skills developed earlier, at lower stages. He constructs three levels of development, each having two stages:

1.   **Preconventional reasoning.** Right and wrong depends on what Mommy or authority says. "I have to do the right thing because the law, the hospital policy, the supervisor said so."

2. **Conventional reasoning**. Right or wrong comes from the family or group. The person wants to maintain existing social relationships or order. "I do the right thing because it's the golden rule; it's good for my family, my profession, my country."

3. **Post conventional (principled) reasoning**. This person thinks above and apart from the herd. She develops a conscience, <u>a priori</u>, without referring to her own situation, that dictates the right thing to do. Justice is the highest value to aspire to, according to Kohlberg. "I do the right thing because it's good for the whole world, and I have reasoned for myself that it is the ideal right thing to do."

The testing required to measure these stages of ethical behavior is intensive and requires a specially trained interviewer. Thus, it's expensive in time and money to do research on his theory.

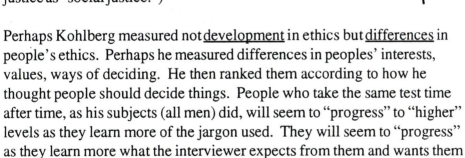

The theory is challenged in particular by feminists, because women tested all seemed mostly to be "stuck" in level 2, and never achieved the "highest" level of an adult! Women consistently cared more for family and friends and decided right and wrong on that basis. They did not "advance" to concern about the ideal of justice for all in an abstract sense. (Or perhaps they didn't agree with the test's definition of justice as "social justice.")

Perhaps Kohlberg measured not <u>development</u> in ethics but <u>differences</u> in people's ethics. Perhaps he measured differences in peoples' interests, values, ways of deciding. He then ranked them according to how he thought people should decide things. People who take the same test time after time, as his subjects (all men) did, will seem to "progress" to "higher" levels as they learn more of the jargon used. They will seem to "progress" as they learn more what the interviewer expects from them and wants them to say.

"Tools" and "instruments" are jargon words for questionnaires and kinds of interviews, not gardening implements. Such tools have been created to test the ethics of various occupations. Watch for bias in their assumptions, design, application, and the conclusions reached.

Consider, for example, the JAND, Judgments about Nursing Decisions, based on nursing's Code of Ethics. The nurse is given a hypothetical situation. She decides what a nurse <u>should</u> do in that ethical case. She then decides what a nurse <u>would</u> do in the case. The right answer is decided according to how close it comes to the Nurses Code of Ethics. This process assumes that all the values in the Code are "right" or ethical. (See Chapter Five, Professionals and Employees, for a discussion of Codes of Ethics.)

Actually, you can't test for ethical behavior with a paper test. All you can test is if practitioners guess the right answer, according to investigator, or the right reasoning, according to investigator, or the right knowledge of jargon, as given in this course.

References: Ketefian, S. "Moral Reasoning and Moral Behavior Among Selected Groups of Practicing Nurses," *Nursing Research,* 1981; 30:171-76.

Piaget, J. *The Moral Judgment of the Child.* New York: Random House, 1965.

Gilligan, C. "In a Different Voice: Women's Conception of the Self and of Morality," *Harvard Educational Review,* 47 (1977), pp. 481-517.

Kohlberg, L. "From Is to Ought: How to Commit the Naturalistic Fallacy and Get Away with It in the Study of Moral Development," *Cognitive Development and Epistemology,* (New York: Academic, 1971).

Lickona, Thomas. "What Does Moral Psychology Have to Say?" in *Teaching Ethics in Higher Education* (cited in Chapter One).

STUDY QUESTIONS

1. What are the occupations of the members of the ethics committee in your agency?

2. How are members selected for your ethics committee?

3. How do ethics committees relate to courts of law?

4. Does the ethics committee at your institution do the following?

- Set policy
- Provide education
- Initiate case investigation
- Receive requests from any person for consultation

- Do case consultation
- Have patients or family present for discussion
- Have an ethicist on staff
- Have a physician consultant
- Decide DNR orders over family disagreement

5. How has the Danforth Amendment affected ethics committees?

6. Does your agency have an Internal Review Board and an AIDS committee to review the work situation of practitioners who are HIV positive?

7. Do you disagree or agree with the following statement (explain your position): "An ethicist is an ethical person who has a Ph.D in ethics and who has no bias."

8. What is the highest value in the two methods of bioethical conflict resolution described?

9. What are the steps in the conflict resolution process described in this section? Explain each step.

10. What is the purpose of the courts?

ETHICS COMMITTEES

Ethics committees are common now in hospital and other agencies. They usually have as members people who are staff of the agency, community representatives, maybe a lawyer, clergy, docs, and nurses. The committee has bylaws, and functions to set policies for staff to use in ethical situations.

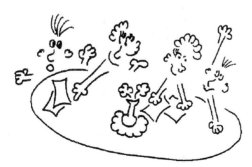

They use the same process to resolve conflicts as ethicists do, and you can do the same. They ask questions, gather information, clarify interests (values), and act as mediator. If the people can't agree after that, should the committee decide the issue?

The members of the committee may have no special qualifications in ethics, but they develop a consensus (a conscience?) of opinion. Maybe they are making ethics. Maybe those ethics will turn to law. Such committees were recommended in the Quinlan case. The New Jersey court in that case mandated the use of ethics committees in "right to die" or withdrawal-of-treatment situations.

Reference: *In Re Quinlan*, 70 N.J. 101, 355 A.2d 1647, *cert. denied* (1976) allowed a respirator to be removed from a patient in a case similar to the Nancy Cruzan situation. But Karen Quinlan lived for years after her respirator was turned off; a feeding tube provided hydration and nutrition.

Some type of case review may be done by the committee, in which the committee hears from all people involved. This, when recommended by the court of law, is delegation to little informal courts of citizens who are closer to the situation.

The analogy can be made to the continuum from law to ethics. The formal law court gives way to a less formal committee, which usually defers to the informal family/patient/physician decision. Government or law usually works better when closer to the problem.

Should ethics committees initiate investigation into cases? Or should they be available to any patient who wishes to appeal to them? Some authorities prefer that an ethics consultation face to face with the patient or family be done before the committee considers the matter. That means the patient is not necessarily present at committee decisions.

Reference: Agich, George J., and Youngner, Stuart J. "For Experts Only? Access to Hospital Ethics Committees," *Hastings Center Report*, September-October 1991, pp. 17-25.

Other writers insist that the patient be involved when committees deliberate.

Reference: Veatch, Robert M. Advice and Consent," *Hastings Center Report*, vol. 19, no. 1 (1989): pp. 20-22.

"Ethics Committees in Hospitals," Georgetown University, Washington, D.C., 1989.

Some criticize <u>any</u> committee review of individual cases. They think the committee should be a forum for discussion of ethical issues; they should make policy and educate. Any clinical analysis of cases and offer of practical advice to the patient's family and practitioner, should be done by an ethics consultant.

Some physicians believe an ethics consultant should be a physician/clinician who has an interest and skill in ethical decision making. Equally, some fear the authoritarian role an "ethicist" might take on, and prefer the joint decision making and increased experience and information available in a committee.

Reference: Siegler, M. "Ethics Committees: Decisions by Bureaucracy, *Hastings Center Report*, 1986; pages 16, 22, 24.

A study from Massachusetts General Hospital showed that consults by ethics committees rose in recent years. There were more cases in which the committee advised Do Not Resuscitate (DNR) orders be written, even against the wishes of family.

Reference: Brennan, Troyen. "Ethics Committees and Decisions to Limit Care," *JAMA*, 1988; 260: 803-7.

Ethics committees may have some fear of lawsuits for their actions, but thus far lawsuits against committees are few. (See Chapter Four, A Time to Die, Withdrawing and Withholding Treatment, the Elizabeth Bouvia case.)

Just as court-made law requires the "ethics court" be the ethics committee, so does another law, the Danforth Amendment, stimulate more use of ethics committees. That law, the Patient Self-Care Determination Act, as of late 1991 mandated that agencies receiving Medicare have a policy for informing patients of their right to refuse treatment. The law requires the institution to decide if it will honor advance directives that require withholding treatment. If so, the ethics committee should help develop that policy.

The law mandates that staff and community be educated about advance directives. The ethics committee should be involved in that also. The ethics committee may also be an "AIDS committee," deciding policy for HIV-infected workers in the agency. (See Chapter Five, Professionals and Employees.)

Reference: "New Law Creates Challenges for Hospital Ethics Committees", *Medical Ethics Advisor*, December 1991, pp. 148-50.

ANOTHER KIND OF ETHICS COMMITTEE

Federal law to protect research subjects (both animal and human) mandates Institutional Review Boards. Review of patient consent is required in advance of research studies; in other situations not involving research, such as therapy by surgery or medication, review of patient consent is not certain. Review may occur only if a malpractice suit is filed.

This is delegation by the Congress, not to administrators but to the people on the Boards. This avoids the necessity of the government agency making decisions on the safety of all research subjects. Again, there is delegation from a formal body, the government agency, to a less formal body, the Institutional Review Board of the institution. And once again, a more local decision results instead of a national one.

Reference: Agich, George, "Human Experimentation and Clinical Consent," in *Medical Ethics*, Aspen, 1989, John Monagle and David Thomasma, eds.

PROCESS THAT ETHICISTS USE TO MAKE DECISIONS: SO CAN YOU

FIRST, WHAT IS AN ETHICIST?

There is no such animal. They're like philosophers—you can only spot one after she's dead. Otherwise we're all philosophers, because we all have a philosophy. We're all ethicists, because we are all deciding, every day, the right things to do. You will see people identified as ethicists, however, and philosophers also. It usually means they work in a position with the title, or that they teach in the field.

There are teachers of ethics and philosophy. The authorities recommend that people who teach ethics have a degree in the field of profession or area they are going to work in, for example in illness care, plus one year of ethics training. Or, the teacher could qualify with an advanced degree in philosophy and one year in the field of care.

The person teaching ethics should "know something about ethics." That is different from being ethical. Any one of us can be, and is, ethical. The role of people called "ethicists" is in dispute. Some people tend to view this person as one of the new priest class. Every time a conflict that has any values to interpret arises, they play "ask the ethicist." That's a foolish idea, but perhaps such a person can ask questions, gather information, and help people see various interests in a case. Maybe they don't need a formal "ethicist" title.

The people who are formally labelled bioethicists are, like journalists, more likely to be politically liberal. There are few conservative bioethicists. This remark, attributed to a bioethicist, assumes that "liberal" and "conservative" is a meaningful label. Often you will note that people so labelled agree more than they disagree. It is usually more helpful to discuss issues than ideology.

Reference: Murray, Thomas H., Ph.D., Director, Center for Biomedical Ethics, Case Western Reserve, in "Physicians, Journalists, Ethicists Explore Their Adversarial, Interdependent Relationship," *JAMA*, 1988, beginning p. 260, at 757.

Ethicists' biases can be detected, if you read carefully. One ethicist cited a number of cases which resulted in patients' deaths, and said "The progressive California decisions just cited were followed by a small number of extremely conservative rulings in New York, New Jersey, and Missouri (the patients all lived in those cases) " (emphasis added).
His characterization of decisions that resulted in death as progressive, while describing rulings that kept the patient alive as conservative (unprogressive), reveals his bias.

Reference: Raffin, Thomas A. Withholding and Withdrawing Life Support," *Hospital Practice*, March 15, 1991, pp. 133-55, at 141.

Can one distinguish between "bioethicist" and "medical ethicist?" A letter to JAMA by two medical ethicists says that medical ethics is not a value-free discipline, meaning that it has bias that practitioners have. This implies that bioethics has no particular values, that it is a pure field of study, objective, without values. (Singer, Peter, Siegler, Mark, and Letter, JAMA, 1988, at p. 789.)

Another medical ethicist admits that the nasty secret—there is no such thing as medical ethics as a discipline.

Reference: Wikler, Dan, Ph.D, Professor of Medical Ethics, University of Wisconsin, Madison, in "Physicians, Journalists, Ethicists Explore Their Adversarial, Interdependent Relationship," *JAMA*, 1988, at 757.

HOW TO DO IT—AN ETHICAL CONFLICT

Other approaches by ethicists all start with gathering information about the case. They start by seeking outside information. The recommendation of this course is to do the opposite, to start with values, the inside information.

As an example of the usual approach, one writer suggests this formula:

1. Determine medical treatment goals.

2. Determine patient preference.

3. Look at Quality Of Life (only if No. 2 is not available). (This has to be done objectively; the patient would assess his own quality of life, subjectively, if he could.)

4. Examine externals (family, impact on others, money issues). Again, he looks at these only if No. 2 is not available (meaning the patient is incompetent). This process considers medical treatment based on what the patient wants. That's rarely a problem; rarely do practitioners treat a competent patient if he doesn't want treatment.

The usual problem in ethical conflict is that no No. 2 (patient preference) is stated, because the patient is not competent. Then the real problem is to assess objectively the quality of life for someone else. Quality of life can really only be done subjectively, by the person who decides whether her life is worth living. The real conflicts come from No. 4, those "externals," who turn out to be one daughter who wants Dad to die, and one who wants him to live.

Reference: Hildreth, Eugene A. "Workup for a Bioethical Problem," *Hospital Practice*, Jan 25, 1990, pp. 86–100.

Another approach to ethical decision making puts heavy emphasis on medical decisions first. Then the patient's wishes are considered, and other values are examined and ranked. In both these schemes, the ethicist starts with a value, implicit or unstated. Both start with the medical aspect of the patient's care: external information. That medical part, though it is never stated aloud, is considered the highest value by it's ranking as first.

Reference: Thomasma, David C. "An Ethical Workup", *Forum on Medicine*, December 1978, pp. 33–36.

A different way to approach ethical conflicts is to start with your own values, the internal information. This can be summarized with some words your parents said before you crossed the street: a warning to stop, look, and listen. Then add one more stop.

STOP, LOOK, AND LISTEN, THEN STOP AGAIN

Stop

When you are confronted with an ethical conflict (any conflict that involves your values) stop and realize it for what it is. Then start this process. Think about your values. Use your values. Decide at the first, before you do anything else, what you intuitively think should happen in this case. Feel what you want to happen here. Realize that you're gathering data, looking, and listening from that point of view.

Admit your values -- your preference -- to yourself, before you do anything else. Remember those sayings: know yourself, and to thine own self be true.

Look and Listen

This part is easy for practitioners; you're good at gathering information, analyzing data, listening to overt and hidden communications. Look at the person, her condition, listen her wishes. Look for the other interested people, listen to their wants. The point is: Having admitted your biases up front before gathering data, you will be able to see if you have really gotten the whole story, or just the part you wanted to hear (the part that supported your bias).

Then Stop Again

Separate your interest as a practitioner from the patient's interest and the agency's interest and the other providers' interests. Put this assessment of interests down in writing for yourself alone to use.

At this point it may be apparent to you which are the most important interests. As we said earlier about easy cases, most of the time they are. If your interest is in less work, the patient's is in more care, the agency's in less cost—which do you think should prevail?

If the patient's interest is in less pain, your interest in having your values "win," the hospital in more money, which should prevail?

What if it seems it's your professional interest against the hospital's money interest? Look at the patient's interest. If the patient is not affected, then what is really your professional interest? Do you really have one? If not, call it your personal interest. That's valid, but do not clothe it with some assumed-to-be-selfless "professional interest."

For example, if the hospital wants to replace licensed practitioners with unlicensed people, it seems to be your professional interest (if you're one of the practitoners) against the hospital's money interest. What is the patient's interest? If you can show that the licensade people give better care (have better outcomes than unlicensed people), then the patient's interest is in keeping licenses. And it's a professional interest or issue for you.

If not, if you can't demonstrate benefit to the patient, then it's not a professional interest. It's a personal economic interest. As already said, that's valid, but not as a patient or professional interest.

The more information you have about the conflict, the better. More information yields a better outcome. At least the result is more likely based on reality. But as noted above in Value Confidentiality, be prepared to deal with the information you seek. Know that if you find the patient's living will, you may also find a revocation of it, signed and sealed at the back.

Often this process of stop, look, listen, stop, is enough. Usually there is someone who didn't hear or know some information. Maybe you. Sometimes just the time involved in the process of gathering all the information will solve the problem. The patient will die without intervention, or get better, the relative will change her mind, or the doctor will decide to try a different treatment.

Don't make a problem if one doesn't exist. Be glad if time solved the problem. If you're so young you don't realize it yet, I promise there will be other problems coming to work on. For example, there's no need to get a court order for treatment or nontreatment if the practitioner, patient and family agree. Some hospital lawyers have not gone to court in years on an ethical conflict case for their facility.

When you come right down to a **conflict** between people who cannot resolve it with information, mediation, persuasion and compromise—that's what the courts are for, despite the practitioner's fear and loathing of courts.

FEAR OF COURTING

Many writers say that courts are inappropriate places for these bioethical decisions. They say the courts are inadequate to decide, because they can't know the wishes of the patient and family and they don't have the medical knowledge. But we have used courts in these situations for years. That's what courts are for—to resolve conflicts between people with different interests. Courts decide an action for people who cannot decide among themselves.

The courts are portrayed as "meddlers" in bioethical situations. Angry people shift and project the anger they feel toward the people who have brought the conflict, onto the court itself. People who feel the court is meddling, really feel the people who are in conflict with their side are meddlers. They may feel that nonfamily members have no business in the situation.

This was true in the Cruzan situation. "Why don't they mind their own business?" was the question. We must remember that a lot of people did mind their own business in the Nazi era. If what we are doing is right, it can withstand the publicity and scrutiny of the legal process.

The problem people have with courts is that courts decide. Somebody wins, and somebody loses. As lawyers know, people should try to stay out of court as long as possible, even when dealing with people you think are meddling. Voluntary compromise means that everybody wins something they wanted. In court, somebody loses it all.

The court is a last resort for solving an ethical conflict. Its job is to resolve a conflict that the parties cannot resolve themselves. Courts are remarkably good at this, despite bad press. Illness issues are no more difficult to understand than any other area of human activity. We'd like to make our special area of expertise mysterious, but engineering, finances, trusts and wills all require expert testimony and evidence from families, just like illness issues, and courts deal quite ably with these complex matters.

STUDY QUESTIONS AND ANSWERS

These are suggested answers. If you have something like these answers in your own words, consider yourself successful. If you have more (quality, not quantity) than these answers, consider yourself excellent.

1. What are three topics that were issues in recent American bioethics that may come back?

    - Who gets dialysis
    - Brain death
    - Patient's right to dangerous treatment
    - Organ transplantation from animals
    - Who should be committed as mentally ill

2. What is an example of a bioethical conflict that predates written history? Imagine and Describe.

    - Like (something from the text, or better if you think of another)
    - Hunters' decision to care for injured
    - Tribe's decision to kill or protect a handicapped baby

3. Which are three professions important in the development of bioethics in America?

    - Clergy
    - Law
    - Medicine

4. What is an example of a bioethical problem that did not arise from, or result in, conflict between people?

    If you can describe one, I want to see it

5. What are your personal feelings about the Nancy Cruzan case (feeding tube removed from young woman diagnosed as being in a Persistent Vegetative State); or the Clarence Thomas–Anita Hill hearing (Supreme Court Justice Candidate accused of sexual harassment by Law Professor)?

    - Whatever you put down is good, so long as you did it and you put some feelings in it
    - (**Not:** "He was guilty," or "she was lying;" but words such as "I thought;" or "I felt;" or "It seemed to me . . .")

6. What is the meaning of "metaphysical," using two words.

   - Not physical
   - Or, meta (outside) physical

7. Is ethics part of the physical or metaphysical?

   Metaphysical

8. What is the definition of "ethics," in one word?

   Customs

9. What is the current German attitude toward bioethics? What is the reason given for it?

   The Germans are afraid to talk about the value of life, for fear they'll commit the same crimes as the Nazis

10. What are the names of the two views of the world, described in the text?

    - Imagine the Ideal
    - Describe the Reality

11. Who are five of the philosophers who represent the View A "Ideal" world? (Any five of the following.)

Plato	Stoics	Hobbes	Kant
Hegel	Engels	Marx	Descartes
Darwin	Maslow	Rousseau	

12. What are the words of Descartes, by which he believed he proved his existence by thought alone?

    "I think, therefore I am"

13. What are five of the "isms" or philosophies related to the View A "Ideal" world? (Any five of the following.)

Platonism	Utopia	Rationalism
Deduction	Evolution	Self-actualization
Socialism	Communism	Fascism
Stoicism	Mind-body dualism	A priori
Categorical Imperative	Christianity	Deontology
Romanticism	Natural law	Collectivism
Natural rights		

14. Who are two of the philosophers mentioned in the View B "Real" world (realists don't get their names on philosophies as much as idealists)? (Any two of the following.)

    Aristotle   Freud   Camus   Bentham   Mill

15. Which are five of the "isms" or philosophies related to the View B "Real" world? (Any five of the following.)

Aristotelianism	Moderation	Existentialism
Humanism	Individualism	Utilitarianism
Teleology	Casuistry	Materialism
Determinism	Induction	Positivism
Emotionism	Intuitivism	

16. What is your view of the world? Is it totally either "ideal" or "real?"

    Whatever your view of the world, as more an ideal to work for or a real place to live, is okay. Most likely, no one's view is totally one or the other

17. Where can you go to get more information on a certain philosophy?

    The local library

18. Do you agree with the statement that there are only seven values in bioethics?

    These are the only the seven the author thinks most important in America now, not the only values, for all times, and all places

19. What is the definition of "beneficence" in taking care of patients?

    • Doing good for the patient
    • Whatever examples you can think of (good therapy, kind care, considerate attitude, etc.)

20. What is one self-interest that practitioners have in being beneficent to patients? (Any one of the following.)

    • They feel good about themselves
    • They want others to see them as good
    • They uphold professional ideals
    • They hope others will help them back

21. What is an example of paternalism in patient care?

    - Giving a patient a treatment without getting her consent
    - Any other example that reveals that the practitioner's wishes come before the patient's

22. What is one reason that practitioners seem less paternalistic at present?

    - Patients are less trusting
    - Practitioners are less willing to take responsibility for them

23. What is the old medical Latin phrase meaning "First, do no harm?"

    - <u>Primum non nocere</u>
    - **Note:** NonEnglish words are always underlined so that in printed material they will come out in italic print)

24. What is one self-interest that practitioners have in being non-maleficence? (Any one of the following.)

    - To feel good about themselves (reasons similar to those listed under beneficence)
    - People won't harm you if you don't hurt them
    - The law will punish you, either civilly or criminally, for harming others

25. What, in your own words, do the values of beneficence and non-maleficence cause professional codes of ethics to suggest?

    Some variation on the idea of continuing competence, and continuing education

26. What is the legal remedy that the patient who is harmed has against a practitioner who fails to be beneficent, or who is maleficent?

    A legal action for damages in a malpractice suit

27. What is the definition of autonomy from the patient's view?

    Any example will do, but the words "freedom" and "choose" or "choice" should be in there

28. Who, for example, is relatively but not absolutely, autonomous?

    - Some description of any person, since no one except a king (maybe) is completely free

- In particular, people who work, patients, children, soldiers, etc.

29. In what situation is a discussion of patient autonomy likely to occur?

   When there is a conflict between practitioner and patient

30. What is the practitioner's self-interest in valuing autonomy?

   We value freedom for ourselves, and the only way to get it for ourselves is if everyone has it

31. How are autonomy and individualism related?

   - Individuals are more autonomous (freer) if the individual is considered the reality, as in individualism
   - When the group or collective is considered real, as in collectivism, the individual's freedom has lower priority

32. What do the scales represent that a statue of Justice holds in her hand?

   - Fairness
   - Lack of bias
   - Weighing without prejudice

33. What is the controversial concept associated with the word "justice?"

   - Distributive justice
   - Social justice

34. Give an example of the concept of "equality" under distributive or social justice?

   Any example in which the actual outcome is equal, no matter what method is used to attain the outcome

35. What can happen if social justice is applied to illness care?

   - (Some variation of this statement) All people would have a share of illness care
   - No one should have more than any other

36. What is the definition of Rawls' Original Position?

   (Something like) Imagine you are making laws, without knowing if you will benefit or be hurt by the law

37. What is the principle that Rawls believes would result from the Original Position?

No person could seek to have more than any other person unless that action would benefit the lowest member of society.

38. What is the definition of the Knowledgeable Position?

- Practitioners know they are in a position, in a system, to help people
- If they do, someday someone in the system will help them

39. What is one self-interest practitioners have in the value justice?

- Treating people justly minimizes the violence people do when treated unfairly
- And treating other people fairly is the only way to hope that the practitioner, too, will be treated fairly

40. What is the self-interest practitioners have in distributive or social justice?

Ideally, everyone will have the same, so the individual will have no less than anyone else

41. Which value in the listed values is protected by the U.S. Constitution?

- Veracity (truthfulness) under the First Amendment freedom of speech
- Probably justice, too, as a whole under the Bill of Rights and other specific sections of the Constitution
- The right to sue, which assures the value of beneficence, is protected also
- Finally, see discussions about the Fourteenth Amendment and liberty to see how the Constitution protects patient Autonomy

42. What is the benefit to the individual and to the system from the value of veracity?

(Some variation on the idea of more information, better results)

43. Why does the word "consent" not need the word "informed" in front of it?

Because consent is not valid (is not consent) unless it is <u>informed</u>

44. What do you think is the purpose of valuing veracity, or free speech?

    (Whatever you answered is valid, because it's what you believe. I believe the purpose of free speech is to gain as much information as possible. I do not think it is to further the purposes of society, no matter who controls the government.)

45. Imagine and describe a conflict you as a practitioner might experience with veracity relative to a patient.

    You probably don't have to imagine, you've had lots. As examples, the patient asks: "What did my biopsy show?", or "I'm not going to die, am I?" or "That pain shot isn't a placebo, is it?"

46. What is the practitioner's interest in the value of veracity?

    • Either to avoid the legal or job penalties of lying, or to be seen as a reliable person
    • To participate in the greater system of veracity which benefits us all

47. What is one of the basic human relationships that underlie the value of fidelity? (Any one of the following)

self	family	tribe	town
school	employer	union	country

48. What is the relationship of the fidelity value to the idea of confidentiality?

    • The patient trusts your loyalty, your fidelity, to him, and believes you will not violate that loyalty
    • He has confidence in you and confides in you

49. What is the self-interest inherent in fidelity?

    If you are loyal to others, they'll be loyal to and benefit you

50. What might be the result as we deal more with strangers in our lives?

    We may have to be less "loyal" in some ways to some groups (our all-white or all-black club) or institutions (our country, right or wrong)

51. What is your view on whether you think the value of life is absolute or relative, and why?

You're right, whatever you said, so long as you realize that "absolute" means that life is always to be valued, and that "relative" means that sometimes life is not to be valued

52. What is the self-interest in the value of life?

- We all value our own life, or we'd have ended it by now
- By extension, we value other life to one degree or another

53. What is the Nazi phrase used to justify killing people?

They were <u>Lebensunwertes Leben</u> (Lives unworth living)

54. How is withdrawing treatment from terminally ill or PUP's different from what the Nazis did?

(Whatever you said is correct, as long as you realize that we can and must think about their actions to make sure we are not doing the same thing)

55. What are the conditions under which we consider a patient's quality of life?

- When the patient is unable to subjectively, for himself, to decide what his quality of life is
- When she is incompetent

56. What is the definition of quality of life?

- You define the quality of life for yourself, subjectively
- If you apply your definition to anyone other than yourself, you are saying that you can assess objectively the quality of life of other people; Hello, God

57. How does the Quality Adjusted Life Years measurement work?

- Don't feel, bad, nobody else knows, either
- If you have this on a test in some other ethics course, the answer should be something like this: A combination of years of life expected to be left to live, factored in some way with illness, or quality of life, of the patient measured

58. Which is the value usually hidden, but always present, in bioethical conflicts?

Money or work

59. Which is economic system in which work is exchanged for work?

Barter

60. Which is the medium used to exchange work more easily, more freely, with more people with more and different goods and services?

Money

61. What are some of the common ideas from the text that are identified with work/money?

moderation   conservation   environmentalism   waste

62. What is the self-interest of the practitioner in the value of work, aside from your own money and work?

Wasting work/money results in higher prices and taxes for me

63. What is the definition of law? (Several answers are possible.)

- Ethics, written and enforced
- Mandated or prescribed or proscribed behavior
- Force
- A guide for human behavior
- Mandatory or prohibited actions
- On a continuum of human action or behavior
- Rules to help us live together
- About extremes of behavior
- Made by people authorized to make law
- Symbolized by the sword Justice carries
- Written down
- Statutes made by rulemakers in the legislative branch
- Regulations made by administrators in executive branch
- Cases made by decisionmakers in the judicial branch
- Minimum ethic, never the highest behavior

64. How can you distinguish ethics from law? Ethics:

- Is not enforced, law is
- Are not mandates, laws are
- Do not have force, laws do
- Are a guide for human behavior, like law
- Do not mandate or prohibit action, laws do
- Are on a continuum of human behavior, like law
- Are rules to help us live together, like law
- Are not usually about extremes of behavior, law is
- Are not made by people with authority, law is
- Are not written, except as opinions, law must be
- Are not statutes, law is
- Are not regulations, law is
- Are not cases, law is
- Of others are potentially unethical by your own ethical standards

65. Why must we use caution when told something is ethical?

In contrast to law, "ethics" or "ethical standards" are not written by people we have authorized to make standards for behavior

66. What distinctions do some people make between "ethics," "morals," and "values?"

- Some writers say morals and values are the standards of behavior that we adhere to now, in the present; the **is**
- They believe ethics is higher, an ideal condition of behavior we should aspire to in the future; the **ought**

67. What is the difference between what some authorities call "moral reasoning" and "ethical practice?"

- Moral reasoning is the <u>thinking</u> about ethics, the deciding
- Ethical practice would be the actual ethical <u>behavior</u> or act of doing

68. What is Kohlberg's theory of moral development?

- Kohlberg theorized that people develop morally just as they develop physically
- He thought there were three levels of development, from lower to higher
- He thought justice was the highest value
- The individual whose highest value is justice is at the highest level of moral development

69. Why do feminists dispute Kohlberg's theory?

    - In testing, women never attain the highest level of moral development because they value relationships over justice
    - The theory places relationships (beneficence, fidelity) at a lower level than justice

70. What are some concerns about theories and tests of morals or ethics? (Any one of the following.)

    - The tests may test the ability to take the test, not the ability to act morally or ethically
    - The "tools" or questionnaires used, may be biased or not measure what they purport to
    - The right answers to the questions may be based on biased assumptions or codes of ethics

71. What are the occupations of the members of the ethics committee in your agency?

    - You received this information from administration at some level
    - If your agency doesn't have an ethics committee, should it?
    - Should you start it?

72. How are members selected for your ethics committee?

    - You received this information from the bylaws of the committee, or a member, or staff
    - Could you be a member?
    - You're qualified now; after this course you'll know more "about" ethics than most of the other members

73. How do ethics committees relate to courts of law?

    Some cases have delegated investigation and decision-making to ethics committees at the institution level

74. Does the ethics committee at your institution do the following?

    - Set policy
    - Provide education
    - Initiate case investigation
    - Receive requests from any person for consultation
    - Do case consultation
    - Have patients or family present for discussion
    - Have an ethicist on staff

- Have a physician consultant
- Decide DNR orders over family disagreement

Note: You had to talk to the staff or a member of the committee to answer this question; you know a lot more about the committee, and probably your institution, than you did before the question

75. How does the Danforth Amendment affect ethics committees?

- They may be involved in the policy making that law requires, or the education of staff and community required in the law
- They also may be involved in deciding what form of Advance Directives to offer their patients (See Chapter Four, A Time to Die, "Advance Directives")

76. Does your agency have an Institutional Review Board, and an AIDS committee to review the work situation of practitioners who are HIV positive?

Same as the first question of this section

77. Do you disagree or agree with the following statement, and explain? "An ethicist is an ethical person who has a Ph.D in ethics and who has no bias."

- You had better disagree and explain that an ethicist is no more ethical than the next person, but has studied ethics to be able to analyze conflicts with ethical aspects
- Either a Ph.D in philosophy with training in illness care, or a professional degree in an illness care occupation with extra work in ethics, qualifies a person to teach
- And bioethicists, like all of us, are biased

78. What is the highest value in the two methods of bioethical conflict resolution given?

- Implicit in both methods of investigation is the importance of the medical information; the patient's physical condition and the practitioner's idea for treatment
- The assumption is inescapable: the highest value is autonomy, not the patient's autonomy, but the practitioner's

79. What are the steps in the conflict resolution process described in this section? Explain each step.

   - **Stop**; acknowledge, admit, and assess your own feelings about the conflict which will affect the information you gather about the situation

   - **Look and listen**; to the patient, the family, the other practitioners, the agency, to all with an interest

   - **Stop again**; separate your feelings as much as possible fromwhat the solution may now appear to be; realize that the issue may not come out the way you wanted it to, and that you can live with that, knowing your own values

80. What is the purpose of the courts? ·

   To make decisions for people who can't decide on an answer between themselves (that's called compromise)

UNIT ONE EXAM

HSM 510
Ethical Considerations in Health Care Delivery

SCANTRON FORM INSTRUCTIONS

Please follow these instructions for completing your Scantron form:

1. Use a #2 pencil **only.**

2. Enter the five-digit Test Number in the box marked **TEST No.** Shade in the corresponding boxes.

   The test number for this exam is: **51001**

3. Enter your Social Security Number in the box marked **SOCIAL SECURITY NUMBER.** Shade the corresponding boxes.

4. Enter your Course Code number in the box marked **COURSE CODE.** Shade in the corresponding boxes.

   The course code is: **510**

5. Print your name, address, and social security number on the lines provided.

6. Enter the estimated number of hours (to the nearest whole hour) you spent on this lesson (this is for our statistical purposes only). Fill in the appropriate boxes.

7. Be careful to darken the entire area within the boxes.

8. Do not make any marks outside the boxes. Completely erase all mistakes. **Do not use whiteout.**

9. Send the Scantron form to CCHS for grading. Your test results will be mailed to you.

If you have any questions regarding your exams or any other questions or comments, please write them on a **Request for Help** form and send it in to CCHS with the Scantron form. **DO NOT STAPLE** anything to the form. Be sure to write your name, SSN, phone number (optional), and Test Number on the **Request for Help** form. GOOD LUCK!!

UNIT ONE EXAM

MULTIPLE CHOICE

Select the *best* answer to each of the following questions. Mark your responses on the Scantron form.

1. Which one of the American bioethical issues below is still in great controversy?

   a. who gets dialysis
   b. whether cancer patients can take laetrile
   c. definition of death as total, brain-stem death
   d. definition of death as persistent vegetative state

2. Bioethical problems arise from, or result in, conflict between _____.

   a. values
   b. people
   c. Institutions
   d. Ideas

3. Metaphysical is _____.

   a. amoral
   b. illegitimate
   c. not physical
   d. the whole world

4. Ethics can be defined as custom.

   a. True
   b. False

5. Quote Descartes' words by which he believed he proved his existence by thought alone.

   a. I Think, Therefore I Live.
   b. I Exist, Therefore I Think
   c. I Am, Therefore I Think
   d. I Think, Therefore I Am

6. Define "beneficence" in bioethical terms.

    a. helping your employer
    b. working for your church
    c. doing good for patients
    d. being kind to your co-workers

7. Identify which item is <u>not</u> a self-interest that practitioners have in being nonmaleficent.

    a. they reduce risk of lawsuit
    b. they reduce risk of criminal prosecution
    c. they feel good about themselves
    d. they will be seen as evil people

8. What is the legal remedy of the patient whose practitioner has failed to be beneficent, or who has been malificent?

    a. lawsuit for malpractice
    b. complaint to the administration
    c. complaint to the practitioner's professional society
    d. lawsuit for breach of contract

9. A synonym for "patient autonomy" is _____.

    a. practitioner autonomy
    b. patient freedom
    c. practitioner autonomy
    d. autonomic choice

10. In bioethics discussion, the term "justice" may be used to mean not only fairness under the law, but also _____.

    a. Communism
    b. Socialism
    c. distributive or social justice
    d. Capitalism

11. Which is the Nazi phrase used to justify killing people?

    a. lives too painful to bear
    b. lives unworthy of living
    c. lives not really alive
    d. lives too expensive to maintain

12. Identify the economic system in which work is exchanged for work.

     a. communism
     b. capitalism
     c. money
     d. barter

13. Identify the medium used to exchange work more easily, more freely, with more people with more and different goods and services.

     a. communism
     b. capitalism
     c. money
     d. barter

14. Which is not a definition of law?

     a. minimum ethics written and enforced
     b. permissive behavior
     c. mandated behavior
     d. prohibited behavior

15. Ethics differs from law, in that _____.

     a. ethics should not be enforceable by the government
     b. ethics is enforceable by the government
     c. ethics is written by people with authority to write it
     d. ethics is mandated or prohibited behavior

16. Which statement is not true?

     a. moral reasoning is the process of thinking about ethics
     b. ethical practice is the process of thinking about ethics
     c. ethical practice is the action of ethical behavior
     d. moral reasoning is reasoning about morals

17. What is the principle reason that feminists dispute Kohlberg's theory?

     a. women were not tested in the study
     b. justice is considered the highest value
     c. women cannot understand the theory
     d. women do not develop to the highest moral reasoning and practice under the theory

18. Describe how ethics committees may relate to courts of law.

    a. there is no relationship
    b. courts have formally delegated authority for decisions to ethics committees in all bioethics cases
    c. courts may delegate some authority for informal decisions to the committee in the institution where the problem arises
    d. ethics committees are like courts, in that they must be selected by the public

19. An ethicist:

    a. has a Ph.D.
    b. must be a physician
    c. is usually unbiased, as she has done extensive reading and work in the field of philosophy
    d. is a title applied to some people who work with bioethical problems

20. List the steps in the conflict resolution process described in this section.

    a. stop, acknowledge your feelings, look and listen, stop again
    b. stop, look and listen to the patient, then decide
    c. look at the problem, listen to the patient, stop procrastinating
    d. look, listen and stop to examine your own feelings

21. When people in conflict cannot compromise, this course suggests _____.

    a. they go to war
    b. they go to court
    c. they go to great lengths to get away from each other
    d. they go fishing

22. Which profession in the list below was not one of the most important in the development of bioethics in America?

    a. clergy
    b. law
    c. management
    d. medicine

23. The concept of ethics is classed as part of the physical, not metaphysical, world.

    a. True
    b. False

24. How many values exist in bioethics?

   a. seven
   b. many
   c. eight
   d. nine

25. Giving a patient treatment that will benefit her, even though she doesn't want it, is an example of _____.

   a. paternalism
   b. beneficence
   c. nonmaleficence
   d. autonomy

26. Absolute autonomy is possible to achieve for some people.

   a. True
   b. False

27. In Rawls' Original Position, you are asked to make laws from the position of not knowing whether you will benefit from the law.

   a. True
   b. False

28. The term "informed consent" has one word too many. Consent is not valid unless it is _____.

   a. understood
   b. informed
   c. express
   d. implied

29. Quality of life is only assessed by another if the patient is _____.

   a. vegetative
   b. unconscious
   c. incompetent
   d. competent

UNIT TWO

CHAPTER THREE
A TIME TO BE BORN

OBJECTIVES

Upon successful completion of the chapter, you will be able to:

1. Identify the values raised in the ethical issues of "A Time to Be Born."

2. Describe the possible genetic outcome of brothers and sisters marrying.

3. Define eugenics.

4. Discuss the question of fairness that occurs in insurance payment for artificial insemination.

5. Describe the religion's objection to artificial insemination.

6. Discuss the fairness question relative to the child born by artificial insemination to a single woman.

7. Define "*in vitro* fertilization."

8. Describe the position of the Catholic Church (and others that oppose it) relative to *in vitro* fertilization.

9. Describe the "fairness" issue relative to insurance payment for *in vitro* fertilization.

10. State your belief about who should get custody or possession of fertilized frozen zygotes when a couple divorces.

11. Discuss why the term "surrogate mother" is applied to a woman who has a baby which she knows she will give to some specific other person.

12. Discuss the two terms in the surrogate mother issue: "womb" and "uterus" and the reason for each use.

13. Discuss the two attitudes: "Surrogate motherhood exploits poor women," and "Surrogate motherhood provides poor women pay for their risk."

14. State some of the possible outcomes of a conflict between a surrogate mother who wants to keep the baby and the people who have "paid for" the baby.

15. Discuss what you think the ethical outcome should be in such a case as above, and why.

16. List the three interests in such a conflict.

17. Agree or disagree with this statement: Technology is the origin of our problems with procreation.

18. Discuss whether better technology has improved our lives in regard to abortion.

19. Discuss this statement: If it's a law, it's ethical.

20. State the name of the famous U.S. Supreme Court case that limited the state's ability to restrict abortions.

21. Identify which subgroup of Americans wish to keep abortion on demand legal during the first three months of pregnancy (as it is now).

22. State whether surveys indicate that Americans agree with the current law on abortion.

23. State why the words "fetus" or "baby" are used when speaking about abortion.

24. State why the words "mother" or "woman" are used when speaking about abortion.

25. State why the words "Pro-choice," "Pro-life," "Anti-abortion," and "Pro-abortion" are used when speaking about abortion.

26. Define the point at which a fetus or baby becomes a person, according to the U.S. Supreme Court.

27. Criticize the statement: Abortions have been done and an ethical conflict about them has arisen only during the last few years.

28. Describe some instances of infanticide during history.

29. Agree or disagree with this statement and state why: Infanticide in former times justifies our present practice of abortion.

30. Describe an example of a society that practices infanticide at present.

31. Define "quickening" and its legal importance.

32. Discuss why English common law of abortion had any effect in the U.S.

33. Describe the state of American abortion law in 1973, before <u>Roe v. Wade</u>.

34. Indicate why it is so important that the Supreme Court in <u>Roe</u> called privacy, and abortion, a "fundamental right."

35. Describe the three stages of pregnancy discussed in that case, with the state's interest at each stage.

36. Define "viability."

37. Agree or disagree with this statement and give rationale: The <u>Roe</u> decision solved all ethical conflicts about abortion.

38. Define the word "right" as used in constitutional law.

39. Distinguish rights from entitlements.

40. Identify who decides what those rights are that are not listed in the written Constitution.

41. Identify a source of rights that has become more important in recent times.

42. Identify the source of unwritten rights in the Constitution, which is being used by the current Supreme Court in place of the right of privacy.

43. Identify the Amendment and right used in the <u>Cruzan</u> case to assure a constitutional right to refuse medical treatment, including food and water.

44. Discuss the right that will probably be involved when a "right to suicide" is at issue before the Court.

45. Identify the original source of state or federal constitutional rights.

46. Discuss whether the legislature or the judicial branch of government should define our rights.

47. Describe the relationship of the power of the federal government to the power of the state government.

48. Discuss some differences in abortion laws in America from those other Western countries.

49. Predict a possible outcome if <u>Roe v. Wade</u> is overturned and state legislatures can pass more restrictive abortion laws.

50. List some of the reasons that women abort.

51. List the reasons that you believe may justify an abortion.

52. Discuss the assumption underlying this statement: Restricting abortion will mean even more black teenage unwed mothers will keep their babies; we must not restrict abortion.

53. Identify a term used to label the attitude that a whole people are better off dead than alive, like the Jews in Germany.

54. Identify the various interests present in the abortion conflict.

55. Discuss the issues around the use of the drug RU486.

56. Distinguish contraception from abortion as a method of family planning.

57. Describe the regulation upheld in <u>Rust v. Sullivan</u> and its potential impact on practitioners.

58. Describe when a father's interest is not one "traditionally protected" and therefore not enforced, according to U.S. Supreme Court Justice Scalia.

59. Name the "ism" or philosophy associated with the value of autonomy or freedom; the philosophy most dominant in the United States.

60. Explain how the term "cesarean" developed for abdominal delivery.

61. List some interests of the woman in any ethical conflicts that affect her concerning the issues in this chapter, "A Time to Be Born."

62. Identify the value that has been found most important when the fetus's safety causes a judge to incarcerate his mother to keep her from taking drugs.

63. Discuss whether having a child is a right, or a privilege which the law may limit.

64. Agree or disagree and discuss this statement: In the future, children will be able to sue their mothers for divorcing their fathers, because they were thereby deprived of support and companionship.

65. Discuss the idea that unequal outcomes, such as different mortality rates for white and black infants, indicates a lack of justice.

66. Define "neonate."

67. Discuss the interest of the newborn with a handicap.

68. Identify the value held by Florida aboriginals living 7000 years ago toward newborns with handicaps.

69. Describe the position of pro-life groups on research and therapy using aborted fetuses.

70. Describe the rationale for allowing aborted fetuses to be used for research and therapy.

71. Distinguish the use of aborted fetuses for research and therapy from the use of bodies of Persistent Unconscious Persons (PUPs) declared "dead."

72. Explain the interest that the state has in all the issues in "A Time to Be Born."

STUDY QUESTIONS

This is not a test. Read the study questions before you begin the chapter. Answer them as you go along or after you finish the chapter. Then look at the suggested answers at the end of the chapter to see if you agree with the answers.

1. Which are the values raised in ethical issues in "A Time to Be Born?"

2. What is a possible genetic outcome of brothers and sisters marrying?

3. What is the definition of eugenics?

4. What is the issue of fairness that occurs in insurance payment for artificial insemination?

5. What is the religious objection to artificial insemination?

6. What is the question of fairness that arises relative to the child born by artificial insemination to a single woman?

7. What is the definition of "*in vitro* fertilization?"

8. What is the position of the Catholic Church (and others who oppose it) relative to *in vitro* fertilization?

9. What is the "fairness" issue relative to insurance payment for *in vitro* fertilization?

10. Who should get custody or possession of fertilized frozen zygotes when a couple divorces?

11. Why is the term "surrogate mother" applied to a woman who has a baby she knows she will give to some specific other person?

12. Which is the correct term in the surrogate mother issue, "womb" or "uterus?"

13. Which statement is correct: Surrogate motherhood exploits poor women, **or** surrogate motherhood provides poor women payment for their risk.

14. What are some of the possible outcomes of a conflict between a surrogate mother who wants to keep the baby, and the people who have "paid for" the baby?

15. What do you think the ethical outcome should be in such a case as above, and why?

16. What are the three interests in such a conflict?

17. Do you agree or disagree with the following statement and why? Technology is the origin of our problems with procreation.

INTRODUCTION

We divide this course into chapters, to provide some stopping places — (and to make the tests shorter). Dividing by time, by chronology, occurs to us humans "naturally." We could do it any number of ways—by issues, by whose interests are affected, and so on. But we choose to divide in a rough way by time of life. We are talking about humans in this course; humans have a limited, finite, life-span. Hence the following division:

I. A Time to Be Born,

II. In Between:

    A. Share of Care
    B. Professionals and Employees

III. A Time to Die.

Ethical issues grouped around the beginning of human life include artificial insemination, *in vitro* fertilization, surrogate motherhood, abortion and use of aborted babies, infant mortality rates, addicted babies, women's reproductive interests and handicapped babies' treatment.

The values in this chapter: First of all <u>life</u> of the fetus or child or woman. The value of <u>autonomy</u> is equally important for the woman or parents or surrogate. The value of <u>beneficence</u>, doing good for the ill or poor or handicapped, will be present. The value of loyalty, to our sex or to our image of ourselves as people, may be raised. And always and forever, the <u>money-work</u> issue underlies and influences all these ethical conflicts.

As a practitioner, we assume you have some grasp of how human reproduction proceeds in a scientific sense; if not, see a basic book on physiology. We will put in some simple explanations for administrators and practitioners whose area it is not.

ARTIFICIAL INSEMINATION

Artificial insemination is the procedure of delivering sperm, semen, to the cervix by "artificial" means, that is, through means other than intercourse. "Artificial" versus "natural" is a <u>really</u> artificial distinction. As generally understood, "artificial" is something that humans cause, that does not come automatically. You can see the difficulty of using the distinction, here. "AIH" is artificial insemination using the husband's sperm, "AID" is artificial insemination using a donor's sperm, and "AIDH" is artificial insemination using donor and husband's sperm. "Ethical" clinics use one donor for only 10 women to reduce the chance of half brothers and sisters unknowingly marrying. Some slight chance would remain anyway.

The care taken to prevent the possibility of brothers and sisters marrying is to avoid the taboo of incest, which violates practically all known ethical codes. Ancient Egyptians brothers and sisters intermarried among the royalty, because their family members were the only immortals. They were gods, and gods can't marry mortals.

In-family marriage tends to emphasize genetic defects. A mother and father who are related have similar genes, so the odds are greater that recessive genes inherited from both parents will be present, combine, and produce the defect carried by the parents.

Usually the semen donor is checked to see that he is free of HIV, Hepatitis B, and other infections. He should be rechecked after several months to verify that he was not latent infected at the first check (sperm is frozen). Also, information is obtained about his family and personal history of health and genetic disease.

There is even a sperm bank of Nobel Prize winners—though some see this as an attempt to do "eugenics." That was a goal of the Nazis, to produce a superhuman race. Would we allow an ideal person to be used "at stud," like a horse, even if we kept a pedigree so that we knew we weren't crossing brother and sister? What if we had a supply of John Kennedy's sperm and a whole lot of people wanted to have him for their child's father? Martin Luther King? Ronald Reagan?

Fertility clinics can produce minor miracles, but there is potential and actual fraud in some cases. A respected physician was charged and convicted for using his own sperm to impregnate as many as 75 women at his clinic. It is possible to inject hormones to make women test positive for pregnancy, to increase the clinic's rate of success and the patient's satisfaction. When the "pregnancy" fails to develop and menstruation commences later, the women could be told that they had aborted spontaneously.

The charges described above were brought against the first American doctor to do amniocenteses, or examination of the amniotic fluid in the pregnant uterus. This procedure will detect conditions of the fetus during pregnancy, which allows abortion for such conditions, which allows controversy about those reasons (see below).

Artificial insemination uses goods and services, so it costs money. Often it must be repeated many times to produce a pregnancy. It is an elective procedure, not necessary to the health of the potential mother or father, except perhaps mentally. Questions may arise as to its payment by insurance. It was proposed in 1994 that all persons be mandated to buy insurance. We are all mandated now to buy insurance for (pay for illness care of) the poor, the elderly, and certain other groups mentioned in Chapter Four, "Share of Care."

The question of justice or fairness arises -- fairness to the other members of the insurance pool -- of using the group's money for elective services. This question would be acute if a basic level of care had been mandated through a national health insurance or system.

The bioethical issue is whether it is "fair" to spend money on something which isn't necessary to life or physical health, and which in the worst characterization is indulgent of the couple (or woman's) desire to propagate their own genes. There are plenty of babies to adopt; if insurance pays, the group must bear the increased cost because people don't want babies of certain color or physical condition.

Some religions oppose artificial insemination on the grounds that it removes the sex act from procreation, and from the expression of love in sexual intercourse in marriage.

With artificial insemination, single women can have babies without having sex or having a man who would then have rights relative to the child (see "Abortion" below). The question is whether this gives women, married or single, equality to have a child. Questions arise about fairness to the child, who will grow up in a single-parent household without the benefit of a father. But this is not different than many other households. We can ask whether the child would be better off not to have been born at all.

If artificial insemination is available for a price, and not paid for by some insurance scheme, then poor people don't have the same opportunity to reproduce their genes as rich people do. Then two levels of care will result again. We could prohibit artificial insemination by anyone. But that involves the government in private affairs again.

The bioethical questions are whether people have a right to have a child, a right to their own genetic child, or a right to a perfect child.

In Vitro Fertilization

Some 10 years ago, the press hailed the ability of medical science to provide means for baby Louise Brown to live. She was the first baby born after conception outside the womb.

In vitro means in glass (*Vitro* is the Latin word for "glass;" *in vivo* is the opposite, meaning "in life"). This fertilization occurs in a glass petri dish like the one you grew organisms in for microbiology. The eggs (the ova), are flushed from the woman's ovaries with doses of drugs that make several ova mature at the same time. The same drugs are used to stimulate ovulation and often result in multiple births when not used with *in vitro* fertilization.

IVF is an even more expensive than AI due to the drugs, the procedure to retrieve several eggs, the fertilization, and the implanting. So the same arguments arise. In addition, the Catholic Church and others oppose the technique; almost always, in order to get at least one viable zygote (the name for the fertilized ovum), four are fertilized at that point several potential humans exist in the dish. Opponents say that.

Only one may survive. All four may be implanted, and if they all survive three may be aborted. Destroying the others, whether implanted or in the dish, raises the same issue as abortion. It can be argued on the other side that no baby would have been born had the procedure not been done. The question comes back to whether it is "God's will" that people have children, and whether the creation and birth of one child justifies the destruction of others.

These fertilized ova can be frozen and thawed to use later, with no apparent damage. If a couple freezes zygotes (an embryo after it's implanted) and later separates or divorces, the custody of the fertilized ova is at issue. They could be considered children, with the attendant legal rules and procedures, or they could be classed as property, to be divided according to those laws.

If either one of the former couple gets "custody" or ownership, the other could theoretically be made to be a parent against her or his will years after donating the cells. Legal outcomes have differed. The issue is still in development because the technology hasn't been available for long.

The issue would seem to be whether; after you have consented to contribute half of a person, you may withdraw that consent. Perhaps some sort of "advance directive" can be made and incorporated in a prenuptial or prepregnancy agreement—"if we divorce then the following should happen to my zygotes. . . ."

The same conditions could be imposed on the abortion choice. Once you've set up the conditions for pregnancy and allowed it to happen, should you be able to change your mind? The abortion issue involves an "involuntary servitude" of the woman's body, in a sense, but this is not an issue in the custody of the zygotes. The custodial parent or owner doesn't force anyone to be pregnant using his or her own body because a surrogate mother can be used. But one can still be made a "mother" or a "father" against one's will.

SURROGATE MOTHER

"Surrogate mother" is the term applied to a woman who has a baby she will not keep. It is the same term applied to the wire forms used to simulate monkey mothers in Maslow's experiments on effects of nurturing, if you remember those from Psych 101.

Interestingly, the term is not applied to women who have babies they intend to give up for adoption to an agency, or to some unknown person. That woman is called the "birth mother" or "natural mother," contrasted to the "adoptive mother." "Surrogate mother" is only applied if the woman knows the person to whom she is giving the baby.

The term implies a woman who deliberately has a baby she intended to conceive, or have implanted as *in vitro* fertilization; and she intended, before she got pregnant, to give the baby to someone else.

Various arrangements are possible—the mother can be artificially inseminated with the sperm of the man who will eventually get the child. It's his genetic child. Or a zygote from a couple can be implanted. It's their genetic child. The couple could be characterized as renting her uterus.

("Womb" is usually used instead of "uterus" in these cases; it is the emotionally loaded "motherhood" word preferred by opponents of the procedure). Or, the couple could be seen as buying the baby, or buying the woman's time and risk.

Some people worry that we might go back to a time, only about 100 years ago, when science thought the sperm contained the whole of the genetic material, and the woman contributed nothing. The woman was merely the carrier or bearer, as in the phrase, "she bore him a child."

This can be seen as exploiting poor women for the benefit of those rich enough to pay. Or, it can be asked, whether it is different from anyone renting his body or mind for work.

Some who approve abortion, and wish the state to stay out of that private area, at the same time oppose surrogate motherhood and approve government intervention in that arena. They worry about the sanctity of motherhood, the relation of the mother to child, and the mental outlook of a woman who would give up her child. These same issues concern persons who oppose abortion.

Not resolved are the issues of what happens when the baby is "defective" in some way—handicapped, mentally deficient, developmentally disabled, or if the baby merely is not what the couple wanted. If the surrogate doesn't want the baby either, he may be given up for adoption. If he can't be adopted, the state (we) have to pay for his care. Possibly the surrogate mother and the potential parents, since they "started" the baby, should contribute.

But by the same rationale, any woman who puts a baby up for adoption would have to pay for the baby's care if unadopted, since she "started" the baby and she could have had an abortion. Her personal moral values were upheld by not aborting, it is assumed.

We have already seen the difficulty when the surrogate mother decides to keep the baby. Some famous cases have thoroughly explored the issues of who the baby is and results have been mixed. In the **Baby M** case the baby was given to the genetic father and his wife, not to the genetic and surrogate mother.

A later case held that motherhood and parenthood of the baby are to be determined genetically. This baby was born as result of in *vitro* fertilization and a commercial surrogate. The Anna J. v. Mark C., 286 Cal. Rptr. 369 (Ct. App. 4th Dist., 1991).

Preliminary studies show that the couples and women involved are happy with the arrangement. They are mentally normal people (as much as can be measured by tests) before and after the event. Several of the surrogate mothers express altruistic motivation, and also express enjoyment of the pregnant state and the feeling of giving life.

Fairly predictably, the women are mostly Caucasian, since there are many babies to adopt in the African American and Hispanic populations. Surrogate motherhood when done for pay is expensive, so the phenomenon tends to be in the population at top of economic ladder.

In the Old Testament there are examples of women giving their babies to another. It was not uncommon in earlier times in America for a childless couple to be given a baby to raise by a relative who had several, an arrangement beneficial to both families.

But now we are not in small groups and families. We have a technology separating and uniting us. A lot of things that seem acceptable when we are a small group (tribal) get complicated and controversial when we are strangers and must rely on laws to make us do the right thing.

The interests here are those of the people who want a baby, and of the woman who will bear the baby. "Bear" means "to suffer," and "bear" means "to carry!" Also, lest we forget, the baby himself has an interest in the proceedings. Some states have passed laws forbidding surrogate motherhood, or forbidding it for pay, or forbidding the rights of the people who paid for the care of the woman during pregnancy.

TECHNOLOGY

Some feminists and some others decry the whole technology around reproduction. Some think the original problem is the technology of contraception. And for some other people contraception itself is an ethical issue. Contraception is a shortened form of the two words "contra," or against, and "conception." We add that the issue is artificial contraception, since abstinence from sexual intercourse is contra conception in a "natural" sense (that distinction is not helpful).

We have not addressed this as a separate issue, since there is not much conflict about it; certainly not as much you will see in the area of abortion (see discussion below). The area of differential fertility (some groups have more babies than others) is controversial in some areas, especially when governments seek to curb that fertility.

Feminists write that contraceptive technology separates sex from procreation and allows choice about when and if to have children. Interestingly, this echoes the reasons of the church's opposition to contraception.

Technology also allows abortion, safely and easily. These technologies of contraception, AI, in vitro fertilization, and abortion, allow a dollar value to be put on children. Technology allows value to be placed on having children when, and in numbers, one can "afford" to have them. That then creates this question: Should rich people be able to have more kids than poor people?

Some people just object to technology. It seems to them that before we had technology, we didn't have these problems. Of course we didn't have these specific problems, but people had problems. The myth of an earlier peaceful plenty time when lions lay down with lambs is just that, a myth.

We are not the first people to cope with technology. Ancient people's ambivalence toward technology can be seen as symbolized in the Greek myth of Icarus, who invented wings made with feathers and wax. He then flew too high (another lesson), melted the wax, and crashed.

The feminist argument is that a woman who has an in vitro fertilized zygote implanted cannot be certain it's really her baby. There could have been a mix-up, accidental or deliberate. By creating the same uncertainty about paternity (maternity) that men have always endured, women will, like men, develop the need to dominate. That argument assumes (first) that males do dominate, and (second) that this reproductive uncertainty is the cause of it.

Another feminist argument against technology in reproduction is that separating a woman from procreation separates her from her original and elemental power of life. It gives men the power to reproduce, which, it's argued, they've always wanted. Technology around reproduction makes children into products, with different prices, different values to society; as is true now with abortion, especially of handicapped babies.

References: **Artificial Insemination, In Vitro Fertilization:**

Sacred Congregation for the Doctrine of the Faith. *Instruction on Respect for Human Life in Its Origin and on the Dignity of Procreation*, in *Origins* 16 (March 1987), 697-711.

Lauritzen, P. "What price parenthood?" *Hastings Center Report*, 1990; 20:38-46.

Surrogate Motherhood:

Callahan, D. "Surrogate motherhood: A Bad Idea," *NY Times*; January 20, 1987.

Hanafin, H. "Surrogate Parenting: Reassessing Human Bonding." Presented at APA Convention, August 28, 1987.

In re Baby M, 537 A.2d 1227-73 (N.J. 1988).

Annas, G. J. "Fairy Tales Surrogate Mothers Tell," *L. Med. Health Care*, 1988; 16: 27-33.

1. Has better technology improved our lives in regard to abortion?

2. Disagree or agree with this statement and state why: If it's a law, it's ethical.

3. What is the name of the famous U.S. case that limited the states' ability to restrict abortions?

4. According to surveys, which subgroup of Americans wish to keep abortion on demand legal during the first three months of pregnancy (as it is now)?

5. Do Americans agree with the current law on abortion?

6. Why do people use the word "fetus" or the word "baby" when speaking about abortion?

7. Why do people use the word "mother" or the word "woman" when speaking about abortion?

8. Why do people use the terms "Pro-choice," "Pro-life," "Anti-abortion," and "Pro-abortion?"

9. What is the point at which a fetus or baby becomes a person, according to the U.S. Supreme Court?

10. Criticize (examine and be critical of) this statement: Abortions have been done and an ethical conflict about them has arisen only during the last few years.

11. What are some instances of infanticide in history?

12. Agree or disagree with this statement and state why: Infanticide in former times justifies our present practice of abortion.

13. What is an example of a society that practices infanticide at present?

14. What is the definition of "quickening" and what is its legal importance?

15. Why did English common law of abortion have any effect in the U.S.?

16. What was the state of American abortion law in 1973, before Roe v. Wade?

17. Why it is important that the Supreme Court in <u>Roe</u> called privacy, and abortion, a "fundamental right?"

18. What are the three stages of pregnancy mentioned in that case, and what is the state's interest at each stage?

19. What is the definition of "viability"?

20. Disagree or agree with this statement, and state what is your rationale: The <u>Roe</u> decision solved all ethical conflict about abortion.

ABORTION

Abortion is the technical word used for expulsion of a fetus, either spontaneously (naturally?) or induced (artificially?). The controversy about abortion is over induced abortion.

This is another birth issue made possible by technology. Before technology made abortion safe and cheap and accessible, the issue was less obvious. Few women had abortions, because they were dangerous, costly, and difficult to obtain; not only because they were illegal, but because the technology was not so prevalent.

This is an issue in which we can most clearly see the overlap of law with ethics. The law in this country that allows abortion is seen as unethical by many. Laws that would restrict abortion would likewise be seen as unethical by many.

The issue of abortion centers around the value of life -- of the child. Also involved is the value of the woman's autonomy. Beneficence may be invoked as a value—no "bad life" for an unwanted child. Finally the value of loyalty may be involved (loyalty to the tribal norm, whatever the norm or custom of our tribe is).

DATA

Abortions were not "illegal" in this country before 1973, but the numbers of abortions have increased since the U.S. Supreme Court announced in <u>Roe v. Wade</u> that abortion could not be restricted by state law during the first three months of pregnancy. In 1973, 744,600 abortions were reported in the U.S. In 1985, 1,588,600 were reported. Nineteen percent of pregnancies in 1973 ended in abortion. In 1985, thirty percent of pregnancies were aborted.

In a democracy, attitudes of the people will eventually determine the ethics and thus the legality of abortion. Among black people, 45% believe abortion should keep the same legal status it has now; 42% believe it should be legal in some circumstances, but with more restrictions than at present; 13% percent believe it should be totally illegal.

Among white people, 49% think abortion should be legal as now; 42%, as in the black population, think that it should be legal but with more restrictions, and 9% think it should be totally illegal. (Have you ever noticed that people are not actually white or black? They're sort of more brown or more pink.)

Among women, 47% want to keep abortion unrestricted legally as now, 40% want it more restricted, 11% totally illegal. Among men: 51% unrestricted, 38% more restricted, 8% totally illegal.

In terms of public approval totally of abortions under various circumstances: over 50% approve abortion for maternal health, fetal defect, of rape. Under 50% approve abortion for financial problems, unmarried status or family size.

About 50% of abortions are done in the first 8 weeks of pregnancy; 90% are done in first 12 weeks, and fewer than 1% after 20 weeks. This 1% is the percentage of pregnancies that the Missouri statute required be tested for viability, that statute being upheld by the Supreme Court in the Webster case.

Twelve percent of abortions done in 1985 were funded by the taxpayer.

References: Abortion data source: The Alan Guttmacher Institute, New York, NY.

"Researchers Amass Abortion Data," *JAMA*, 1989; 262:1431-32.

"Abortion in Context," *Family Planning Perspectives*, 1988; 20:273-75.

The law is a minimal, agreed-on compromise about an ethical issue. That it is law for all does not mean that all find it ethical. The current law that prohibits states from restricting abortion in the first trimester is a good example. People who believe this law to be too low a minimum behavior unethical wish to make the law more nearly conform to their ethics. When and if they do, the law will then seem too high a minimum ethic to other people who favor abortion as a choice.

Abortion for any reason is legal during the first three months of pregnancy everywhere in the U.S. A majority of people believe it should not be (see survey above). Men are the only subgroup in which a majority wish to keep the law as it now exists.

WORDS, WORDS, WORDS

As noted above, the words for the cells before fertilization are "ovum" and "sperm." After they unite, the cell is called a "zygote." When implanted in the uterus, it starts growth through cell division and is called an "embryo." When the practitioner can see with ultrasound at 8 weeks or hear heartbeat with a Doppler stethoscope at 10 weeks, the term used is "fetus" until the time of delivery. In lay speech, we talk about the "baby" in utero. The word "baby" has a whole load of connotations, such as "person" and "human being."

Some people insist that the only correct word to use at any time before birth is "fetus." Some people insist "baby" is the only correct word. "Fetus" has been a less emotionally loaded word than "baby."

You often hear the word "woman" used in place of "mother" in abortion discussions. The word "mother," like "baby," has many connotations. Traditionally, "mothers" do not kill their "babies." (But see below under history—some have.) Politically, it sounds bad to have "mothers aborting babies." It stirs less emotion to say that "women abort fetuses." Perhaps it is more nearly the truth. Perhaps not.

The terms that the proponents and opponents use are great examples of using words for political impact. Pro-abortion? Anti-abortion? Pro-choice? Pro-life? "Pro-life" sounds good—who could be anti-life?

"Pro-abortion" doesn't sound good and isn't accurate, because these people are not automatically in favor of abortion. They favor the right to choose abortion, therefore, call themselves "Pro-choice." Some people in the Pro-choice movement seek to justify their position by talking about the bad lives of kids who would be "better off aborted;" that would be qualified as an Anti-life position.

The Pro-life people are usually Anti-abortion, and probably wouldn't have a problem being seen as against abortion; though some of them favor some abortions at some times under some circumstances. But "Anti" anything sounds negative and as discussed before, pro-life is a great public relations term.

We are "pro" crazy, by the way. A new word has been created: "Pro-active." That is supposed to be the opposite of reactive, which must be bad, old, conservative, reactionary. But it's an unnecessary adding of "pro-." The opposite of reactive is "active," pure and simple. The "pro" does add emphasis, and it remains to be seen if it's useful enough to stay in the language or if it is a fad. Remember "awesome?"

Resource: Orwell, George. "Politics and the English Language," in *Selected Writings*, 1946, pp. 75-89.

Words are especially important in law. Live human things, whether called fetuses or babies, have no rights under the U.S. Constitution unless they are deemed persons. The fetus does not become a person under the Supreme Court's decisions on abortion until somewhere between viability and birth. Other kinds of law recognize some earlier personhood, or at some least limited remedies for injury to the fetus.

For example, legal action can be brought for manslaughter for damages, and for criminal acts to "viable" fetuses (another loaded word; see the discussion below under Legal History regarding viability.)

HISTORY

Termination of pregnancy before delivery has been going on for a long time; since women first got pregnant. There have always been spontaneous abortions, also called miscarriages. And there have always been some induced abortions, using drugs, violent falls, or other physical interventions, such as insertion of various materials through the cervix into the uterus.

The ancient Persians knew of abortifacients and punished abortions under the criminal law. Part of the Hippocratic oath from ancient Greece reads: "I will not give to a woman a pessary to produce abortion; I will not give to a woman an abortive remedy."

Both Plato and Aristotle discussed and approved of abortion. The ancient Greeks, the Pythagoreans, were against suicide and also opposed abortion because they believed the embryo was "animate" from conception. St. Augustine, a churchman from the sixth century, distinguished between *embryo inanimatus*, and *animatus*. He wrote that the embryo was formed and alive at 40 days for a male, and, at 80 days for females. Aborting an *embryo inanimatus* presumably would not have been a sin.

Infanticide has also been a part of history, and is sometimes cited to justify the present practice of abortion. Plato recommended killing infants that were born defective or handicapped more severely than would fit into his ideal world. Some societies have controlled birth rates by killing children of the wrong sex or wrong characteristic or handicap, at birth.

In Roman times, a sort of a free baby market existed in which unwanted newborns were left at a place commonly understood to be where one could get a child. The word underlined exposition may have been wrongly interpreted as meaning that these children were left exposed to the elements. Some authorities believe the interpretation should be that the babies were on exposition, or exhibition, at this baby market. The children would be taken and raised by slaves or the poor or others who didn't have children.

People actually wanted children at that time in history; they were a source of labor and thus added to the family's wealth more than their cost. This was true in rural America until this century. The exposition in Rome may have been infanticide, but it also may have functioned as an adoption agency when demand for infants was present.

During the middle ages babies usually slept with their nursing mothers some were suffocated when the mother "overlay" them. The poor or people with too many children always had the option (and took it) of putting children in the monastery or church. The incidence of infanticide during that time too may have been overstated.

Even if infanticide in prior times was common, that probably does not justify abortion for our society today. If we believe abortion is a solution to a problem we have now, we should be able to face that decision squarely. We need not rely on the fact that "everybody else did it, too." Herod killed all the baby boys in Israel, trying to get Jesus. That would not justify our killing all the adult men in Iraq to get Saddam Hussein.

The Chinese, whose effort to control their population includes limiting couples to a maximum of two children, order abortions for women pregnant for the third time. It is also common practice in that country, which values boy babies for many social reasons, to kill the second baby at birth if she is a girl. Infanticide is not just in the far distant past, it exists now. If we want to justify it we need only look to the East.

Reference: Post, Stephen G. "History, Infanticide, and Imperiled Newborns," *Hastings Center Report*, August-September 1988, pp. 14-17.

LEGAL HISTORY

Most of the states in the U.S. inherited the common law of England as their first law in the early 1800s. Texas, whose abortion restriction law was struck down in of Roe v. Wade importance, established English common law principles in that state in 1840. Under that law, aborting a "quick" child was a capital offense. Abortion before quickening was not indictable. Quickening occurred when the mother could recognize movement, between 16 and 18 weeks. One can imagine that quickening as a concept is related to our use of "viability" in American law.

Reference: Coke's Institutes, Blackstone.

In the U.S., the laws criminalizing abortion were passed in the mid- and later-1800s with the purposes of discouraging illicit sex, protecting maternal life from the usually septic techniques, and protecting prenatal life. The Texas statute which was struck down in Roe v. Wade was passed in 1854.

By the 1950s, all states prohibited abortions unless to save the life of the mother. Alabama and the District of Columbia allowed abortions for danger to the mother's health.

By 1973, a trend in the state legislatures toward liberalizing the abortion statutes had resulted in 14 states changing their abortion laws to allow abortions under some conditions, (see the numbers of abortions performed in 1973, above). In 1973, the Roe decision struck down the Texas statute, saying it violated personal, marital, familial, and sexual privacy.

The Court found a right of privacy in the U.S. Constitution. The right was not written specifically, but was said to be in the "penumbra" (shadow of a shadow) of all the rights written in the Bill of Rights.

The Roe decision did not grant an unqualified right to abortion. It did say that privacy, which includes abortion, is a "fundamental right." That means that a state would have to have a compelling interest in order to pass a law restricting abortion in the first trimester, first three months of pregnancy. The state would have to prove that it passed such a restriction because it had a compelling state interest in the outcome it was seeking, the law directly resulted in that outcome, and that there was **no** less restrictive way to achieve that outcome.

In constitution talk, this means that the state can't pass a law restricting abortion in the first three months. The state has no interest which is that compelling, and almost always there can be found some less restrictive way to achieve the state's goal.

In the second trimester (second three months) the state can regulate abortions in the interest of the mother's health. That is, the state can require abortions be done by a doctor, in a hospital, and so on.

In the final trimester the state can consider the fetus or baby's interest in living. In summary:

> First trimester; no state interest.
>
> Second: State can protect mother's health interest in life.
>
> Third: State can protect fetus or baby's interest.
>
> However the Court is moving away from the "trimester rule.".In 1979, the Webster case upheld a Missouri statute requiring doctors to assess for "viability" before performing an abortion, if the pregnancy was in its 20th week or later. The normal gestation period is 40 weeks; the lower limit of survival outside the womb, and therefore "viability," is 24 weeks. The rationale for the 20-week restriction is that if the date of the last period date is mistaken, the estimate of gestation can be off by four weeks.

At 24 weeks gestation, 25% of fetuses survive; at 25 weeks, 60% live; at 26 weeks, 80% live. By gestational age of 29-30 weeks about 90% will live.

Reference: Werner, Carmen, Pediatric's Amarillo, Texas

Subsequent decisions through the years, political activity, and new state laws, have challenged the prohibitions in Roe. Some state statutes have restricted where abortions are done, required procedures to notify parents and husbands, required some delays, and required explanations of the development of the fetus and alternatives to abortion. Some states have passed laws restricting abortion to cases of rape or incest.

These will be considered by the Court, too, unless Roe is expressly overturned by the Supreme Court. Some people, even some in favor of the right to choose abortion, hope Roe will be expressly overturned (instead of continuously restricted), because then state legislatures will be free to make their own laws in this area.

STUDY QUESTIONS

1. What is the definition of the word "right" as it is used in constitutional law?

2. Illness care, housing, and social security are examples of _____ (not rights.)

3. Who decides what those rights are that are not listed in the written Constitution?

4. Which source of rights has become more important in recent times?

5. What change is the source of unwritten rights in the Constitution, which is being used by the current Court in place of the previously identified right of privacy?

6. Which Amendment and right was used in the Cruzan case to assure a constitutional right to refuse medical treatment, including food and water?

7. Which is the right that will probably be involved when a "right to suicide" is at issue before the Court?

8. What is the original source of state or federal constitutional rights?

9. Which branch of government, legislature or judicial, should define our rights?

10. What is the relationship of the power of the federal government to the power of the state government?

RIGHTS, RIGHTS, AND MORE RIGHTS

Proponents and opponents of abortion use the word "rights" freely. Since the word "rights" is so misunderstood, some explanation is in order.

In legal terms, rights are limits on the freedom of the lawmaker, legislator, regulator, or judge, to make law. Such limits are listed in constitutions, either state or federal. The "rights" to illness care, housing, or social security are properly called entitlements, not rights.

The United States Constitution lists certain rights. Those rights limit the laws that states and the federal government can make. One of the Amendments to the Constitution, in the Bill (list) of Rights, carefully says that the list of rights is not all-inclusive. This means that there may be other rights than those listed. The list of rights in the Constitution does not mean that those are the only rights people have.

Someone must decide what those other rights are. The Supreme Court does that in deciding if laws made by the states or the federal government go beyond those limits (rights) listed or implied in the Constitution. Your state constitution also has a list of rights, probably more numerous than the federal. State courts too decide if lawmakers have exceeded limits (violated rights) in the state or federal constitution.

In recent years, state constitutions have been used more often than in the past to protect people from lawmakers. Several state constitutions specifically list a right of privacy. Florida's does (Section 23, Article 1, Constitution of the State of Florida, adopted 1980).

The courts of Florida have held that a law that limits abortions violates the Florida Constitution's listed right of privacy. In addition, Florida state courts have held that a law preventing feeding tube removal violates that right of privacy also. See "Withdrawing and Withholding" in Chapter Six, "A Time to Die."

In the U.S. Constitution there is no "right to die" listed, nor any right to abortion or to suicide. A right of privacy has been implied in the Constitution by the Supreme Court in the past. The court used that implied right to limit lawmakers' ability to make laws restricting abortion and birth control.

The Court presently is not writing opinions that speak of an implied right of privacy. Instead they have relied on the right of liberty guaranteed in the 5th and 14th Amendments, when they want to limit lawmaker power.

Those two Amendments also guarantee a right to life (and property). The Court has thus far has not ruled that a fetus at all stages of life is a person. Therefore, states may not prohibit abortions completely as long as the fetus is not "viable" (implication: not a person).

The Court in June 1990 declined to find an unlimited "right to die" implicit in the right to liberty, in the Cruzan case (noted earlier and later in this course). They allowed states to make their own decisions on what level of evidence to require that the person would refuse treatment.

They did assure, for the first time, that the right to refuse treatment is based on the Constitution -- the right of liberty in the 14th Amendment. That refusal can include food and water. The finding of a Constitutional right to refuse treatment means that no state law can override that right. Many state "living will" laws will be unconstitutional by this standard, since they prohibit the withdrawal of food and water even if requested in advance by a competent patient.

The current debate on a right to "assisted suicide," is more important to nonphysician practitioners than to doctors. After assisted death or euthanasia were legalized doubtless nonphysician practitioners, not doctors, would be employed in them and asked to "assist death" or to "kill." (The word used depends on your view of the activity.) Further, any practitioner whose patient suicides would be inculpated in that suicide if it were legal.

The issue of whether states may prohibit such activities can be argued under the issues of a right of liberty/privacy. Cruzan held that people have a right to refuse treatment under the right of liberty. Perhaps they have a right to end actively their lives. Then state laws punishing suicide, attempts and assistance, would be unconstitutional.

The state's interest in protecting the citizen's life, even against her own hand, would be subordinate to her right to do what she wished with her life. These are precisely the issues in the abortion and Cruzan cases: Where does the individual's liberty right (autonomy) end? Where does the people's interest in protecting life (sanctity of life) end?

All these questions revolve around the issue of what is it to be human, to be a person. When does a fetus become a baby—a person? When does a woman become a vegetable—a nonperson (dead?). When, if ever, does the government (the State, the Society, We) have an interest or a duty to intervene and protect life?

WHO SHOULD DECIDE?

A simpler question is whether these issues should be decided by courts (the judicial branch) or by legislatures (the legislative branch). Ultimately rights, which are limits on government action, are decided by the will of the people. Either they are written in the original Constitution or in Amendments to the Constitution by the elected representatives of the people.

Justice Oliver Wendell Holmes, Jr., said, "All rights tend to declare themselves absolute to their logical extremes." Rights are not absolute. The right of free speech does not extend to telling defamatory lies about another, and the right to practice religion does not extend to sacrificing children in the ritual. How far rights do extend is interpreted by the courts, under our present system.

Rights are designed to protect the people, individuals, from the laws of the those in power, elected by the majority. Are laws, which <u>force</u> us to act or not act in some way, better made by judges or legislators? The legislative process has more information input and therefore should make laws more likely based on reality.

But lawmakers unlimited by a Constitution with rights for individuals can result in a tyranny of the majority. A majority can be legal and at the same time unethical, because the law can be set at a <u>very</u> minimum ethic. The good Germans and Austrians who voted overwhelmingly for Hitler are a bad example.

Think about it. As with any part of our system, we can change it if we choose. You may get to vote on it one day.

POWER

To understand the abortion legality fight, we must know who has the power to make abortions legal or illegal. The states, in our system of government, have original and complete power. All the powers the federal government has, were granted to it; remember the 13 original colonies (states) were independent countries.

Through their federation, joining together, the colonies granted some power to their joint (federal) government, and put some limits on it too (the Bill of Rights in the U.S. Constitution). The people of the states, through their legislatures, have the power to make laws restricting abortion.

The federal power over abortion law is asserted by the U.S. Supreme Court. The Court decided in <u>Roe</u> that the Bill of Rights in the Constitution effectively prohibits the states from making abortion illegal during the first trimester (first three months) of pregnancy.

STUDY QUESTIONS

1. What are some differences in abortion law in America and elsewhere?

2. What do you think would be the outcome if <u>Roe v. Wade</u> is overturned and state legislatures could pass more restrictive abortion laws?

3. What are some of the reasons that women abort?

4. Which, if any, from that list of reasons do you believe justify an abortion?

5. What assumption do you think underlies this statement: We must not restrict abortion, for then even more black teenage unwed mothers will keep their babies.

6. What is an emotional term used to label the attitude that a whole people like the German Jews, are better off dead than alive?

7. Whose are the various interests present in the abortion conflict?

8. What are the issues around the use of the drug RU486?

9. What is the difference between contraception and abortion as methods of family planning?

OTHER GOVERNMENTS

Most of the other industrialized countries now do not prohibit abortion. Ireland is an exception, and now some of the Eastern Bloc countries, which after liberal abortion laws under Communism have turned to more restrictive abortion regulation. Many of those countries are Catholic. The religion and its expression, including feelings against abortion, were repressed under Communism.

Only in the U.S. is abortion allowed for any reason during the first trimester. Most countries require physician certification that the abortion is for a reason other than birth control. Some countries forbid abortion after the first trimester. Some require delay and furnishing information to the woman seeking the abortion. This is like the parts of Pennsylvania law upheld in 1992 by the Supreme Court.

The U.S. is the only country in which liberalized abortion law was made by judicial decision (a few state courts in Australia took that power route, too). Abortion legality has not been established in the U.S. by legislative vote and the usual compromise process. If the Supreme Court overturns <u>Roe v. Wade</u> (see "History"), states will be able to enact further limits on abortion. Some states will do so, and some will not. The process of legislation, halted in 1973, will begin anew. The problem to some is that state laws will vary, so women will be able to get abortions in some states, not in others.

People who are unable to afford travel to another state will not be able to get an abortion in their own state. The court's decision will not change the situation that even now, women in some states have little or no access to abortion (few clinics do the procedure in some states.)

No matter what the outcome at the Supreme Court level, people will still disagree about the abortion issue. The <u>Roe</u> decision did not stop the disagreement, and the overturning or continued reduction of its scope will not stop the disagreement either. The issue must to be debated, compromised, and agreed upon finally before law is written.

This is the difficult, painful, unsatisfying, democratic process. It means that nobody gets to win it all, as people do in court. It means that everybody gets to win a little, as people do when people don't go to court -- when they agree on a solution even if it's not exactly what each side wants.

WHY TO ABORT

Shall the <u>reason</u> for aborting be a factor in allowing abortion? Through amniocentesis and other tests, we can know a lot about a developing fetus, early enough to choose an abortion if the news is bad.

What is "bad" news? That she is a baby with developmental disability? That she's anencephalic? That she has a genetic defect that will cause her pain or that may mean she will have a defective baby herself? That she has a gene for homosexuality? That she's a she?

Since 1973, when the Supreme Court made first trimester abortion on demand legal nationwide, that legality has carried with it the freedom to abort for any reason. If proponents want the government off women's backs and out of their bedrooms, can they then ask the police to protect babies who are aborted for any reason?

Prenatal diagnosis was first made available in the sixties to detect fetuses with gross chromosomal defects. Now couples may have genetic testing to determine whether they carry genetic problems likely to be passed on to their children. A project is underway to map the entire human genome structure; this may make possible diagnosis of many other problems, in utero, or before pregnancy, in the parents of potential babies.

Genetic reasons given for to abortion are many and increase daily. Tests are available to the woman who is pregnant to determine whether her baby has Down's syndrome or fragile x, both of which cause mental retardation, or another genetic condition that might be undesired in her child. In most cases, the results are available early enough to abort.

Amniocentesis is necessary to make determinations in many of these conditions. And amniocentesis is available only if the practitioner will do it; practitioners vary on their willingness to do amniocentesis, depending on the age of the mother and the reason she wants the test. Usually practitioners limit amniocentesis to mothers 35 and over, because they are the group most likely to have Down's syndrome babies.

This is an ethical issue for the practitioners (the subject of patient demand and practitioner autonomy is discussed in the next chapter, "Professionals and Employees").

A survey of doctors in various countries revealed that 78% of doctors surveyed would do amniocentesis on an anxious 25 year old, with no medical indication for the amniocentesis. There is a 0.50% risk of losing the baby as a result of the amniocentesis, but only a 0.13% risk of having a Down's baby by a mother that young.

As we know more about genetics, chromosomes, diseases, and babies before birth, the numbers of conditions that can be prevented multiply the condition is not prevented, actually, but the birth of the baby is. Should it be?

In a large study of 27,000 pregnancies, 84% of the amniocenteses done were indicated due to risk of a chromosomal disorder. The median maternal age was 36 years.

Of amniocenteses done, 1.5% revealed chromosomal abnormality. 73% of those pregnancies were terminated. Severity of the genetic disorder affects decision; autosomal abnormalities (mental retardation) cause termination in

92 to 95% of cases. Half or less of babies identified as having sex chromosomal abnormalities were aborted. A high proportion of couples finding abnormalities terminate the pregnancy; the degree of clinical severity predictably influences parental decisions.

Reference: Vincent, Victoria A., et al, "Pregnancy Termination Because of Chromosomal Abnormalities: A Study of 26,950 Amniocenteses in the Southeast," *Southern Medical Journal*, 1991; 84:1210-12.

Amniocentesis and other tests for genetic abnormalities, and legal abortion for those conditions is available. Should we encourage or even mandate women to have such tests and such abortions if they test positive?

Is it "right" to allow a handicapped child to be born if it can be aborted? Is it right for the child who may suffer, right for the society that might have to pay for its care?

Is it "right" have children who carry chromosomes that will in the future present a risk of genetic defect? In Nazi Germany, people with the possibility of genetic defect transmission were forcibly sterilized, so the issue of aborting their children never arose.

Reference: "Biomedical Ethics and the Shadow of Nazism: A Conference on the Proper Use of the Nazi Analogy in Ethical Debate," *Hastings Center Report*, 1976, August, Special Supplement, p. 20.

Could we admit that it is for the parent's own good? That the energy and strength and money cost of a handicapped child are more than some people can bear? More than the society can bear? If so, then we should say so, and not lie to ourselves about whose interests we are protecting.

Could we be honest enough to say that economic or cosmetic or purely personal reasons for abortion are enough? Women who have abortions often cite as reasons the economics of having a child. As noted earlier, children are no longer economic assets, contributing wealth to a family; they are enormous economic costs, almost luxuries.

Can we admit that there are sexual reasons to abort? In India, pregnant women who have an amniocentesis or sound ultra frequently choose to abort when they find the baby is a girl/female. The feminists of India are particularly offended by this, as are others. They call for a ban on abortion when done for that reason. Of course, if abortion is freely available for other reasons it is a simple matter to lie.

Reference: Wertz, Dorothy C., and Fletcher, John C. "Ethics and Genetics: An International Survey," *Hastings Center Report*, July/August 1989, pp. 20-24.

In the above survey of geneticists about amniocentesis, 34% of U.S. doctors would test for the sex of a fetus. The hypothetical conditions given the doctor were that the couple wishing amniocentesis already had four daughters, and planned to abort if the fetus turned out to be the fifth daughter instead of a desired son.

But if we prohibit discrimination against the handicapped that are born (see the discussion of the Americans with Disabilities Act, in the Professionals and Employees Chapter), is it not also discrimination against the unborn handicapped, to allow them to be selectively aborted?

It is said that we differ from the Nazis in that we do not have in mind a "super" or pure race as an ideal to strive for. But when we abort babies that are not ideal, are we acting differently?

If abortion is allowed, the value of autonomy for the woman is placed above the value of life of the fetus. Abortion on demand is just that; abortion for any demand. If the state (we) will not interfere with a private decision to abort, then we probably may not interfere with whatever the reason to abort.

GENOCIDE?

Statistics are cited that many more babies are being born to unwed mothers. Some quote these data to justify keeping liberal abortion laws. The fear is that if abortion were less accessible, even more unmarried women would keep their babies.

The change of attitude toward being pregnant and single has many causes we don't pretend to understand. Some must be rooted in the relatively greater ability now of women to work and take care of their children without a husband. There is not the economic necessity that there may have been in earlier times. In some situations in welfare families, it is an economic necessity <u>not</u> to have a husband, in order to qualify for or keep benefits.

Some writers sound as though they think the unwed teens who are delivering and keeping their babies, should be aborting those babies. Since many of unwed teens are black, we must examine whether there is some unseen, or perhaps even unrecognized, value judgment in preferring abortion for those girls. The value implicit is that children are better off aborted than born to and kept by teenage unwed black mothers.

On the other hand, the argument that these babies should not be aborted because they can be adopted, only holds if there is a market (demand) for the babies. Are all the black babies adoptable? All the handicapped?

Does the baby have a right to be born wanted? If not, is he better off not being born? That's a "quality of life" issue more difficult than that for Cruzan or Quinlan (see Chapter Six, "A Time To Die"). Is a life begun with a poor child–mother, or in a foster home or an institution, worse than no life at all?

And if it is, could we ever consider infanticide for those children? Can they sue their mother for the psychological harm done them? For wrongful life?

A related issue is whether a child should be conceived deliberately and brought into the world for the primary purpose of providing a bone marrow transplant for her sister (this has happened already). The assumption here is that the big sister's survival is more important than any "suffering" the little sister's life might cause her. If you believe that life itself is a higher value, then the little sister got a good deal because she got life she wouldn't have otherwise. And big sister got to keep living.

Any discussion beyond the individual interests (woman/mother, fetus/baby) is about society's interest—each of our interests. Is it better for us to have unwanted children born or aborted? Which will save money? Which will result in the kind of society, kind of people, we want to be? Is there some not-so-subtle elitism here? Can we call it genocide?

While we gnash our teeth at how low our morals have fallen, we can look at our history and take comfort that we're no worse than our ancestors. A large percentage of babies born in Connecticut in the 1700s were illegitimate also.

HOW TO ABORT AND WHEN

The physical techniques of abortion somewhat limit the timing of abortion. The technique most used early in pregnancy is dilating the cervix and suctioning out the contents of the uterus. Later the doctor does a dilitation with curettage [French for using a curette scraper to scrape out the lining of the uterus].

Still later when the fetus is too large to dissect with the instrument and remove through the minimally dilated cervix, a solution is injected into the uterus through the cervix and labor is induced, causing the contents (baby, fetus) to be expelled (delivered vaginally). A variation of this late abortion is to deliver the fetus except for the head, which is decompressed by suctioning out the contents of the skull so it will collapse and be more easily removed through the partially dilated cervix. All these require some anesthesia, and sterile equipment, and skilled practitioners.

State laws that require an abortion to be done in a hospital would have the effect of limiting the availability of abortions. Fewer places for abortion would be available, with the desired end being fewer abortions performed. Advocates of such laws say that women deserve the protection of abortion procedures done under strict standards of care.

The contraception method of intrauterine devices (IUDs) work by causing an "abortion," probably causing the fertilized egg to fail to implant after entering the uterus from the fallopian tube. Some abortion opponents are doubtless opposed to this method of contraception for that reason, while others oppose all contraception except abstinence on religious grounds. (See the discussion of contraception under "Technology," above.)

Still other people oppose abortion but not contraception. As in labeling any diverse group of people, it is hard to characterize all anti-abortion or pro-choice people. Pro-choice leaders do fear that "losing" the abortion right at the constitutional level will encourage opponents of birth control to mount forces against that technology as well.

A drug has been used in Europe and now in the U.S. to accomplish abortion without the necessity of the above techniques. The drug is given orally; then 24 hours later prostaglandin is injected, causing uterine contractions and expulsion of the contents of the uterus (whether baby or not). The drug must be given under supervision; complications are possible but not usual.

The drug, RU486, can be used during the first weeks of pregnancy; it was developed in France and has been used there. The drug maker is the Hoechst Company, which will seek to market the drug in this country. Any company marketing the drug might provoke a boycott of its other business by people who are pro-life, anti-abortion.

Questions around this issue are whether it is ethical for people to enforce their own moral vision, keeping a drug off the market, by a boycott or threatened boycott. By the same token, an ethical question is whether one should enforce moral attitudes by boycotting lettuce because it was picked by nonunion people, or whether it is ethical to influence the pro-life owner by boycotting his pizza chain, to change the allegedly sexist attitude of a brewery management by boycotting their beer.

Another issue in the abortion debate is late abortions. Of the 1.5 million abortions per year, 1% (about 15,000) are done after the 20th week, by saline injection or by the technique described above. The babies delivered without decompressed skull may be born alive. If they breathe spontaneously, shall the practitioner support them or allow them to die?

A practitioner in this field must do some "values clarification," -- some thinking about his role. Is your patient the woman, who does not want a live baby? Does your responsibility extend to the child? State law may require one or the other, but law does not in this case (nor in few others) solve the problem of the practitioner's ethical choice.

STUDY QUESTIONS

1. What was the regulation upheld in Rust v. Sullivan and what is its potential impact on practitioners?

2. When is a father's interest not an interest "traditionally protected" (and therefore not enforced) according to U.S. Supreme Court Justice Scalia?

3. What is the "ism" or philosophy associated with the value autonomy (freedom) -- the philosophy most dominant in the United States?

4. What is the origin of the term "cesarean" for abdominal delivery?

5. What are some of the interests listed of a woman in an ethical conflict?

6. Which value has been found to be the most important when a judge incarcerates a pregnant woman to keep her from taking drugs?

7. Is having a child a right, or a privilege which the law may limit?

8. Agree or disagree with the following (discuss): In the future, children will be able to sue their mothers for divorcing their fathers, because thereby they were deprived of support and companionship.

9. Do unequal outcomes, such as different mortality rates for white and black infants, mean lack of justice?

10. What is the definition of "neonate?"

11. What is interest of the newborn with a handicap?

12. What value can you speculate was held by Florida aboriginals living 7000 years ago, toward newborns with handicaps?

13. What is the position of pro-life groups on research and therapy using aborted fetuses?

14. What is the rationale for allowing aborted fetuses to be used for research and therapy?

15. How can the use of aborted fetuses for research and therapy be distinguished from the use of bodies of Persistent Unconscious Persons (PUPs) declared "dead?"

16. What is the interest that the state or government has in all the issues in "A Time to Be Born?"

FREEDOM OF SPEECH VIOLATED OR EMPLOYER POLICY IMPLEMENTED?

The policy of the Republican administration under President George Bush was against abortion. Regulations were made by the Department of Health and Human Services in February 1988, requiring health professionals in Title X (Family Planning Services and Population Act) to tell any pregnant woman requesting information on abortion that the project does not consider abortion a method of family planning (contraception, birth control).

Prior to this, state statutes that mandated what practitioners must say to women before abortions had been struck down on grounds that they violated the privacy right within the practitioner–patient relationship. The Court in some narrow majorities in those days was finding a privacy right in the "penumbra" of the Bill of Rights, though it is not specifically written there.

When this regulation was challenged, the Supreme Court upheld it in Rust v. Sullivan, 59 U.S.L.W. 4451,500 U.S. 173 (1991). The court did not find a privacy interest here, as it also did not in Webster (see above). The federal government did not have to show a "compelling" need for the regulation, only a reasonable or "legitimate" need, since the Court decided no fundamental right was at stake. Also, the government did not have to show that there was no other possible way to achieve its end. This issue is discussed in Chapter Five, "Professionals and Employees."

Practitioners worried that the decision jeopardized the confidential relationship of practitioners to patients. They also worried about their freedom and responsibility to give women information about abortion when they thought indicated. Contrary arguments: This is not an unusual exercise of employer control over policy; such regulations about what patients are told or what treatment is to be provided are necessary to the agency's interest.

The Administration changed its regulation again in March of 1992, allowing physicians but no other practitioners to counsel patients about abortion in such clinics. This distinction between professionals raised further ethical issues: Is professional autonomy more important for physicians; are they more ethical than other practitioners; is the patient-practitioner relationship more important in that profession than others; is it "just" that physicians have the freedom to practice and not other professionals. The election of Bill Clinton in 1992 resulted in further changes in the regulation -- it has been withdrawn. What if a new regulation required practitioners to <u>counsel</u> about abortion? Could they refuse?

Actually abortions do control (prohibit) birth. They are not contra (against) conception; they do not prohibit conception, but deal instead with its consequences. Evidence exists that women do use abortion instead of contraception as birth control. Only 43% of women seeking abortion had been using birth control prior to the pregnancy. (Data from Guttmacher Institute.)

THE FATHER'S INTEREST

The value we discuss in the father's interest is justice -- his fair treatment under the law.

The father has an interest in the abortion decision. The issue is how much, and whether his interest takes precedence over the mother's interest in being free from pregnancy and a child. As an analogy, the father has an interest, and even some legal remedies, when his child is placed for adoption. He has some interests in visitation and contact with the child (if the child is not aborted) just as he has some financial responsibility.

This will be true unless we come to believe the family unit is the mother and children, with occasional visits by a series of fathers and uncles. This is a pattern of behavior in some human groups, particularly in aboriginal tribes. It has not been the mainstream custom of the United States.

To the contrary of the father's rights or interest is the case decided by the U.S. Supreme Court, <u>Michael H. v. Gerald D.</u>,491 U.S. 110 (1989) in which Justice Scalia wrote a plurality opinion. (In a plurality opinion the Justices reach a "majority" <u>decision</u>, but there is no "majority" <u>opinion</u> as to how or why the decision was reached.) The court upheld a California court in its decision to refuse to grant a paternity hearing to a man who had a daughter with a married woman.

Justice Scalia held that the only Fourteenth Amendment liberty interests to be upheld were those "traditionally protected" and that states had not given such protections to an "adulterous natural father."

INTEREST OF THE WOMAN

This society values greatly the right of the individual, we are a very plural nation, compared to others. We are not of one tribe. Our individuality is inevitable, a product of that plurality -- not a choice someone has made. That individuality is the base of the value we place on autonomy. The value most important for the pregnant woman in the abortion issue is the value of autonomy (the woman's freedom to be pregnant or not; to choose to live her life as she sees fit).

This individuality, and the resulting autonomy and freedom extended to the "right" to choose abortion, are a particularly sensitive issue now, as women are gaining rights and status they seem not to have had before.

Because women are the sex that gets pregnant, responsibilities and limitations fall on them. It's been said that if men got pregnant, abortion would be a sacrament (a sacred ritual in the church). At least if men also got pregnant, we could discuss abortion without the added load of potential sex discrimination.

Women have been forced to undergo sterilization in some societies: In Nazi Germany, because they carried undesirable genes; in America, because they were mentally retarded (in the 1970s, by doctors one of whom later was nominated for Surgeon General in the Clinton Administration). They have been forced to undergo Cesarean sections because the life of the baby they were carrying was in danger, even though that surgery put their own lives in danger.

They have been kept on life support for weeks though brain damaged, so their babies could develop longer. Truly, in that situation the woman was only a life-support system for a baby.

There's a tradition of "fetal rescue" at the woman's expense. The Greek god of medicine, Asklepios, was cut out alive from the womb of his dead mother (it is said). We assume she was dead when they started. And 600 years before Christ, the Lex Regia, law of the king, mandated that when a woman died the infant must be delivered abdominally. After the Emperors came into power, they called the law, Lex Cesarea, hence the word for Cesarean delivery. (Another theory is that "cesar" means "to cut"!)

The closer to full development and birth, the more the interests of the baby are valued and the mother's interests decline in importance.

Reference: Steinbodk, Bonnie, "The Relevance of Illegality," *Hastings Center Report*, January-February 1992, pp. 19-22.

ADVOCATE FOR WOMEN?

Women have an interest in not being pregnant if it is not to their advantage at any particular time.

Women have an interest in having a baby as free as possible from conditions that will make the baby's life, and therefore her life, difficult. Raising a "normal" child is expensive and difficult enough, and adding the burdens of physical or mental problems is something any woman has an interest in avoiding—any man, too.

A woman has an interest in having a baby of the sex that she wants, when she wants. She's doing the child an enormous gift to give him life. The odds of any individual sperm penetrating an egg are literally millions to one. She should be able to choose the sex of child she will bear.

Why does that penetration (and union and following cell division) entitle that particular zygote to life? It could have as easily been a sperm with an x (girl) as a y (boy) chromosome. Why does the existence of that particular tiny parasite have to limit her life and forever deny her the privilege of buying little pink dresses?

Does the woman who gives up her baby for adoption have any interest in where the child goes? Several examples of Indian women being refused the ability to give their child to nonIndian couples are documented. If the mother gives up her child to obtain a better life, should she have some ability to decide with whom the child lives, or does her giving up the child cut off all her rights?

The woman's right to work in a job that potentially could damage her child if she conceived was upheld by the Supreme Court. Critics of the company said it used that policy as an excuse to keep women out of higher-paying jobs they were qualified for. They said the real purpose of the policy was to minimize the risk to the company of lawsuit.

The Supreme Court said that to exclude pregnant or potentially pregnant women from jobs that might harm their babies was discrimination because of their possible or actual pregnancy. And that's against the law—the Federal Pregnancy Discrimination Act of 1978. International Union v. Johnson Controls, 111 S.Ct. 1196 (1991).

INTEREST OF THE CHILD

The child has interests, also. The child has an interest in autonomy, and most importantly in life, though its interests can't be self-expressed. How we decide whose interests "win" depends on how much we value the interests of the woman versus the interests of the baby. Our decision may rest on how much we value adults versus how much we value children. Make no mistake, the value of money-work is very much a consideration in these situations. Consider the money required to care for a baby born addicted or AIDS infected; the money required to care for a severely handicapped neonate; the money required for prenatal care to decrease some of the preventable complications of pregnancy and childbirth.

The fetus has an interest in not being born addicted. When does that interest win over his mother's (bearer's) interest in taking the drugs she wants or feels she needs? Should she be prosecuted for child abuse? Jailed to prevent her drug use? If she's had treatment available, offered, and refuses?

The media has called much attention to the plight of "crack babies," infants addicted to cocaine. More recently commentators have said the harmful effect on the baby of addiction may have been overstated.

CRIMINAL LIABILITY

The fetus has an interest in not being born with damage from alcohol. A Missouri woman was charged with second-degree assault and child endangerment when her son was born with blood alcohol content reported to be in excess of 0.10, the legal level for intoxication. The county prosecutor said he charged the woman after doctors gave information to police about the incident.

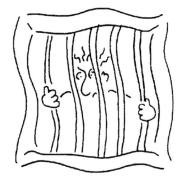

Reference: "Mother Charged with 'Assault' in Birth of

Intoxicated Baby," *Missouri Lawyers Weekly*, December 9, 1991, p. 1.

This is similar to more widely reported occurrences of babies being born addicted to crack cocaine or other drugs. Several of these cases have been brought in Florida. Delivery of cocaine (through the umbilical cord) and contributing to the dependence of a minor are the usual charges. Pensacola authorities began arresting mothers who use cocaine in an effort to encourage pregnant women to seek drug treatment before giving birth.

Many in the medical community believe that such prosecutions will drive pregnant mothers away from seeking treatment for themselves or their babies. While such cases publicize the dangers of crack addiction in babies, or fetal alcohol syndrome when the mother drinks to excess, social welfare people fear the same publicity about prosecution will deter the mothers from getting help.

Addicted mothers present particular problems. If they are unable to help themselves (to choose) some people say the society (we) must choose for them to protect their children. They base this on a need to reduce harm to the child, but also to protect the society from increased costs of the birth of a damaged child and presumably more abuse.

Related to this, technology in contraception allows the government to do a "forced sterilization" that is reversible. A judge can (and has) order a woman implanted with a timed-release birth control drug. In the particular case, the woman was found guilty of child abuse and the judge's motive was to prevent a potential child.

Recent cases allow lawsuits by child against parent. In former times, the family was seen as a unit, so no individual could assert a claim against another -- particularly not a child against her parent.

Many states now allow suit for harm in civil liability, or prosecution for criminal act done to a "viable" fetus. In a state like Missouri, where a statute declares that the life of each human being begins at conception (Section 1.205 RSMo, 1986), the question of viability is a difficult one.

In most states, prosecutors will only prosecute for criminal activity directed against a live "person." Personhood has generally been held to be at the age of viability, when the child can survive outside the uterus. But civil liability (money damages) might lie for injury to a nonviable fetus that was then born damaged or dead at term. A situation could arise that resulted in damages for <u>injury</u> to a nonviable fetus that survived; but no liability if <u>death</u> resulted.

Under state civil and criminal laws, unborn children do have some property rights, rights to inherit, and have personal rights which are sometimes recognized by the appointment of a guardian ad litem. That is Latin for a guardian appointed for the duration of the litigation or court case.

Reference: "Drunk Driver Gets Manslaughter for Viable Fetus' Death," and "'Viability' the New Battleground for Civil Suits, Too," *Missouri Lawyers Weekly*, December 9, 1991, pp. 1, 16-17.

The baby has an interest in not being exposed to harmful chemicals *in utero* because his mother chose to work in a dangerous place, or felt she had to. But a company cannot discriminate against a woman to protect her baby (see the *Johnson* case above). In *Johnson*, the interests of the women were valued over potential interests of the children.

Now children are suing parents for negligent or intentional harm. They can sue for physical abuse, failure to safeguard, and in the drug-abusing mother, for negligent or intentional exposure to harmful drugs. Many of these mothers have no money, so the issue is not going to come up right away. More and more, but it is possible; some suits have been instituted for alleged child abuse that is remembered many years later.

Certainly the baby could sue a drug manufacturer who supplied a defective drug to her mother, causing an injury to the baby. By the same reasoning, a baby could sue a mother who exposed her unborn child to drugs or alcohol, thereby causing damage. Assault, battery, and outrageous conduct are possible claims; in addition, some courts have held parents responsible for negligence in the supervision of their children.

With advances in technology permitting treatment *in utero*, and in future genetic correction of problems, the child has an interest in treatment if needed *in utero*. If the mother refuses, again rises a conflict of interests between the mother and child. The same issue arises when during labor the practitioner recommends a Cesarean for a compromised fetus. Cases and practitioners are split on whether surgery may be done to protect the child without the woman's permission.

The baby has an interest in being born into a system that gives her the best chance she can have to live, whether she's white or black. Black babies on average weigh less at birth, regardless of the social status of the mother or the amount of prenatal care given. Research is needed to determine the cause, since lower birth weight is associated with higher infant mortality.

This racial difference accounts for most of the reason that the U.S. has relatively higher infant mortality rates than European countries with homogeneous populations. In turn, that explains the somewhat shorter life expectancy in the U.S. than in Europe. The infant mortality rate directly affects life expectancy numbers. See Chapter Five, "A Time To Die," for explanation.

References: Murray, Jann, and Bernfield, Merton, "The Differential Effect of Prenatal Care on the Incidence of Low Birth Weight among Blacks and Whites in a Prepaid Health Care Plan," *NEJM*, 1988; 319:1385-91.

Oechsli, Frank, "Prenatal Care and Low Birth Weight among Blacks and Whites," *NEJM*, April 13, 1989, p. 1010.

NEONATES NEED LIFE, TOO

Increasingly, the newborn child is referred to as a "neonate." This is the Latin term for "newborn;" it may be an attempt to sound more scientific than saying "newborn baby." It also has the effect, intended or not, of considering the newborn still not quite human (not quite a person). This attitude may make it easier to deal with children that are born severely handicapped.

Francis Crick, the Nobel Prize winner, proposed that society might have to consider that no neonate should be declared legally human until it is a few days old and has passed a genetic test. The infant wouldn't be human, so it wouldn't be the same as killing to "dispose" of it.

The interest of the newborn is in living. Some writers on the subject say that the child has no interest that should be considered. It has no experience, no thought process, and so people from the outside must evaluate its fate.

Some might say a severely handicapped newborn such as an anencephalic has an interest in dying if she's born severely handicapped. What if she's born a little handicapped? In the Baby Doe case of a few years back, a Down's syndrome baby was born with a birth defect that is easily corrected. This defect, esophageal atresia with tracheo-esophageal fistula, would always be corrected on a mentally normal baby. Baby Doe was allowed to starve in a hospital nursery at the parent's request (Stevenson, Derek et al., "The "Baby Doe Rule," *JAMA* 1986; 255: 1909-12.)

That situation prompted a federal regulation requiring whistle-blowing. What are the newborn's interests if she's born as a result of abortion? If she's born unwanted? (See the discussion of "Teenage Mothers.") Some writers have suggested the decision about whether the newborn be treated, cared for, or fed should be left to the wishes of the "parents" who would have to deal with the child.

Evidence exists of prehistoric Americans' attitude toward handicapped newborns: an archeological site in Florida (Windover) revealed a burial site with skeleton of a carefully buried child. Examination by experts revealed that the child had been born with spina bifida, a handicap that can be very difficult to care for even with the resources we have today. The child had been cared for and lived until a teenager.

USE OF ABORTED FETUSES

Another issue around this area is experiments on abortuses. The first question is why the term "abortus" is used, and not "aborted baby" or "aborted fetus." I have no answer; perhaps it is again an attempt to remove emotion by removing the name.

In 1988, the federal government banned the use of tissue from fetuses for research and transplants as a condition of receiving federal money (private groups can and do use fetal tissue for research). Use of fetal tissue from spontaneous abortions and abortions necessary to prevent health risks to the mother are not at issue; the use of fetuses from elective abortions is. The 1992 change in president changed this regulation too.

References: Martin, Douglas K., "Abortion and Fetal Tissue Transplantation (and Commentary same issue), " IRB, A Review of Human Subjects Research, 1993; 15: No. 3, pp. 1-5.

Pro-life people believe that the use of the tissue is immoral; that to benefit some from the death of others is wrong. They say the use will be another factor encouraging women to have abortions, if they believe that their fetus can benefit research. But if women are not told their fetus might be used, they have not given truly "informed consent" to abortion.

Reports of benefits to research on Parkinson's, Huntington's, and diabetes caused some members of Congress to propose legislation lifting the ban. They cited the benefit to individuals and the whole society from use of the tissue.

We make an analogy to the idea of using people who are declared dead; we might make use of their bodies for the good of humanity. There's a move to change the definition of "dead" to include people diagnosed as in a Persistent Vegetative State. Proponents have proposed that such "dead bodies" then could be used for donation.

As researchers gain more information about genetic problems in utero, there may be more pressure to have aborted fetuses available for use in transplanting genes. Then might poor women become pregnant and abort for economic reasons -- to sell genes to rich parents for their own babies?

Resources: *Medical Ethics Advisor*, January 1992, pp. 5-7.

Robertson, John A. "Rights, Symbolism, and Public Policy in Fetal Tissue Transplants," *Hastings Center Report*, December 1988, pp. 5-12.

Nolan, Kathleen, "*Genug ist Genug*; A Fetus Is Not a Kidney," same issue, pp. 13-19.

INTEREST OF THE STATE–SOCIETY–US

When we say "state" we mean "society" (read *other people*) -- all individuals as a group. "Society" also is a word, a construct, a concept; it means what we want and agree on. The interest of the "state" (that is, all of us) is in preserving the lives of people without defenses. It is the original enforcement of the ethical and religious mandate "do unto others."

The question, always, is where to draw the line. When does the state intervene in family life? The autonomy of the family, of the parents, is not absolute; the law prohibits child abuse, drug abuse, homosexuality, not abortion (some), nor birth control. No interest is absolute; it depends on what we want and think is right. Rights are only words; the reality depends on what people are willing to tolerate or fight or enforce.

STUDY QUESTIONS AND ANSWERS

These are suggested answers. If you have something like these answers in your own words, consider yourself successful. If you have more (quality, and quantity) than these answers, consider yourself excellent.

1.   Which are the values raised in the ethical issues in A Time to Be Born?

- Life
- Autonomy
- Beneficence
- Loyalty
- Money-work
- Any other you can justify

2. What is a possible genetic outcome of brothers and sisters marrying?

   More likely occurrence of recessive gene defects

3. What is the definition of eugenics?

   Selecting people for reproduction by their genetic material, to produce a superior people

4. What is the issue of fairness that occurs in insurance payment for artificial insemination?

   Whether it is fair to require all people buying insurance to pay for a procedure that is not "necessary"

5. What is the religious objection to artificial insemination?

   - It separates procreation from the act of sexual intercourse
   - The primary purpose of sex is for procreation, under the Church's view

6. What is the question of fairness that arises relative to the child born by artificial insemination to a single woman?

   - Whether it is fair to create a child who will not have or know its father
   - (But this is common in single-parent families now)
   - Whether such a life is worse than no life at all

7. What is the definition of "in vitro fertilization?"

   Union of the ovum and sperm in a glass petri dish, outside the woman's body

8. What is the position of the Catholic Church (and others who oppose it) relative to in vitro fertilization?

   - The same objection as in artificial insemination
   - It removes procreation from intercourse

- In addition, when such fertilization is done, several ova are fertilized
- In the church's view these are human lives of which some are then destroyed

9. What is the "fairness" issue relative to insurance payment for <u>in vitro</u> fertilization? The same arguments exist as do for artificial insemination:

- Whether others also paying insurance premiums should have higher premiums for a procedure which is not necessary to the insured's life
- The expenses of the procedure make the argument much more compelling

10. Who should get custody or possession of fertilized frozen zygotes when a couple divorces?

- You should have answered some version of "it depends"
- It depends on all the usual custody questions in a divorce, who'd be the better parent
- Whether the usual rules of custody prevail
- Again, realizing that these may or may not be like "children" or more like property
- Or, even more than children, since one "parent" may not want to be a parent any more

11. Why is the term "surrogate mother" applied to a woman who has a baby she knows she will give to some specific other person?

I don't know either, but there's some reason people want to distinguish this woman from one who gives her baby to an adoption agency -- something to do with money, and intent.

12. Which is the correct term in the surrogate mother issue, "womb" or "uterus?"

- It depends on how you want to influence emotion
- Condemning "rent-a-uterus" isn't nearly so effective as condemning "rent-a-womb"

13. Which statement is correct: Surrogate motherhood exploits poor women. Surrogate motherhood provides poor women pay for their risk.

- Neither is more correct; both are value judgments
- Both are valid feelings which you need to be able to identify in yourself first, before you investigate anything else

14. What are some of the possible outcomes of a conflict between a surrogate mother who wants to keep the baby, and the people who have "paid for" the baby?

- The surrogate mother could be considered the "birth mother," and get to keep the baby
- Or the parents, if they are the genetic parents, could be considered the "natural parents" (Anna J. Case)
- Or the surrogate mother could be the genetic mother, but the genetic father and his wife could be considered "better parents" because they seem more stable and have more assets (Baby M Case)

15. What do you think the ethical outcome should be in such a case as above, and why?

- Whatever you answered is valid, because there are no "correct" answers in ethics
- You should have mentioned or discussed the issues of who makes the better parent, who the baby "belongs" to, and what is fair in the case, to parents and to baby and to surrogate

16. Whose are the three interests in such a conflict?

- The surrogate mother's
- The parents'
- The baby's

17. Do you agree or disagree with this statement and why? Technology is the origin of our problems with procreation.

- You had better disagree
- Technology makes more things possible, but people had problems before technology

18. Has better technology improved our lives in regard to abortion?

- This will depend entirely on how you feel about abortion
- If you believe that the woman's choice is the primary good, then safer and easier abortions are good
- If you believe abortion is wrong, then the technology that makes it easier is bad

19. Do you disagree or agree with this statement and why? If it's a law, it's ethical.

    Your answer should compare the legal with the ethical, mentioning that law is a minimum ethic, that legal does not mean very ethical, nor vice versa, certainly

20. What is the name of the most famous U.S. case that limited the state's ability to restrict abortions?

    Roe v. Wade

21. According to surveys, which subgroup of Americans wish to keep abortion on demand legal during the first three months of pregnancy (as it is now)?

    According to a Guttmacher survey, men

22. Do Americans agree with the current law on abortion on demand?

    If you believe surveys (and some skepticism is in order about what people say on surveys), a majority of Americans think abortion laws should be more restrictive than they are,

23. Why do people use the word "fetus" or the word "baby" when speaking about abortion?

    To appeal to the emotion, using "baby;" or to avoid the emotion, using "fetus"

24. Why do people use the word "mother" or the word "woman" when speaking about abortion?

    • To appeal to the emotion, using "mother;" or to avoid the emotion, using "woman"

25. Why do people use the terms "Pro-choice," "Pro-life," "Anti-abortion," "Pro-abortion?"

    Each is used to appeal to the emotion

26. What is the point at which a fetus or baby becomes a person, according to the U.S. Supreme Court?

- Not even Constitutional scholars know, because the justices don't know, either
- This makes you realize that you're as smart as they are
- And you realize they are as human as we are

27. Criticize (examine and be critical of) this statement: Abortions have been done and an ethical conflict about them has arisen only during the last few years.

You should have mentioned some of the examples of abortion known in history, from Persian and Greek times

28. What are some instances of infanticide during history?

- The ancient Romans sometimes "exposed" children, though some of those were probably found and adopted from the area where they were customarily left
- During the middle ages, mothers "overlay" nursing infants

29. Agree or disagree with this statement and state why: Infanticide in former times justifies our present practice of abortion.

- Whatever you believe is correct, but
- You should discuss why we can or cannot and should or should not justify our present ethics and actions with past people's behavior

30. What is an example of a society that practices infanticide at present?

The Chinese, who abort the third child conceived, and often kill the second if she is a daughter

31. What is the definition of "quickening" and what is its legal importance?

- Under English common law, it was defined as the point in pregnancy when the mother could feel movement of the fetus
- Abortions performed before that point were legal; after, illegal

32. Why did English common law of abortion have any effect in the U.S.?

HSM 510: Ethical Considerations in Health Care Delivery

139

- Because many of the English legal theories, and actual common law of England, was made law in American states
- Thus the English law was American law, too, unless and until specific statutes changed it

33. What was the state of American abortion law in 1973, before <u>Roe v. Wade?</u>

Several states had liberalized their abortion laws and several more state legislatures were in the process.

34. Why is it important that the Supreme Court in <u>Roe</u> called privacy, (and abortion) a "fundamental right?"

Because in constitutional law terms, that means a state can almost never pass a law restricting that right

35. What are the three stages of pregnancy mentioned in that case, and what is the state's interest at each stage?

- **First trimester:** State has no interest; no restriction of abortion will be constitutional
- **Second trimester:** State has an interest in protecting the mother's health
- **Third trimester:** State has an interest in protecting the fetus or baby

36. What is the definition of viability?

Ability to survive outside the womb or uterus

37. Disagree or agree with this statement, and state your rationale: The <u>Roe</u> decision solved all ethical conflict about abortion.

- Conflict existed before <u>Roe</u>
- Conflict has existed since <u>Roe</u>
- And if <u>Roe</u> is overruled, conflict will still exist about abortion
- It is a fundamental issue, about how we value life and how we value autonomy

38. What is the definition of the word "right" as used in constitutional law?

A right is a limit on the power of lawmakers to make laws that restrict what are considered basic human freedoms

39. Illness care, housing, social security are examples of _____, not of rights.

   Entitlements

40. Who decides what those rights are that are not written in the Constitution?

   The judges of the courts, federal and state

41. What is a source of rights that has become more important in recent times?

   State Constitutions

42. What is the source of unwritten rights in the Constitution being used by the current Court in place of the previously found right of privacy?

   The court is using the liberty interest as written in the 5th and 14th Amendments—"life, liberty and property"

43. What is the amendment and right used in the <u>Cruzan</u> case to assure a constitutional right to refuse medical treatment, including food and water?

   The 14th Amendment right to liberty

44. Which is the right that will probably be involved when a "right to suicide" is at issue before the Court?

   The same, the 14th Amendment right to liberty

45. What is the original source of state or federal constitutional rights?

   The will and belief of the people, through elected representatives who wrote the first constitution, or who write Amendments

46. Should the legislature, or the judicial branch of government, define our rights?

   • The legislature has more input, is more "democratic," but is in more danger of having the majority dominate the minority
   • The judiciary is not as responsive to the will of the people, because they're not usually elected, they are isolated; but at the same time they're insulated from the temporary whims of the electorate

47. What is the relationship of the power of the federal government to the power of the state government?

    • The original power rests in the people through the state governments
    • The states granted some power to the federal government, and kept all the rest
    • In this century, more and more power has been given to or taken by, the federal government from the state governments

48. What are some differences in abortion laws in America and elsewhere?

    • America is the only Western country in which abortion without restriction is available during the first trimester
    • Like most other Western countries, America does not prohibit abortions generally
    • The U.S. is the only Western country where abortion was legalized by the judiciary, not the legislature

49. What do you think would be the outcome if Roe v. Wade were overturned and state legislatures could pass more restrictive abortion laws?

    • Your prediction is valid, as long as it is based on some reasoning
    • My prediction is that some states will pass restrictive laws, some won't
    • Abortion may be more difficult to obtain for women who can't travel

50. What are some of the reasons that women abort?

    • Genetic defects
    • Economic reasons
    • Handicapped fetuses
    • "Wrong" sex
    • Whatever else you thought of is fine as long as you can defend it

51. Which if any from that list of reasons do you believe justify an abortion?

    • This is purely your personal belief
    • Realize that what you and all of us believe will get translated into what the society believes is an "ethical" reason to abort and these reasons may even become the legal reasons for allowing abortion

52. What assumption do you think underlies this statement: We must not restrict abortion, for then even more black teenage unwed mothers will keep their babies?

   • Somewhere in there is a belief that it is bad to be the baby of a black teenage unwed mother
   • It may believed to be so bad that it would be preferable to be aborted than born to such a condition

53. What is an emotional term used to label the attitude that a whole people like the German Jews are better off dead than alive, ?

   Genocide

54. Whose are the various interests present in the abortion conflict?

   • The woman's
   • The child's
   • The father's
   • The society's (mine)

55. What are the issues around the use of the drug RU486?

   • The drug can provide abortions more safely and easily
   • Therefore abortions would be safer, with less pain and fewer maternal lives lost
   • But making abortion safer and easier results in more abortions, with more pain and fetal lives lost
   • Preventing the marketing of the drug in the U.S. with threatened boycott is ethical or unethical, depending on your view of abortion

56. What is the difference between contraception and abortion as a methods of family planning?

   Contraception prevents conception; abortion prevents birth

57. What was the regulation upheld in Rust v. Sullivan and what was its potential impact on practitioners?

   • The regulation required that a question asked by a woman to a federally funded family planning practitioner about abortion, be answered by the statement that the agency does not consider abortion to be family planning

- The impact was on the freedom of the practitioner to give information to patients, and the power of the agency to intrude on the practitioner-patient relationship

58. When is a father's interest not an interest "traditionally protected" and therefore not enforced, according to U.S. Supreme Court Justice Scalia?

    - When the father's interest is in his child with a woman married to someone else
    - The law will not protect the interest of an "adulterous natural father," said Justice Scalia

59. What is the "ism" or philosophy associated with the value of autonomy or freedom; the philosophy most dominant in the United States?

    Individualism

60. How did the term "cesarean," for abdominal delivery develop?

    - No, not because one of the caesars was delivered that way
    - The term was first Lex Regia
    - It was a law of the king
    - When the caesars became kings, the law was called Lex Cesaria, law of the caesars

61. What are some interests of a woman in an ethical conflict described in this chapter, "A Time to Be Born?"

    - In having a healthy, as near perfect as possible baby
    - In not having a baby at all if she doesn't want
    - In having a baby of the sex she wants
    - In having her baby go to the family or kind of home she wants for the baby if she gives the baby for adoption
    - In working at a job she wants, regardless of any damage to a potential child

62. Which value has been found most important when a judge incarcerates a pregnant woman to keep her from taking drugs?

    The value of the baby's life, and his interest in being born free of drugs, is obviously put over the mother's autonomy and her literal freedom

63. Is having a child a right, or a privilege which the law may limit?

    - Because we see that people can be deprived of their children (through abuse or neglect charges) and kept from having more (through sterilization or forced birth control), we see that it is a privilege which can be curtailed by the state
    - Either it's a right or it's not; and anyway no rights are absolute

64. Agree or disagree and discuss: In the future, children will be able to sue their mothers for divorcing their fathers, because thereby they were deprived of support and companionship.

    - Either answer is OK, as long as you discussed the trend to allow suits by children against parents for wrong
    - This kind of suit may be at the far end of the spectrum
    - It will probably happen first in California

65. Do unequal outcomes, such as different mortality rates for white and black infants, mean a lack of justice?

    This viewpoint is directly from the philosophy of social distributive justice discussed in Unit Three

66. What is the definition of "neonate?"

    Latin term for "newborn"

67. What is interest of the newborn with a handicap?

    - The newborn's interest is in living; we project our feelings onto them, that they have that interest, since they can't speak for themselves
    - Other people project that they have no interest since they have no thought (remember the Cartesian maxim: "No mind = no person")
    - Still others believe that severely handicapped newborns have an interest in not living (in dying)

68. What value can you speculate was held by Florida aboriginals living 7000 years ago toward newborns with handicaps?

    From the skeleton of a child with spina bifida that had been cared for until death as a teenager, we can speculate that they valued life for newborns with handicaps

69. What is the position of pro-life groups on research and therapy with aborted fetuses?

   • They believe it is wrong to benefit from the loss of life
   • Further, they believe that if women thought their fetuses were to further research and therapy for illness they might be encouraged or at least not discouraged from abortion

70. What is the rationale for allowing aborted fetuses to be used for research and therapy?

   • Since the fetuses are to be aborted anyway, whatever good can come from their use is a bonus
   • This is called "begging" or assuming the answer to a question (the assumption is that the abortion question is settled)

71. How can the use of aborted fetuses for research and therapy, be distinguished from the use of bodies of Persistent Unconscious Persons (PUPs) declared "dead?"

   • The aborted fetuses are certainly dead
   • The PUPs are only defined dead

72. What is the interest that the state or government has, in all the issues discussed in "A Time to Be Born?"

   • The interest of the state (us) is in protecting persons who cannot protect themselves
   • The question is, when shall that interest come first over some other person's interest?

UNIT TWO EXAM

HSM 510
Ethical Considerations in Health Care Delivery

SCANTRON FORM INSTRUCTIONS

Please follow these instructions for completing your Scantron form:

1. Use a #2 pencil **only**.

2. Enter the five-digit Test Number in the box marked **TEST No.** Shade in the corresponding boxes.

   The test number for this exam is: **51002**

3. Enter your Social Security Number in the box marked **SOCIAL SECURITY NUMBER**. Shade the corresponding boxes.

4. Enter your Course Code number in the box marked **COURSE CODE**. Shade in the corresponding boxes.

   The course code is: **510**

5. Print your name, address, and social security number on the lines provided.

6. Enter the estimated number of hours (to the nearest whole hour) you spent on this lesson (this is for our statistical purposes only). Fill in the appropriate boxes.

7. Be careful to darken the entire area within the boxes.

8. Do not make any marks outside the boxes. Completely erase all mistakes. **Do not use whiteout.**

9. Send the Scantron form to CCHS for grading. Your test results will be mailed to you.

If you have any questions regarding your exams or any other questions or comments, please write them on a **Request for Help** form and send it in to CCHS with the Scantron form. **DO NOT STAPLE** anything to the form. Be sure to write your name, SSN, phone number (optional), and Test Number on the **Request for Help** form. GOOD LUCK!!

Unit Two Exam

Multiple Choice

Select the *best* answer to each of the following questions. Mark your responses on the Scantron form.

1. Define eugenics.

   a. creating average people
   b. creating better people
   c. creating genetics
   d. generating creation

2. Define "*in vitro* fertilization."

   a. fertilization in glass
   b. fertilization in life
   c. artificial insemination
   d. surrogate motherhood

3. Fertilized frozen zygotes are _____.

   a. given to the custody of the mother
   b. given to the custody of the father
   c. people, having a right to life
   d. in court cases, either property or people, depending on the view of the judge

4. Either the word "womb" or "uterus" is used when discussing surrogate motherhood largely because _____.

   a. one is the correct term
   b. people prefer one or the other
   c. the law requires one's use, and not the other
   d. one or the other raise the right response emotionally

5. Technology is the origin of our problems with procreation.

   a. True
   b. False

6. If it's a law, it's ethical.

   a. True, because all laws are ethical
   b. False, because no laws are ethical
   c. True, because ethics are laws
   d. False, because some laws are such a minimum ethic

7. Either the word "fetus" or the word "baby" is used when speaking about abortion, largely because _____.

   a. one is the correct terms
   b. one or the other raises the right response emotionally
   c. the law requires one's use, and not the other
   d. people prefer one or the other

8. Either the word "mother" or the word "woman" is used when speaking about abortion, largely because _____.

   a. one is the correct term
   b. one or the other raises the right response emotionally
   c. the law requires one's use, and not the other
   d. people prefer one or the other

9. "Quickening" under English common law is related to what concept in American Constitutional and state statute law?

   a. trimester
   b. animatus
   c. viability
   d. infanticide

10. In Roe v. Wade, the Supreme Court divided pregnancy into stages. What are the stages called, and whose interests are protected at each stage?

    a. trimesters; none, woman's health, child
    b. trimesters; woman's health, state's interest, child
    c. semesters; woman's interest, child's
    d. semesters; woman's interest, state's

11. Which statement is false about Roe?

    a. ethical conflict about abortion existed before the case
    b. ethical conflict about abortion existed after the case
    c. Roe solved the ethical conflict about abortion
    d. overturning Roe will not solve the ethical conflict about abortion

12. As used in constitutional law, the word "right" means:

    a. entitlements to programs
    b. natural rights
    c. human rights
    d. limits on government

13. Which amendment and right was used in the <u>Cruzan</u> case, and will probably be used in future abortion decisions.

    a. 14th Amendment, right to liberty
    b. 14th Amendment, right to life
    c. 14th Amendment, right to property
    d. right to privacy in the penumbra of all the Bill of Rights

14. If <u>Roe v. Wade</u> is overturned and state legislatures can pass more restrictive abortion laws, which is <u>unlikely</u>?

    a. some states will restrict abortion further
    b. abortion will be illegal everywhere
    c. some states will not restrict abortion further
    d. legal abortions will still be available

15. What is the potential impact on practitioners from <u>Rust v. Sullivan</u>?

    a. practitioners can be required to modify their practice
    b. practitioners can't be required to modify their practice
    c. practitioners can be required to lie to patients
    d. practitioners have complete autonomy in the patient relationship

16. Name the "ism" or philosophy associated with the value autonomy or freedom, the philosophy most dominant in the United States.

    a. utilitarianism
    b. collectivism
    c. individualism
    d. romanticism

17. Identify the value that has been found most important when the fetus's safety causes a judge to incarcerate his mother to keep her from taking drugs.

    a. mother's life
    b. baby's life
    c. baby's autonomy
    d. mother's autonomy or freedom to take drugs

18. Unequal outcomes, such as different mortality rates for white and black infants, indicates to some people a lack of _____.

    a. distributive or social justice
    b. justice
    c. health care
    d. illness care

19. The 7000-year-old skeleton of a teenager with spina bifida leads to speculation that Florida aboriginals of that time believed _____.

    a. that newborns with handicaps had some value
    b. that some lives were unworthy of life
    c. that newborns with handicaps should be put out of their misery
    d. it's just a skeleton; no speculation is possible

20. Regarding research on aborted fetuses, the following is the most nearly correct statement from all points of view _____.

    a. it is wrong to benefit from the fetal death, and it encourages abortion
    b. the fetuses are dead anyway; a use which could benefit many should be made of them
    c. one's position on the issue depends heavily on one's underlying position on abortion
    d. we should stop using innocent fetuses and start using tissue from people in Persistent Vegetative States

21. Regarding the use of the drug RU486, the following is the most nearly correct statement from all points of view _____.

    a. the drug is good; abortions would be safer and easier
    b. the drug is bad; abortions would be more frequent
    c. boycotting the drug company which makes it is unethical
    d. one's position on the issue depends heavily on one's underlying position on abortion

22. Identify the original source of state or federal constitutional rights.

    a. the legislature
    b. the judges
    c. the people
    d. the law

23. Why should brothers and sisters marrying, which is possible if many women are artificially inseminated with the same sperm donor, concern all practitioners?

    a. their kids might have genetic defects
    b. their church would consider it a sin
    c. the law would consider it a crime
    d. the judgment of history would be that we as a people were incestuous

24. The future result of continued rights for children could include a lawsuit against the parent for some version of "bad parenting."

    a. True
    b. False

25. Having children is a _____.

    a. right, guaranteed by the constitution
    b. right, guaranteed by natural law
    c. privilege, since the law can limit contact with and even conception of children
    d. pain

26. Which is correct?

    a. surrogate motherhood exploits poor women
    b. surrogate motherhood provides poor women pay for their risk
    c. surrogate motherhood allows babies to live that wouldn't otherwise
    d. the answer you give will depend on your own value judgments

27. Which party does not have an interest in a conflict arising from surrogate motherhood?

    a. the court
    b. the surrogate mother
    c. the potential parents
    d. the baby

28. The terms "Pro-choice," "Pro-life," "Anti-abortion," "Pro-abortion," are used more to convey information than to appeal to the emotion.

    a. True
    b. False

29. Abortions have been done, and ethical conflict has arisen about them, only during the last few years.

    a. True
    b. False

30. Before <u>Roe v. Wade</u>, several states had changed their law to make some abortions legal, and several more states were in the process of doing so in state law.

   (a.) True
   b. False

31. Illness care, housing, social security are examples of _____.

   a. institutions
   b. benefits
   c. rights
   (d.) entitlements

UNIT THREE

Chapter Four
Share of Care

Introduction

The next topics group issues in illness care in between "A Time to Be Born" and "A Time to Die" . These next two chapters will discuss issues that fall in between birth and death. As you have already figured out, all the issues cut across all the lines. This division is purely arbitrary to meet our need to classify and group things. It makes the tests shorter, too.

Objectives

Upon successful completion of this chapter, you will be able to:

1.   Describe why the ethical issues in the "Share of Care" chapter are important to you personally.

2.   Define the problem with the existing system of illness care as you see it.

3.   State the percentage of illness care expenses now paid by taxpayers through state, local, and federal governments.

4.   Name the values most often mentioned when share of care is discussed.

5.   List the three specific things that are protected from taking without due process of law, under the 5th and 14th Amendments to the U.S. Constitution.

6.   Name the value that these Amendments exemplify.

7.   State the maxim or saying that best characterizes social justice.

8.   Identify the philosophy that advocates the greatest good for the greatest number.

9.   Identify the value that keeps us from forcing people to do things we believe are good for them.

10.   List the three factors of the economy of illness care.

11. Explain what happens to the cost when the demand for a service goes up and the supply stays the same.

12. Explain what happens to the supply of technology in illness care if the demand or share of care goes up, and the government controls the price or cost at the same level.

13. Define GNP.

14. State what percent of a country's gross national product is too high a percentage when it consists of illness care.

15. State why people confuse health care with health and life, and the absence of health care with illness and death.

16. State how many people are uninsured for illness care in the U.S.

17. Distinguish "uninsured" from "unhealthy."

18. Distinguish "uninsured" from "uncared-for."

19 Discuss the way insurance works.

20. Discuss the values involved in refusing to pay for patients who have "self-inflicted" diseases.

21. Identify the philosophy that allows us to force individuals to buy insurance they don't want, if it is considered better for society.

22. Use a schematic to illustrate the contract between patient and practitioner. Use a schematic to illustrate the relationship when the payment is made indirectly, by a third party.

23. Discuss why indirect payment causes more use of care.

24. State why increased money available for care stimulates increased use of technology.

25. Describe why technology is more likely to be paid for than other kinds of care.

26. Discuss why increasing the money available, or seemingly available through the "free" care attitude resulting from indirect payment, causes inflation in the industry.

27. Discuss the effect of indirect payment on malpractice suits.

28. Describe how limits on illness care have been set in the past and are set presently.

29. Describe some "socially just" illness care systems already functioning in the U.S.

30. Describe the intended consequences of the Medicaid program.

31. Describe the unintended consequences of Congress' adding more requirements each year to the benefits under Medicaid.

32. Describe the intended consequences of the Medicare program.

33. Describe the unintended effect of the Diagnostic Related Group cap on reimbursement to hospitals for Medicare.

34. Identify the good news about the VA.

35. Identify the bad news about the VA.

36. Describe the main differences between Hawaii and Massachusetts regarding employer-mandated insurance.

37. List the three principles of the Oregon reform of Medicaid.

38. Describe the criterion for determining which care will be paid in Oregon.

39. Describe the philosophy or ethic that underlies the Oregon plan.

40. Describe your feelings about the Oregon plan for Medicaid reform.

41. Relate your feelings about the plan to your philosophy of life.

42. Define "monopsony."

43. Describe how Canada holds down costs in its national health system.

44. Describe how the European national health systems solve the problem of two levels of care.

45. Describe how Great Britain holds down costs in the National Health Service.

46. Explain the sequence of cost shifting for nonpaying people's illness care.

47. List the three groups most vocal in the request for national "health" insurance.

48. Describe three major proposals for illness care reform.

49. Describe one major problem with a national health system.

50. Describe the major problem with a "play or pay" employer-paid health insurance system.

51. Describe the major problem with a tax credit for purchase of individual health insurance.

52. Differentiate buying insurance from gambling in Las Vegas.

53. Differentiate a tax credit from a tax deduction.

54. Discuss the ethical question of malpractice insurance.

55. Discuss your reactions to the Modest Suggestions at the end of this chapter.

STUDY QUESTIONS

This is not a test. Read the study questions before you begin the chapter. Answer them as you go along or after you finish the chapter. Then look at the suggested answers at the end of the chapter to see if you agree with the answers.

1. Why are the ethical issues in the "Share of Care" chapter important?

2. Why might they be more important to you personally than any other issues in the course?

3. What is the problem with the existing system, assuming you think there's a problem?

4. What is the percentage of illness care expense paid now by taxpayers through state, local and federal governments?

SHORTEST CHAPTER, MOST IMPORTANT

This is the shortest chapter, with only one large issue. The big debate is about what kind of illness care system we have now and what we will have in this country in the future. The debate will not be solved this year, or the next, no matter what programs are tried. There are some basic ethical issues.

This topic will probably have more effect on your life as a practitioner and patient than any other in the course. You will have something to say about what kind of system the U.S. has; your voice can be heard through elections, referenda, committees, participation in your agency, and so on.

Discussions and decisions about what kind of system we will have may seem far away. They are, however, close to home. The issues are who will be paid, how much, for doing what, for whom. You will see that it matters very much if you have a patient who needs medication or intensive care and she happens to be a month older than the age that disqualifies her for that care in your hospital.

It matters if your friend has AIDS, and the government panel has decided that quality-of-life numbers and longevity don't add up to justify any treatment other than nursing care. Or if your mother's Quality Adjusted Life Years numbers and longevity expectation don't even justify nursing care. . . .

Or if paying for all these things because the legislators couldn't face the hard choices meant that everything was paid, for everyone, by the taxpayer. Congress did just that when faced with the hard choice about who should have dialysis. It was a scarce resource until we paid for it for everyone who needed it.

If Congress and the state legislatures decide you will pay for everything for everyone, then you will have to dig deep into your pocket. You may deny yourself and your family some other necessities to pay for more "health care."

Or if your occupation is one of those considered to be less medically necessary than present use indicates, and you lose your job. What if two-thirds of the workers are to be laid off at your hospital, and all over the country, since the standards and payment system are national?

It matters, very much, to us as practitioners, citizens, and future patients.

Is There a Problem?

Even to ask the above question may seem to be heresy. Many people think or assume there is a problem with our system of illness care. Some people want to change the system, because their part of the industry has a problem. Whatever change they want will benefit them.

Are the people unhappy with the present system? In a survey by the Health Insurance Association of America, 76% of people surveyed said they were "very" or "somewhat" satisfied with their own insurance. But 67% said the system either needs significant change or is beyond repair, and 24% more said the system needs "some change." There was no agreement on what change was needed. See the discussion in "Proposals."

IF THERE IS A PROBLEM, WHAT IS IT?

If change is needed, what is the problem? Is it lack of availability, or share, of illness care? Does the care cost too much? Is it the quality (or lack of quality) of care? Related to this, is it the wrong kind of care—technological and tertiary versus preventive and primary?

There will be changes in the system. As practitioners and as citizens you will be involved in causing and dealing with the changes. What follows is some information about the economics and the ethical implications of the changes.

THE MARKET

In order to understand what the ethical issues are, we must understand the economic system. In a pure market system, people pay directly for goods and services they want, like lawyers and hamburgers. When you don't have the money you don't get the stuff.

Some people believe "health care" is different since we equate "health care" with health and with life itself (see the "Myths" section to correct this misconception). We do value life, at least our own. It seems wrong to allow people to do without illness care if they don't have money to pay for it. But, theoretically, everyone in the U.S. has the money to pay for care.

People who don't spend money for illness care or insurance, prioritize. They choose to use the money for something else. If they are so poor they would have to choose food over care, for example, they would theoretically be eligible for Medicaid (see discussion about Medicaid to correct that misconception). Few are rich enough to buy all the care that is available, just as few are rich enough to buy some cars that are made.

The U.S. does not have a pure market system. We modify the market by supplying people with minimal support to live. We do not let people starve, as some believe a pure, untampered market system would do. There are minimal payments to the poor, such as food stamps paid for by the taxpayers. If poor people are threatened with losing their liberty, lawyers are provided for them paid for by the taxpayers.

There is no pure market system in illness care, either. Through federal, state, and local governments, taxpayers have already chosen to pay for 42% of the illness care in this country. Some groups - the poor, elderly, veterans, American Indians, and military groups, receive illness care paid for by the taxpayers. The question to be decided in a future care system is how, and how much, will be paid that way.

Reference: "Health Spending," *The Economist*, November 16, 1991, p. 127. [1989 data.]

STUDY QUESTIONS

1. Which are the values most mentioned when share of care is discussed?

2. Which three specific "things" are protected from taking without due process of law under the 5th and 14th Amendments to the U.S. Constitution?

3. These Amendments are examples of which value?

4. What is the maxim or saying that best characterizes social justice?

5. Which philosophy advocates the greatest good for the greatest number?

6. Which is the value that keeps us from forcing people to do things that we believe are good for them?

"JUSTICE" AND AUTONOMY AND MONEY

The big ethical issues in this conflict are justice and autonomy. The autonomy value can be seen when patients are asked to give up their freedom to choose practitioners. The autonomy for practitioners is compromised by restrictions on what care is given to whom.

Social justice is the most often mentioned value in any discussion of share of care. The value really is beneficence—doing good for patients. The good is done with a socialistic illness care system. But you will constantly hear this referred to as social justice, or simply justice.

Here, one can see the Marxist "distributive justice" ideal in its most appealing form: All people should get an equal share of a good. When people don't get illness care, it's seen as unfair. Fairness is always a justice issue.

This chapter discusses justice, and the special meanings of distributive or social justice. The word "justice" means fairness under the law. That is, that people are free to do what they want, unless and until they break the law. At that point, the process of the law must be applied fairly, equally, without bias for or against any individual.

In particular, justice implies the right of individuals to the results of their work—their property. To take someone's property is stealing. The time and work used to get that property is stolen.

This is the promise and guarantee of the 5th Amendment to the U.S. Constitution, which limits the federal government. It is the same promise as the 14th Amendment, which limits the state governments. These Amendments say that people will not have their life, liberty or property taken without "due process" of law, without it being fairly done.

The use of the word "justice" in any other sense, especially with a modifier, is code or jargon for a different social system. Such a system would provide beneficence, its promoters believe. Clothing the idea with the word "justice" lends the idea instant status, power, and credibility. Everyone is "for" justice and "against" injustice. Relating your idea to justice, even using the word in the name of the idea, is an effective technique to gain support.

In ethics discussions in particular, the word "justice" is used when speaking of or advocating distributive or social justice. These ideas are not related to justice as the word is correctly used, but are about a "just" or equal outcome, the end desired.

SOCIAL JUSTICE

We have all heard, "The end justifies the means." That says, if the outcome is what we want, "just" or fair or equal, then whatever means we used (whatever process or whatever we had to do to get the result we wanted) was justified; was a just thing to do. So if it comes out that Billie and Sammy have the same number of cookies (the end or result we want), it doesn't matter that Billie knocked Sammy down and took a cookie, or that Big Mother took one from Sammy and gave it to Billie. At least Sammy has 1 cookie still, equal with Bullie (I mean Billie).

Reference: Rawls, John. *A Theory of Justice.* Harvard University Press. Cambridge: 1971.

JUSTICE:

Sammy and Billie had the same opportunity to make cookies and Sammy chose not to make some. Whatever the result or end or outcome, the result is fair. If Billie made 2 cookies and chose not to share them, it is her right to keep the cookies resulting from her labor. If anyone interfered with Billie and her possession of what she had worked to make, it would be unjust stealing.

MARKET VS. SOCIAL JUSTICE

Practitioners have the worst of both worlds now. They do not have either the advantages of the market nor a socially just system. A pure market system would let every practitioner negotiate his own price, and have none of it set nationally. With a national system of payment, in which someone other than the patient pays, this is not possible.

A socially "just" system would compensate all equally, equitably, as in comparative worth. The nationally set compensation now, by Medicare, is not based on comparative worth. It is based on a "market" in illness care that doesn't exist. The government, which is the "buyer" of that part of the care, sets the prices it will pay, not by supply and demand, but by itself.

Paying nurse practitioners 85% of the payment that physicians get for the same work is not socially just. Nor is it socially just to pay licensed practical nurses less than registered nurses for some of their work that is the same as RN's.

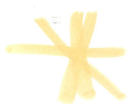

Rural hospitals and rural workers including doctors are paid less than their counterparts in the cities for the same work under Medicare. This is based on a nonexistent market price. It is not the market, because it's set by "national" bureaucrats, not by local supply and demand. But neither is it "just," if we mean social justice (distributive justice, equal pay for equal work, comparable pay for comparable worth).

In a socially just, comparative worth system we would have to figure out who decides, how much, how to compensate for what (education, skill, experience, empathy?). A bureaucracy would be needed to do that, a central authority with law and force behind it. They do it now, but not on any social justice system.

References: Ginzbert, Eli, "Health Care and the Market Economy—A Conflict of Interest?" *NEJM*, 1992, 326:72-74.

ETHICAL ISSUE

The availability of illness care is an ethical issue. It is not to be merely an economics issue as is the availability of cars. We don't classify other issues the same way: We don't worry about access to cars, or distributive justice in where and how people are going to buy Cadillacs, or whether the poor have to drive Hyundais.

Illness care seems different. Some people believe that illness care is more like police or fire protection than it is like food or legal services. They believe it should be available to all on an equal basis. They will tolerate differences in food, housing, and other goods and services, but they believe different levels are intolerable in the service of "health care."

We cannot or will not afford the very best for all. If we are going to have one level for all, it will be less than the best available. We cannot and will not buy a Mercedes for everyone.

Does anyone really <u>need</u> a Mercedes, or Mercedes illness care (all right, Cadillac)? Perhaps not. The best will have to be denied to all, if something less than the best is given to all. That's the way social justice must work. Everybody gets something, some better than they had before. But nobody gets the best possible. Such "social justice" would produce a uniform system, a system poorer in quality. Some would say it's better to be equal even if misery results (Socialists make all equal: equally miserable).

PREVENTIVE CARE IS AN ECONOMIC, NOT AN ETHICAL ISSUE

Some argue that everyone should have free preventive care, not because it is beneficent (socially just) but because it's a good investment. They say there's no ethical conflict here, just money. (But money and work are values we use in ethics).

People who get preventive care -- immunizations for children, good diabetes care, and other healthy people, need less expensive secondary and tertiary care. Primary care for those people is called a good investment; in the long run it costs less to care for them early. "Pay me now or pay me later" is the argument. Healthy people are an asset to an economy, because they are more productive, etc.

Proponents say that these arguments are pragmatic and don't involve beneficence or justice for preventive care. In Chapter Two, you saw that such arguments proposing the greatest good for the greatest number was a utilitarian philosophy.

If more money is spent on prevention, less money is available now for critical care, so the interest of people who need tertiary (third-level) care is at stake. Thus this is not a value-free, nonethical stance.

(Take care to look for studies that show that prevention actually works -- reduces complications. We all "know" preventive care is good for you but does the data bear it out?.

Further, what if people won't get preventive care even if it's available? There are some studies that show they don't. (You have probably had patients who have been counseled to stop smoking). Will the ethical value of autonomy of the individual permit us to make people take care of themselves? They'll certainly be more productive, less costly to the state. Now we see the obvious utilitarian philosophy: We could right now make laws to force people to stop smoking, drinking, eating potato chips, having anal sex, and working late. The cost of care would be a lot less, but so far we've not decided to make such laws.

STUDY QUESTIONS

1.   What are the three factors to the economy of illness care?

2.   What happens to the cost when the demand for a service goes up and the supply stays the same?

3.   What happens to the supply of technology in illness care if the demand or share of care goes up, and the government controls the price or cost at the same level?

4.   What is the definition of GNP?

5.   What percent of a country's gross national product is too high a percentage when it consists of illness care?

THREE ECONOMIC PARTS OF CARE

There are three economic factors of health care:

DEMAND (BY THE PATIENT; "ACCESS") (THE "SHARE" OF CARE)

Availability. It's wrongly called "access to care." It's the patient demand for care. Demand is how many patients want care, and what kind of care they want. That's determined very much in this country by what is paid for. Most people do not expect to pay out of their own pockets for their care. A word about "access." People generally have access to care in this country now. Practitioners are located within reasonable distance of most people. Some of them don't have the money or don't spend the money to pay for care. We have access to a car dealer in the same way. We may not be able to or want to pay for the car.

Here we are not talking about access unless we change the definition of access. This changing the definition of a word is pretty common practice, as you've noticed by now. Instead of access, we are really talking about share, distribution of care, as in distributive justice. We don't merely want access to a practitioner, we want an appointment. We don't want access to a car dealership, we want a car.

SUPPLY (FROM THE PRACTITIONER, OR QUALITY)

The second factor is the quality, the adequacy, the level of care. The level of care really means how much technology is available, since the actual adequacy or excellence is hard to measure. If quality is hard to measure, we simply don't measure it. We substitute something else, like technology.

COST

As with all else, there is the cost, the amount of money and time and energy to be "spent" for care.

All three, demand (patient want), supply (technology), and cost, are related. The law of economics is this: If demand for a product or service goes up, and the supply stays the same, the cost must go up. That's the law of the market.

$$\uparrow\text{DEMAND} \quad + \quad \updownarrow\text{SUPPLY} = \quad \uparrow\text{COST}$$

Then what happens in the free market is that the higher cost will cause the demand to decrease. People buy fewer strawberries when they are expensive.

$$\uparrow COST \ + \ \updownarrow SUPPLY \ = \ \downarrow DEMAND$$

This doesn't work as well in illness care, because there's more of a constant demand—people can't decide when or if to be sick. And more important, the cost does not go up for the person with taxpayer or private insurance (See "Myths" below).

If the government tries to control the cost, the providers, the practitioners in our case, will make or give fewer goods or services because the low controlled price gives them no incentive.

The law of the market will still work. The attempts to control economies in eastern Europe and the former Soviet Union are examples. So is Medicaid: The government controls the price the practitioner will be paid. The result is that few practitioners will work for such low fees. The supply of care available to the patient is limited.

$\uparrow$ DEMAND OR SHARE OF CARE + GOVERNMENT $\updownarrow$ COST CONTROLS =
$\downarrow$ SUPPLY: FEWER PRACTITIONERS WHO WILL TAKE MEDICAID PATIENTS

Increasing the cost (the amount of money available) will increase the technology. Government spending on Medicare and other taxpayer-paid systems, and private insurance, have increased the technology available. The price for the technology has gone up, too.

$\uparrow$ PAYMENTS FROM TAX AND INSURANCE \$
+ SAME DEMAND = $\uparrow$ SUPPLY OF TECHNOLOGY

A system of care that provides more care for more people is another way of saying it increases patient demand. This increases the total cost. When you buy more at the store, you pay more money.

$\uparrow$ DEMAND BY PAYING FOR MORE PEOPLE +
KEEP THE SAME   SUPPLY OF TECHNOLOGY $\uparrow$ COST

If our goal is to reduce the cost, we will have to care for fewer patients at the same level of technology.

WANT TO $\downarrow$ COST + SAME $\updownarrow$ SUPPLY OF TECHNOLOGY?
= REDUCE $\downarrow$ DEMAND - - FEWER PATIENTS CARED FOR

If we think the present system doesn't provide a share of care for enough people, and we want to keep the present level of technology, the cost will have to go up. Again, as above:

IF YOU ↑DEMAND BY PAYING FOR MORE PEOPLE + KEEP THE SAME ↕ SUPPLY OF TECHNOLOGY = ↑COST

What if we want to do both—increase demand (shares) and decrease cost at the same time? Then there must be a decrease in supply of technology. We will have less technology for each patient.

↑DEMAND + ↓ MANDATED COST =↓ SUPPLY OF TECHNOLOGY

Those are the choices that the law of economics leaves us.

Changing the amount of one will change the other two directly. Increasing the share of care, meaning that more people can have care, increases the cost. Say we increase the share, and the cost is made to stay the same with caps on spending or limitation of practitioner fees. Again as above:

↑DEMAND (SHARE) + ↕ COST (CONTROLLED)
= ↓SUPPLY OF TECHNOLOGY (or hours of care)

Then the quality (the level of technology) must decrease. Maybe we use too much technology. It's easy to decide that we should decrease the use of technology—until you or yours are one of the few who will die without it.

ABOUT COSTS

A word about GNP, the Gross National Product. In other countries you may see this called the GDP, the Gross Domestic Product. The GNP is all the production of this country, with a dollar number attached to it and added up. This is not like your personal budget, not like how much you spend. It's more like what you earn, what all the products you made during the year were worth. So the portion of the GNP for illness care is not what we "spend," but what we produce or make in illness care. You will see "spend" everywhere, because very few people understand the GNP.

In 1991, the illness care portion of the Gross National Product care was 12%. This represents a large industry, a lot of product. Is 12% too much? In most other areas of life, producing a lot is good. We produce and use a lot of care. We produce and use more health care in the U.S. than any other country produces and uses. Canada's number is approaching 10%, with most other industrialized countries at about 8%. All but a few increased their share of GNP in the area of illness care between 1980 and 1990. The U.S. increased from about 9% to 12% in the same period. But comparing GNP across countries is fraught with inaccuracy. Not everyone calculates production the same way.

Reference: "Health Spending," *The Economist*, November 16, 1991, p. 127.

Even if we accept the GNP comparison, does this mean we produce too much? If we produced less care than any other country, would that mean we produced too little? Is there some magic rank in GNP for illness care that will make us a "moral" nation?
Part of the "too much" problem is that people feel they don't have any control over what they spend for illness. When they spend a lot of money for a car, it is not "too much." They decide to spend or not. But people don't really decide to spend for illness care. The spending is forced. People are forced to pay money for Medicare and Medicaid through taxes that have risen in the last few years. Their premium for illness insurance rises yearly. The only alternative is to go without insurance.

Using less care themselves, as individuals, does not cut their costs at all. This is unlike individual restriction in driving less or turning off the electricity. Actually, people are penalized for using less care. They get less of the money back that they paid for insurance, compared to people who use the care. The question remains: is it ethical to force people who do not and never will use the care, to pay for insurance for care?

IMPLICATIONS FOR THE PRACTITIONER

The other side of the coin: you as practitioner are part of this production and use of care. This is your industry they are talking about. Cutting back nationally on illness care is cutting back in your industry. You are bound to feel some effect. There would be fewer jobs, less pay. A large industry in the country would be in depression or at least recession. The whole economy would feel the drag, as it does when the military-industrial complex is downsized.

Few of you would resist reform of the system just because such reform might lower production and use of illness care (your industry). Few would resist needed change, only because such change would hurt us practitioners economically. But individuals must be aware of trends for their future as practitioners. They must know of the effect such a depression in illness care would have on the economy as a whole. As reform proposals are discussed, the economic impact on the industry must be remembered.

THE DILEMMA

We are now at the point where the cost is greater than many want to pay. At the same time, many believe the share per person (demand) is not high enough. Decreasing cost, and increasing shares, are not possible at the same time unless quality (supply) is to be drastically decreased.

We can have it cheap: low-tech care for many, or high-tech care for few. Or we can have it expensive: for a lot of money, we can have high-tech care for all. We do have choices.

References: "Access to Health Care," American College of Physicians, *Annals of Internal Medicine*, 1990; 112: 641–49.

STUDY QUESTIONS

1. Why do people confuse health care with health and life, and the <u>absence</u> of health care with illness and death?

2. How many people are uninsured for illness care in the U.S.?

3. What is the difference between "uninsured" and "unhealthy?"

4. What is the difference between "uninsured" and "uncared-for?"

5. How does insurance work?

6. What are the values involved in refusing to pay for patients who have "self-inflicted" diseases?

"HEALTH CARE" IS THE SAME THING AS HEALTH

We have confused "health care" with health. That's an example why the words we use to describe things **are** important. If we were to call what we do by its proper name,"illness care", we would never confuse what we do, illness care, with health. After they are told illness care is "health care," people then believe "health care" will make or keep them healthy. In reality, "health care" does not make or keep people healthy. It cares for their illnesses.

People wrongly assume that the lack of "health care" (really illness care) results in illness—and even further, with death. So in their minds, lacking "health care" quickly translates to being "sick" and "dead."

If something is essential to life, and is in short supply, we ration that thing. We give it out in shares. We let each person have only a certain amount. As we saw above, people wrongly see "health care" as something essential to life. In reality, illness care is essential to life in only a few unusual situations. We may die for lack of a heart transplant. We will not die for lack of hemorrhoid surgery. Because we have decided all "health care" is essential to life, we are unable to tell the difference. At that point it seems logical to ration (give shares of) all illness care.

MILLIONS AND MILLIONS

The "37 million uninsured" cited as the number of Americans uninsured is an arbitrary number. Nobody has counted the uninsured. This is an estimate, based on an extrapolation from a small study. Writers in the *New England Journal of Medicine* in 1986 were using figures like 28 million uninsured. The rise in population since then has come to far less than that would justify. Current estimates would mean over a 33% rise, and nothing like that has been documented.

What has happened is a lot of writing -- a lot of speculating with little data, and some opportunities for change to benefit some special interest groups. A recent article estimates that 25% of our population is uninsured or underinsured. This would be more like 60 million people. That writer says "more than 30 million uninsured." The writer quotes another author who says that we fail to give effective medical care to about a third of our population.

This totals up to 80 million or more people. Maybe no one is insured, or receives "effective medical care." It depends, like anything else, on what you think is effective. Talk, especially number talk, is cheap. When you see statements like this, ask where the numbers come from.

References: "Insuring the Uninsured Is Not Enough," *AIM,* 1991; 151:860-862.

Brown, E. Richard, "Health USA: A National Health Program for the United States," *JAMA,* 1992;267:552-58.

MORE MYTH: UNINSURED MEANS UNHEALTHY, UNCARED FOR

Uninsured cannot be equated with "unhealthy" or "uncared for."

UNHEALTHY?

A study by the Oklahoma Medical Research Foundation shows that 18.9% of people in Oklahoma are without health insurance (the fourth highest of all states in 1989). This "uninsurance" is similar to other Southern states. And at the same time, Oklahomans were ranked the 21st healthiest people in the nation. This was thought to be due to a cleaner environment, with less risk of heart disease, fewer motor vehicle deaths, and less violent crime (before the Oklahoma City bomb).

This more holistic view of health takes into account physiological, psychological, and environmental factors. "Health insurance" will not make those people, however many or few are insured, healthier.

Jerry Nida, Senior Medical Consultant for the State Department of Health, asserted that people can be healthy without having health insurance. "Access to care takes care of a person's illness status. But not a person's health status." (Quoted in the January 15, 1991, issue of *Physician's Financial News*, p. 36.) Health is not the same thing as illness care, "health care," or even "health insurance."

But within a whole population, the uninsured <u>are</u> more unhealthy. One factor in that statement is that people who are already ill with some diseases are less likely to be able to buy insurance. By definition, the "uninsured" category includes people who are sicker.

The utilitarian's question remains whether more insurance will make people healthier. If it will not, that is the end of the utilitarian's question. Her goal is healthier people, not "cared-for" people. If insurance will not make people healthier, but will get them more care and comfort, do we still need to give them insurance? Is this an ethical question?

Reference: Blendon, R.J., et al, "The Uninsured and the Debate over the Repeal of the Massachusetts Universal Health Care Law," *JAMA*, 1992;267:1113-17.

Uninsured does not mean "uncared for." All uninsured can get care. This is largely the reason that the hospital industry supports mandatory insurance. They (and you) are caring for the part of the uninsured who don't pay now, and we are doing it without compensation. The term "self-pay" is shorthand in the hospital industry for "no-pay," though some uninsured do pay for their own care.

The uninsured, whether they are paying for their care or not, see practitioners and are admitted to hospitals about as frequently as people who are insured. In 1989 in Massachusetts, the uninsured under 65 had 5.2 visits to physicians on average. The insured had 5.5 visits, not a statistically significant difference. Of the uninsured, 8% were hospitalized, of the insured 7%; this is also not statistically significant. The uninsured do get care.

Reference: The Blendon article cited above.

Some people choose not to be insured; they choose to pay for their care out of their pockets if and when they need it. For a lot of people it's cheaper than buying insurance. The average healthy person will never actually need the amount of money he spends on his health insurance premiums. He pays for other sicker people, because that's the way insurance works. He pays so that **if** he gets sick, he'll have money to pay the bill. The average person who doesn't get sick and doesn't buy insurance will not spend as much for health care as you or your employer pay for premiums for a year. Some people prefer to play the odds they won't get sick. "No insurance" does not mean sick, and it does not mean "no care" for people who are sick.

At last resort, poor people will get care when they present to an emergency room, since the federal anti-dumping law now in effect requires it. Certainly, people without insurance (either private or tax paid) are more careful about buying care. The money they spend on illness care decreases the amount they have for food, or housing, or fun. This is budgeting (prioritizing, choosing). It keeps their costs down. It may be that they fail to get preventive care that they need.

If self-paying people choose not to pay for preventive care, they are making that decision themselves. Suppose preventive care is paid for by all. We would then have to decide if it would be right to force people to get it. Could we refuse to pay for complications that were preventable? Let the diabetic's leg rot because she hadn't watched her diet and taken her insulin?

Even without paid-for care to justify our moral condemnation, people suggest that we limit care for "self-inflicted" diseases. Suggestions are made that we limit care for people whose life-style contributed to their illness. For example -- no liver transplants for alcoholics, no lung cancer care for smokers, no AZT for people who become infected from risky behavior after the mode of transmission of AIDS was known. But that assumes we can be sure the behavior caused the disease.

If people "self-inflict" poverty by being lazy or stupid, shall we deny them food stamps? If they "self-inflict" failure to pay for their retirement, shall we deny them social security payments? The "self-infliction" theory is broader than just illness care.

STUDY QUESTIONS

1. Which philosophy allows us to force individuals to buy insurance they don't want, if it is better for the society?

2. Illustrate the contract between patient and practitioner with a drawing.

3. Illustrate the relationship when the payment is made indirectly, by a third party.

4. Why does indirect payment cause increased use of care?

5. Why does increased money available for care stimulate increased use of technology?

6. Why is technology more likely to be paid for than other kinds of care?

7. Why does increasing the money available for care (or seemingly available through the "free" care attitude resulting from indirect payment) cause inflation in the industry?

8. What is the effect of indirect payment for care, on malpractice suits?

The Myths That More Insurance and Indirect Payment Solve The Problem

The presence of private and government insurance of illness care encourages use of care (demand). That then increases cost. If the goal is to decrease cost, more insurance will do just the opposite. If the goal is to increase share (demand), there is no way to decrease cost without decreasing quality (supply).

There is a short-term way to decrease everyone's average cost and to increase the share for those "37 million uninsured." It is to require them to pay for insurance, or to require someone else to pay for them. This will increase the cost (the money available) and will not greatly increase the demand.

As we noted above, most of those "uninsured" will not need much care at first, being younger and relatively healthier than the average. However, they will immediately become the "underinsured" and require more insurance.

There is an ethical problem regarding the autonomy of the individual. Can we force someone to buy something she doesn't want to spend money on? We've done that before when balancing the interests of the individual against the greater good.

The Effect Of Indirect Pay For Care

The myth that more insurance (government or private) will solve the problem is a pervasive one. Even renowned economists propose forced insurance in the private or public sector as the solution to the illness care problem.

Reference: Friedman, Milton, "View from the Forum: Commentary by Milton Friedman," *Courtlandt Forum*, January 1992, pp. 27-40.

Indirect payment for illness care, from taxpayer or private insurance, interferes with the practitioner-patient contract. One of the first, fundamental concepts of law involves contract, in which two parties agree that each will do something. It has been postulated that this is the beginning of civilization, when there is the ability to force another to keep his promise. With illness care practitioners, the contract looks like this: the patient promises to pay, and the practitioner promises to provide service.

Patient ⟹ Gives $$ ⟹ Practitioner

Practitioner ⟹ Gives Care ⟹ Patient

In the present system of payment for illness care, the patient does not directly pay for care but instead pays a third party, who pays the practitioner. The connection (the contract between the two) is interrupted.

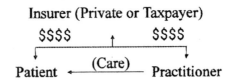

Insurer (Private or Taxpayer)
$$$$ $$$$
Patient ⟵ (Care) ⟶ Practitioner

Demand

Under the present system, nobody is sure exactly who is responsible to anybody. Consequently, nobody **is** responsible to anybody. The patient doesn't know how much his care is going to cost he never values the care on a scale of priorities. He doesn't know how much care he should expect. Consequently, he expects an unlimited amount.

The practitioner giving the care doesn't know how much is required. He has no agreement with the patient on how much care the patient has agreed to buy. Consequently he gives "some" amount. No matter how much he gives, he may feel it wasn't enough.

No limit is set on how much the patient wanted. The practitioner even feels free to give more than the patient may want, He gives the amount <u>he</u> thinks the patient needs. This immediately puts the decision on what care and how much care in the hands of the practitioner, not the patient.

When and how one pays for service determines how much is used. It affects the demand. If an employer or the government or an insurance company pays for service (not the patient) it will seem to the patient that the care is free. "It's already paid for", or "someone else will pay", and more is used. People eat more at a one-price buffet and drink more at an open bar.

If payment is to be directly out of pocket, use of care is restrained depending on how much it is valued. The need or desire for care is ranked in some list of priorities. With direct pay, the law of supply and demand works: more use (demand), causes higher cost for the individual. He then decreases his use (demand).

If there is no cost to the individual for more service, because someone else will pay the bill, the demand continues. The patient has no incentive to use costly services sparingly and wisely. The patient never has to choose. Individuals can make such choices; unlimited care is not necessary or even beneficial.

Supply (Quality)

If the care made for better health, it might be worth all the cost. "Free" care (paid for later in higher premiums and taxes) has not necessarily improved the effectiveness of care. It has increased the amount of care given, and especially the amount of technology.

Technology can be easily quantified, documented, and reimbursed by the indirect payers. Activities like patient teaching are more subjective and less easy to reduce to numbers. They are less likely to be paid.

Seemingly unlimited money for care, through government spending and insurance reimbursement, has induced industry to develop new technology. This allows medical scientists to use new techniques. Many of the new procedures cost hundreds or thousands of dollars each. Special techniques may be valuable in appropriate situations. But their application to all patients because they are considered "free" is disastrous.

Quantitatively, there is more technology available in Florida than in all of Europe. Longevity from age 45 has not significantly increased since the 1920s, however. And people live no longer here than they do in western Europe.

The indirect payment encourages spending money for technology. American patients are guinea pigs as a result. Long-term studies may continue 10-15 years before showing some new technique is no better or is actually worse than conservative treatment. By then, or before, a new technique will be introduced and the cycle repeated.

Although many techniques are not necessarily better medically, they are documentable, compensable, and mandatory. Practitioners make more money if they use them. If they don't, they believe they may be liable if sued. More technology does not necessarily equal better care.

But its use is a clear and predictable result of paying indirectly for care. The resulting belief is that the care is free; there is unlimited money to pay for it. Patients and practitioners alike make this error.

Cost

Care of the sick accounts for a growing percentage of our gross national product. That percentage has grown every year, often faster than the average rate of inflation. The supply of services is limited because the number of practitioners is limited. The demand is unlimited when the care appears to be free.

Indirect pay for care, by insurance and government, works much like the inflation in Spain after the discoveries in 1492. Gold poured into Spain. Services and goods were limited, and it seemed there were apparently unlimited resources to pay for them. The same happened with the increasing payment for illness care by taxpayer and private insurance. With seemingly free care, it would be an economic anomaly if we didn't have high inflation in the industry.

Here the only limitation on spending is what the people are willing to pay after the fact. They pay indirectly in taxes or insurance premiums or out of pocket for services, which are inflated in price by the seemingly unlimited money available. People who are not wealthy now can't afford **not** to buy insurance. Indirect payment causes the "free" care attitude. That has removed prices from any market forces of restraint.

Blamed for part of the increasing cost of care is the profusion of malpractice suits, awards, and insurance in the industry. These are in some measure also created by the "free" attitude toward care of the sick. Patient expectations are elevated. People complain of malpractice when their expectations are not met.

For example: Mr. Patient enters the hospital with indirect pay. The patient does not ask the doctor that only the necessary be done. It's obvious to all that there's no limit on cost. The doctor must order every test and procedure that could conceivably have any relationship to the case.

From the patient's view, there is no reason to refrain, no economic reason. There is good reason to do everything. The standard of practice, the legal minimum the practitioner must meet to avoid liability, becomes limitless. Any failure has no excuse, at least no economic excuse.

This attitude encourages lawsuits for any result less than perfect. The ensuing defensive medicine, malpractice insurance premiums, and lawsuit proliferation all add to future costs.

The Result - Changed Under Management Care

The combination of "free" care, unachievable standard of practice, and technology all affected patients directly. They might be patients just because their hospitalization is "free." They might not want hospitalization, but the nursing home or their doctor has a duty to send them to the hospital. The standard of practice is limitless.

They would be admitted to the hospital and get tubes in their arms and their bladders and their noses and any other available orifices. They would get some new ones, too. Technology and unlimited care is available, reimbursable, and expected.

Patients lost control. They must spend most of their care money on the last year of their lives, more on their dying than on their living. Practitioners can't help them. The care is paid for, and therefore there's an obligation to do it. It's unrealistic to expect the practitioner to be willing to forego the income from unlimited care. Even if she did, the standard of practice is unlimited care. The practitioner must try to meet that impossibility or worry about liability.

There is no contract. Nobody knows who's responsible to whom for what. More insurance, more indirect payment for the people now uninsured will not improve the system. It could make the problem even worse.

Reference: Hall, Jacqulyn, and Werner, Harold, "U-Pay Later: At Last a Free Lunch," *Academy of Senior Professionals Update*, Summer 1989, pp. 14-17.

STUDY QUESTION

How have limits on illness care been set in the past and presently?

RATIONING

The "R" word. People charge that we would ration care under any system other than this one. Or that we ration care under this one and wouldn't under another. The word has a high inflammatory value. It conjures up visions of lines of patients waiting for care—queues (the British word for "lines", pronounced "cues") of people with ration cards in their hands. Visions arise of the gray-coated, gray-faced people of Eastern Europe queuing for milk, or the bread lines of the U.S. depression; and of queuing for appendectomies or heart transplants.

The word ration is from Latin, "ratus," meaning to count, to measure, and to reason (as in rational). A ration is a portion, originally a portion of a scarce commodity. In some places at some times, it was thought unfair to allow some scarce commodity to be bought at a high market price by those with enough money, while others were denied. Thus, butter and sugar were rationed during the Second World War, and the price was controlled. This rationing is still commonplace in countries with socialist system for example Cuba.

The basis of the concept is in fairness. Rationing is the ultimate in distributive justice, where each person is allowed only so much of a good and no more. Rationing of goods during wars has always implied a limit on what individuals can have, not a guarantee that they can have them. You still had to have the money to buy the sugar, you didn't get it free.

The limiting factor was not money, though, since the price was controlled low. The limiting factor was the number of ration coupons you had. Theoretically, they were distributed equally (fairly, justly).

Rationing connotes administrative control, lack of freedom, ability to pay, yet lack of goods. The "rationing" that we have now of illness care is not rationing, but limitation. Limits are set by practitioners who decide what patients need (as opposed to what they want). The "want" question will be dealt with in the "Professionals and Employees" section.

Limits are set by providers who won't, or can't (or at least don't) provide care unless they're paid. That limit exists whether the patient pays in cash or with insurance or taxpayers' money. Limits are set by the individual without insurance as to how much she can or will buy.
Limits are set by insurance companies as to how much they will pay and for what care. The same limits are set by the taxpayers through their legislators and government agency employees. That is not rationing, unless you define rationing as limiting.

You can argue with where or how or by whom limits are set, but a system without some limits, made individually or system wide, is unimaginable.

The opposite of limitations would be everything for everyone, instantly. That is not a reality in housing, food, or any other area of life. If having less than everything all the time is rationing, then everything is rationed.

We have always limited care in this country by income and geographic access. Now we may need to limit care more systematically, even limit care we know to be beneficial, because even the limits we have had don't keep down the cost enough. (See the discussion on Oregon's Medicaid reform in the next section.) Managed care is another way of limiting care, by limiting what will be paid for.

References: Hadorn, David C., and Brook, Robert H., "The Health Care Resource Allocation Debate: Defining Our Terms," *JAMA*, 1991; 266:3328-31.

New England Journal, 1990; 322: 1809-18, various titles and authors.

STUDY QUESTIONS

1. What are some "socially just" illness care systems already functioning in the U.S.?

2. What are the intended consequences of the Medicaid program?

3. What are the unintended consequences of Congress' adding more requirements each year to the benefits under Medicaid?

4. What are the intended consequences of the Medicare program?

5. What is the unintended effect of the Diagnostic Related Group cap on reimbursement to hospitals for Medicare?

6. What is the good news about the VA?

7. What is the bad news about the VA?

8. What are the main differences between Hawaii and Massachusetts regarding employer-mandated insurance?

9. What are the three principles of the Oregon reform of Medicaid?

10. What is the criterion for determining which care will be paid in Oregon?

11. What is the philosophy or ethic that underlies the Oregon plan?

12. What are your feelings about the Oregon plan of Medicaid reform?

13. How do your feelings about the plan relate to your philosophy of life?

ANOTHER "R" WORD: REFORM

Before we look at other countries' systems and some state solutions to health care, we can look at the socially just illness care already given in the U.S.

EXISTING SOCIAL JUSTICE IN AMERICAN ILLNESS CARE

The U.S. and state taxpayers pay for systems now that provide "social justice" in illness care for some. These people have "access" to care and it is paid for.

The people in our country who already enjoy access (social justice, equality in "health care") are the old (Medicare), poor (Medicaid), disabled (Medicare again), war veterans (VA), Native American Indians (Indian Health Service), and people in the military (CHAMPUS, Civilian Health and Medical Program of the Uniformed Services).

We can use these examples of "socially just" illness care, provided at taxpayer expense, to see what benefits and problems they demonstrate. They might provide lessons for examining the idea of expanding such programs to cover all the people of the country. The VA, Medicaid, and Medicare offer particularly good examples of intended and unintended consequences.

$$$$$$$$$

First, the costs of the care is so expensive that taxpayers fund them at minimal levels. The U.S. and state governments set payment to practitioners at low levels. Often the people in the program can't get care, though it's paid for. The payment for service may be set lower than the cost of providing the service. The practitioner who cares for such patients at payment lower than cost will be bankrupt.

So they don't do it, or they take a few. This amounts to a certain amount of charity work that the practitioner contributes to the system. A laudable effort, but it cannot be counted on to continue and to expand.

Because we have these social justice care systems, we can contentedly say that the old, poor, disabled, veterans, abo-Americans and military are provided for. We can ignore the reality of whether or how well they work. We can then say that the only people we now have to worry about are the "xx million uninsured."

Medicaid continues to cost more money and provide less service for fewer people. The federal Congress yearly requires state governments to provide more services to poor people in their states in order to qualify for matching federal funds. The intended consequence is that poor people will have good illness and illness prevention care.

An unintended consequence results because some of the state legislatures are required by their constitutions to balance income and expenses. None can print their own money like the feds. So every year they cut some poor people off the Medicaid rolls to save enough money to give the rest of the people the newly required care.

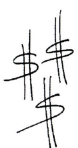

As noted above, the payment for services for Medicaid is poor in most states. Few practitioners can afford to care for many Medicaid patients, so the supply of care is limited.

Medicare was started in 1965. The intention was to provide low-cost illness care for people over 65. Adjusted for inflation, such people pay about twice as much out-of-pocket for their care as they did then. Medicare premiums rise yearly also, along with the deductible that the over-65 must pay before receiving benefits. As a result, the cost of premiums rises for "medigap" policies, which cover expenses that the government doesn't pay.

The Medicare payment system to hospitals changed in the mid-80's, when Diagnostic Related Groups limited payment for certain conditions to an average cost of an average patient for an average course of treatment. The intended consequence was to encourage hospitals to be efficient.

Immediately, the nonaverage healthier patient was a profit maker, the nonaverage sicker patient a loss maker for the hospital. The unintended (but foreseeable) consequence was that patients were discharged sicker, quicker. A new for-profit industry, the home care industry, developed to meet the need. This was federally paid, too. Save any money?

The intent of reducing payment for dialysis is to save money. The response by providers is to do more dialysis in shorter time to make up for the reduction in payment. The unintended consequence: short-time dialysis patients have dramatically increased risk of mortality. Avoiding mortality was the purpose of the dialysis in the first place.

Reference: Held, P.J. et al, "Mortality and Duration of Hemodialysis Treatment,"*JAMA*, 1991;265:871.

Another example of a "social justice" experiment is described in the introduction. The intent in Massachusetts was to provide low-cost care to the elderly by requiring physicians to accept Medicare payment as a condition of being licensed in the state. The unintended consequence was that many physicians left the state, and the elderly had even less care than before.

Measures have been proposed to return control of Medicaid to states and to put Medicare funding into the private sector (through HMO's -- managed care -- and Medical Savings Accounts). These measures will change those systems to be less socialist and more like private enterprise.

THE VA EXAMPLE

THE UP SIDE

The good news about the socially just VA system is that it has successfully contributed to education of practitioners, at the same time benefiting from affiliation with medical and other practitioner schools. Money for research has been rewarded with results for better care, especially in geriatrics.

The VA is remarkably efficient. It has implemented DRG's (diagnostic related groups) in which a set amount of money is paid to the practitioner (provider) for each diagnosis. This encourages practitioners to get patients out earlier to save money. The VA budget, adjusted for yearly inflation, has remained nearly flat. The VA has increased efficiency, reduced average stay on acute services, and seen an increase in the number of patients treated.

In 1985, the Reagan administration considered "mainstreaming" the VA. That would have meant dismantling the system and using the money to purchase private insurance for veterans, who would then use private hospitals and practitioners. After the study, that administration decided keeping the VA hospital system would cost less than private insurance. The VA does not pay the 20% overhead for administrative costs which private insurance reaps. The U.S. private system of purchasing "health" insurance has administrative costs of 20% of the total bill. That means that 20% of every dollar is used, not for practitioner care of the patient, but for paperwork. That is higher than overhead in the VA or the national health system of Canada.

Those systems, where all eligible are paid for, work more like our social security for old people. The clerk sees the name, and automatically pays. So costs for administration are less.

Government management is not always more inefficient than private management. Incentive makes the difference. If government workers have incentive to be efficient, they will be. If private workers do not, they won't be. There is nothing inherently lazy or wasteful about government or its employees. But most of the time, government systems are set up without incentives for individuals to be efficient.

THE DOWN SIDE

Cost-cutting would probably occur in other health systems as it has in the VA. Staffing levels are lower in all departments than the private sector. In 1987, the overall U.S. staff-to-patient ratio was 4.29 staff per patient. The VA ratio was 3.2 staff per patient. Nurse staffing levels on acute services was 50% of comparable community hospitals; respiratory therapist staff numbers were one-third those of community hospitals. The author of one study thought the VA ratio of respiratory care practitioners was about right.

Physician services were 9% of the VA budget. The cost of physician services accounts for 19.5% of illness spending in the U.S., and 15.7% of such spending in Canada. The VA got that lower medical care cost from less staffing, lower salaries, flat reimbursement. Maybe we don't need all those doctors in the private hospitals. Or nurses. Or respiratory care practitioners?

The socially just VA system now limits care by income level, due to a Congressional mandate. Veterans in the middle class without private insurance lose. They also limit care by queue like Canada and Britain do, putting people on waiting lists for care. But the VA doesn't exclude the needy, or the high risk, or veterans with costly illnesses.

The VA, in response to proposed health care reform, instituted much reorganization in the direction of reducing cost and increasing efficiency. As government continues to "downsize", the future of this large government entity is in question.

Reference: Smith, Charles, and Wolcott, Mark, "Veterans Health Care: Lessons for a National Health Care System," *Annals of Internal Medicine.* 1991; 115:907-09.

HAWAII: YES

Hawaii passed a law in the 1970s which provides that employers pay for a minimum health insurance for their employees. The system works pretty well from their perspective. There are some reasons: Hawaii is a "boom" tourist economy, with practically no unemployment. Therefore, few people are not covered by the employer insurance, and the money to pay for it is available.

Second, the ethnic and environmental situation of Hawaii is unique. There are no ghettos, no pollution, less crime and violence, no ice and snow to fall on. The people are mostly Asian, Caucasian, and native Hawaiian and have better health profiles than people in many states. They see the doctor more often, and go to the hospital less. The hospitals sometimes have a 48-hour wait for admission, and a nurse shortage.

Finally, it is an island. If any other state passed such a law, the easy access across its borders might raise costs from people crossing to get the benefits.

Reference: Holoweiko, Mark, "Health Care Reform: What Does Hawaii Have to Teach?" *Medical Economics*, January 1992, pp. 158-74.

MASSACHUSETTS: NOT

The legislature in Massachusetts adopted an employer-paid mandatory health insurance in 1988, as part of then-Governor Dukakis' presidential campaign. The implementation has been delayed several times, most recently until 1995 (it was delayed again). Massachusetts has all the problems Hawaii does not, the most obvious and important being its much poorer economy.

It is anticipated that many small employers, mandated to pay several thousand dollars per employee for insurance, will fire enough employees to make up the dollar difference. See the problems anticipated with the "play or pay" proposal, below.

PEOPLE OR PROCEDURES

The Oregon example is a "socially just" system that does not exist yet. But it is more than just an idea, like the other solutions seen below.

The state of Oregon has run out of money to pay for Medicaid (at least they do not have enough money to pay for all the benefits that the federal government requires states to provide in order to receive the matching money from the feds). The people of Oregon could tax themselves more for Medicaid, but they have chosen not to do so.

As required benefits were added by the feds, the states keep spending down by making the requirements more difficult. That is, fewer and poorer people are covered for all the required benefits. Oregon leaders decided that limiting care this way was unfair. It meant that a few people were covered for a lot of care, while a lot of people were not covered at all.

THE PRINCIPLES

I. They decided to tell the truth. Care was limited under the old system. It would be limited under the new system, too. But it would be limited in a rational, systematic way, a different way. Instead of covering a few people for a lot of things, they want to cover a lot of people for a few services.

II. The premise is that more care does not necessarily mean more health. (See the above discussion under "Myths" for the present confusion that "health care" equals health.) Oregon leaders know that's not true.

III. They hope to be able to decide what are the most effective kinds of care, the care that does result in less illness.

In order to accomplish this, they compiled lists of diseases or conditions, paired with the treatment for those conditions. They then rank the items on the list, from highest priority to lowest. Each year at budget time, the legislature decides where to cut off the list.

The number of patients covered will not change, but the line separating treatments paid for, from treatments that will not be paid for, will change depending on money available.

So far 709 pairs of Conditions and Treatments are identified; 587 were budgeted for during the first two years. Top priorities on the list were services for children and expectant mothers, acute conditions with high expectations of recovery, and preventive care.

Examples of conditions and treatments not covered: No. 588 on the list, a laminectomy for intervertebral disc disorders; No. 689, cochlear implant for sensorineural hearing loss; No. 695, medical therapy for benign polyps of vocal cords.

CRITERION FOR CARE

Care is limited informally—by choice, by geography. Distribution of care is not uniform; patients and practitioners choose to live in different areas. Oregon leaders restrict care systematically according to condition and treatment. They decide which treatments result in less illness and are most cost effective. That requires some line drawing, which Oregon is prepared to do.

Oregon is using as its criterion for ranking, a combination of quality of life and longevity. (See discussion of the Quality Adjusted Life Years in Chapter Three.)

Quite clearly, the people who will receive the most care under the plan are those who are younger and healthier to begin with. The younger will get care before the older, because the younger will have more years to live. The healthier will get care before the sicker, because the healthier will have better "quality of life." At some point we will have to examine why we care for people at all. Is it because they are relatively healthy and don't need much, or because they are sick and need the care?

Eventually, it can be seen that if they have data that people over 70 do less well with bypass grafts, Oregon may pay for them only for people younger than 70. If babies born weighing under 3 pounds do not do as well as babies over that weight, Oregon may treat them less intensively.

If they have data that handicapped persons live fewer years, have more medical costs, and contribute less to society, Oregon may pay for fewer procedures for them. If people have diseases that are probably self-inflicted,

Oregon may pay less for their treatment, such as smoking related diseases, cirrhosis of liver, AIDS, heart disease. Oregon puts AIDS treatment at a low priority because such patients do not live as long as some others.

THE PROCESS

The proponents of the Oregon plan had 12 public hearings, 47 community meetings, and a telephone survey of 1000 people, plus uncounted consultations with experts to try to come up with this list. Because the list does not include all the benefits mandated by the federal government, Oregon asked for a waiver of the requirements for five years. The Bush Administration denied the waiver in 1992, saying the plan violated the Americans with Disabilities Act. Vice President, Albert Gore, attacked the plan as unethical.

More people were covered; all 2.8 million of Oregonians would be covered; 450,00 estimated to be uninsured. Before only 150,000 were on Medicaid in Oregon; half of those are under the official poverty line of about $12,000 for a family of four. In stages, eventually all the poor would be covered under Medicaid.

CRITICISMS

All of the following are criticisms addressed to the program in Oregon:

- Cruel

- Irrational

- Impractical

- Taking from the poor to pay for poor

- No ranking of illness care among other spending in Oregon before this was done

- Oregon should pay more in taxes to pay for more care (Gore's position)

- Utilitarian

- Sacrifices the individual for the faceless mass

- Failure to investigate other ways to solve the problem

- Pits potential organ transplant patients against pregnant mothers and indigent children

Reference: Rothenberg, Leslie S., and Franklin, Cory, "Commentaries: That Which Is Wanting," *Hastings Center Report*, 1988; December, pp. 34-36.

STUDY QUESTIONS

1.   What is the definition of "monopsony?"

2.   How does Canada hold down costs in its national health system?

3.   How do the European national health systems solve the problem of two levels of care?

4.   How does Great Britain hold down costs in the National Health Service?

OTHER COUNTRIES: CANADA

Notice below under "Solutions" the big three who wanted national health insurance: business, hospitals, and the insurance industry. Note that none of them called for a national health **system**, like Canada's. Canada's provinces (like our states) are the primary payors and administrators of the system. The taxpayers of Canada pay the premiums. The governments are the insurance companies.

Administrative costs are lower because there is only one insurance company paying. There is no quarrel about what the limits are. There's no bureaucracy to see if you qualify; if you're Canadian, you're covered. The government is the only payor of the bills. In economic terms, having only one buyer in a system is called a "monopsony." The opposite, only one supplier, is a "monopoly." As discussed in the licensure section of Professionals and Employees, neither condition can

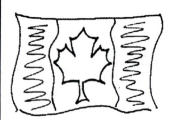

exist without government force. That's why American insurers aren't eager for the U.S. to adopt a Canadian plan; they'd be out of business.

Canada has provided availability (demand) of care for nearly everyone. By keeping the supply (quality, technology) of care low, the costs have risen slowly. The government will not pay for everything for everyone on demand.

Limits on supply are achieved by limiting the amount of technology available. For example, there are more CAT scanners in Seattle than in all of Canada. There are some 250,000 Canadians on waiting lists for operations. Physical facilities are in deteriorating condition in some cases for lack of funds.

Canadian physicians are generally self-employed. They are reimbursed at a set rate by the government of the province. That rate is periodically negotiated by their medical society, which functions more like a union in Canada than the American societies do. The AMA and state associations in America de facto (in fact, not in law) negotiate with Medicare and Medicaid through lobbying, but not formally.

Canadian physicians' incomes are not greatly lower than Americans' since, although fees per patient are lower, the volume of patients seen is higher. Patients are not allowed to consult specialists directly. This is the same situation that patients in HMO's or managed care plans experience in the U. S.

Malpractice suits exist in Canada, though the judgments have been lower than in the U.S. This is largely because of legal system and societal differences in the two systems. The cost of malpractice insurance has risen dramatically there.

References: Danzon, Patricia M. "The 'Crisis' in Medical Malpractice: A Comparison of Trends in the United States, Canada, the United Kingdom and Australia," *Law, Medicine and Health Care*, 1990,18:48-58.

Coyte, Peter C., et al, "Medical Malpractice—The Canadian Experience,"*NEJM*, 1991;324:89-93.

There are limits to care in Canada, of technology in particular. The costs have risen steadily despite this control. That's why U.S. business isn't eager either about the Canadian system. Costs now threaten to force more limits on care. That's why the hospitals don't think it is an answer, together with the fact that all the hospitals are owned by the government and all administrators employed by it. The Canadian system has become so obviously costly that it is not seen as a desirable option for this country.

The United States provides a safety valve for Canadian citizens' illness care. The Canadians can and do come to the U.S. and obtain treatment they would not be able to get in Canada. This tends to pacify those who would otherwise be vocal critics of the system. The provinces are in process of cutting costs (services) still further.

References: Orford, R. R., "Reflections on the Canadian and American Health-Care Systems," *Mayo Clinic Proceedings*, 1991; 66:203-06.

Kirkpatrick, David, "Practicing Medicine Above and Below the 49th Parallel," *AIM*, 1991;151:2150-53.

European Solutions

Most of the other industrialized countries (except South Africa, it is always noted) have a national health system. Unfortunately, they have problems too. They are all in some ways like Canada's. Almost all have universal coverage, (share, availability of some level of care). All limit the quality or level of care provided, some by limiting the amount of technology available.

Some schemes allow private insurance and private care. That results in one level of care under government payment and at least one other level for people with more money. It is charged that this country has such levels now. From the experience of other countries, we can see that a national health system would not change that.

Illness care is reported as a smaller part of the GNP or GDP in other countries than in the U.S. Those figures are slippery; not all countries report finances the same way. Watch carefully when statistics about the "health" of the countries are compared. Remember that other countries, especially European ones, are often are composed of heterogeneous, all-Caucasian populations. Their social welfare systems, which have a great impact on health, are quite different from ours. Those countries usually do not cope with sizeable minority populations whose values and health practices differ from the majority.

Systematic and avoidable differences exist among social, ethnic, and geographic groups within and across Europe. The goal of the Europeans is one group of united states. Sound familiar? But differences in health status, access to care, use of care, and quality of health care exist.

These sound like American problems, though all of the European countries have some form of national health insurance or system. Writers believe that the focus should be on infant health, working conditions, and equity in care. Like the Oregonians described above, they want to use a cost-benefit analysis to decide what care to give.

Great Britain limits care in their national health service. The practitioners assist in this limitation, telling patients, for example, that they "don't need" some unavailable technology, instead of "you can't have it." There is little or no process for people to have input into what procedures are paid, what care is denied. The waiting list or queue is used to ration; about one million patients are waiting for procedures. Patients over age 65 are usually denied kidney dialysis or transplants.

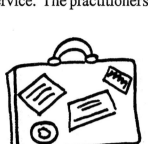

One region of the National Health Service identified five conditions that will not be treated through the Health Service. They were varicose veins, benign lumps, wisdom teeth removal, tattoo removal, and treatment for infertility. The public in England learned about it only through a leak to a newspaper. Contrast this to the Oregon decision-making process, outlined above.

References   "London Perspective: The Oregon Trail Reaches Britain," *The Lancet*, 1991;338:1133-34.

Whitehead, Margaret, and Dahlgren, Goran, "What Can Be Done about Inequalities in Health?" *The Lancet*, 1991;338:1059-63.

STUDY QUESTIONS

1.   What is the sequence of cost shifting for nonpaid illness care?

2.   What are the three groups most vocal in the request for national "health" insurance?

3.   What are the three major proposals for illness care payment reform?

4. What are the major problem with a national health system?

5. What is the major problem with a "play or pay" employer-paid health insurance system?

6. What is the major problem with a tax credit for purchase of individual health insurance?

7. What is the difference between buying insurance and gambling in Las Vegas?

8. What is the difference between a tax credit and a tax deduction?

9. What is the ethical question of malpractice insurance?

10. What are your reactions to the Modest Suggestions at the end of this chapter?

JUST DO IT

To figure out who wanted reform and why, you have to know who's going to benefit and how. The cost of care went up and up after the indirect payment of care started under Medicare. Nonpayors' care was paid before by charging paying patients a little more. "Nonpayor" is not the same as "uninsured," since some "uninsured" pay for their own care.

Soon the government and private insurers paid more of the total bill than individuals. Together, indirect pay for care accounts for about 73% of all the illness care. The indirect payors didn't want the cost of the nonpays shifted onto them. They stopped paying that cost, as much as possible. Further cost of the nonpay's care then shifted onto the providers—the hospitals and practitioners. They're now subsidizing some of the care for the whole system.

The insurance companies are getting costs shifted onto them, because they insure the employees of the big businesses. And mandating insurance for a whole pool of uninsured people will surely bring in a lot of money.

From the above you can see that three major entities would want national "health" insurance: the indirect payors, government and insurance companies; big employers who already pay for their employees insurance; and providers. Government doesn't exist as a group, except in the form of politicians, so we won't discuss their interest. The three biggest beneficiaries of national health insurance would be big business, illness care providers, and insurance companies.

Business started paying health insurance premiums during World War II as a way of attracting scarce workers while avoiding wartime wage controls. Most big business pays for insurance for their workers already. They want to get some of the cost off their backs and make their bottom lines look better. They will call for national illness insurance, waving the flag of international competition.

Hospitals and other practitioners call uninsured patients "self-pay," which translates to no-pay, though not all uninsured are "no-pay." Hospitals and independent practitioners want all people insured, so they'll get paid for some of the care they now have to give without receiving payment. Did you wonder why AMA would support national health insurance?

Insurance companies want national health insurance to increase their premium dollars and spread the risk. Immediately an enormous pool of young, healthy people who need little care will be paying, either from their own pockets, their small business employers', or the taxpayers'.

How To Do It?

Reform proposals come in three groups. A national health system like Canada's or Britain's (also called a single payer system). Or a mandate that employers pay costs for insurance (Democrats). Or a tax credit for individuals to purchase their own insurance (Republicans). Since failure of the Clinton Reform proposal in 1994, "reform" (or change) has come about through managed care and general decrease in money available for care.

National Health Service

If a national health system were implemented, it might produce more freedom for practitioners, not patients. A national health system or service is not a new idea.

The Federal Social Security Administrator under President Truman in 1948 proposed a system of universal illness insurance. President Kennedy spoke in favor of a program of limited national health insurance in 1962. Medicare, which had been proposed in some form since the "New Deal" of Roosevelt, passed into law in 1964. President Nixon proposed extending Medicare to all during his term.

A national health system like Canada's was endorsed by 56% of the respondents in a survey. (See descriptions above for problems and advantages of that solution.)

A national health system like Canada's is estimated to cost over $250 billion per year. But a report of a Republican joint economic committee staff said it would cost $81.5 billion per year for a government single payer of the bills, no private insurers. But the Government Accounting Office (GAO) at one point said a single-payer national insurance program would save $3 billion a year. Take your pick of numbers.

SOLUTIONS

What would it cost to insure the uninsured, if there are 37 million of them? The GAO said $18 billion. The staff of a Republican congressional committee said $37 billion. A little math: **if** there are 37 million uninsured, and coverage is bought for each one with current coverage costing employers about $3,700 per year, then it has to cost a lot. Even a minimum cost of one thousand dollars per person per year is $37 billion. What is your own coverage cost, per year, including what you and your employer pay? Multiply that by 37 million (or any other number).

PLAY OR PAY

A "play or pay" plan, in which employers pay for employee insurance or pay taxes and the taxpayer pays for the unemployed, was favored by 67% of those surveyed. Critics point out that this would cost jobs, because employers would fire or would not hire low-paid employees, who would cost $3,000-$4,000 per year more than at present. But politically such a plan is attractive because it seems that the employer is paying the bill.

A "play or pay" plan, in which employers pay for employee insurance or pay taxes, is estimated to cost $36 billion for taxpayers (for the unemployed) and would cost employers $30 billion more. (See the Massachusetts and Hawaii examples for advantages and problems.)

MORE OF THE SAME, ONLY MORE

Expansion of the existing system is proposed to be done with tax credits for purchase of health insurance. In response to a survey, 87% supported keeping the existing system with some expansion. That is, presumably, tax credits for insurance premiums. President Bush had made such a proposal, along with price controls on the costs for the Medicare and Medicaid programs.

This would finance purchase of such insurance at the direct benefit of the insurance industry. Twenty cents of every dollar of benefit from that industry is spent for administration, not practitioner care.

The present system gives tax-free income to workers for health insurance premiums (tax deductions for premiums). This results in $3,000-$4,000 in yearly income that workers can't control themselves. The workers have no choice about spending the money.

That money is not added to the worker's income and taxed; it is deducted from the employer's profit as expense. This results in a 15 to 31% bonus on that money, depending on the worker's income level (tax rate).

That is money that the government does not receive as tax income. The money has to be made up through more taxes on other people on other income. Workers are subsidized by the tax code to buy health insurance. They have no choice, usually, in what insurance is purchased by their employer.

The purchase of that insurance is encouraged by its tax-free status. No other kind of insurance premium goes untaxed; you cannot deduct the cost of your car or house insurance from your income before you pay taxes. The net result is that the "health" insurance industry is subsidized by the taxpayer.

ABOUT "MANAGED CARE"

For "Managed Care" read "Limited Care". That' all there is to it; HMOs reduce cost by limiting care. The insurer (HMO) goes to the employer or customer and says, "I'll give care cheaper than the traditional fee-for service insurance." Then the insurer (HMO) says to the providers (hospitals and doctors), "I'll guarantee you patients if you'll accept a discounted fee."

A WORD ABOUT INSURANCE

Bet. The word about insurance is "bet." You bet that you will get sick. The insurance company bets you won't. It's not really a pool as we have sometimes said. It's a contract. The company is in business; if you don't get sick, you don't get paid. They make a profit and they are not holding the money for you. You are not guaranteed to get back benefits equal to the premiums you put in.

Another survey by Aetna Life & Casualty Co.: 60% of Americans surveyed prefer a private-sector approach (so do the insurance companies). They want health insurance available to all. They agree that no unnecessary and expensive procedures should be performed. They did not, however, give a list of unnecessary procedures.

The people surveyed want to make it harder for attorneys to sue physicians. Let me explain something: Attorneys do not sue practitioners; patients sue practitioners. Attorneys represent patients. Attorneys are the patient advocates after practitioners get through with them. Some people must truly believe that if we got rid of all the lawyers, people would just live together happily ever after without suing each other. Perhaps we need another "Myths" section here.

Giving tax credits for buying "health" insurance will decrease tax revenue to the government, a cost to the government. For the same cost, we could just give the uninsured vouchers for illness care. People would spend these directly with the practitioner and hospital like food stamps are with the grocery stores, avoiding the 20% loss in bureaucracy. These would then be redeemed by the government.

This is how a tax credit works. A tax credit is given to the individual who buys insurance. Note that this is not a deduction to income, which is a 15 to 31% bonus on the money depending on your tax bracket. Instead this is a tax credit, a 100% bonus on the money; whatever you paid for the insurance decreases your taxes by exactly that much. The insurance premium is free to you. You would have had to pay that amount in taxes anyway if you hadn't bought the insurance. Would you rather pay the government $3000 a year and get nothing, or pay Aetna $3000 a year and get coverage for illness?

The government revenue goes down as a result of the money going to the insurance company instead of the government. The insurance company gets a profit on the insurance premium. 20% of the money for care is lost in bureaucracy to the insurance company.
The hospital and independent practitioner who've been losing money on the uninsured get paid now. The employers who've seen their cost of health insurance go up as costs are shifted to them, get a reprieve.

This takes money right out of the treasury and gives it to insurance company. Right out of the treasury to help the hospital make a profit. Right out of the treasury to help big business' bottom line.

MALPRACTICE INSURANCE COSTS

The cost for malpractice insurance is a separable and significant part of reimbursement for practitioners under Medicare reimbursement under the 1992 Relative Value Resource Based System. This outlay of money could provide lots of care if not paid to insurance companies.

Is there a moral issue in paying insurance companies profits, instead of paying patients for care? Is the payment of malpractice insurance premiums an "escrow" account or fund kept for people who are injured? Malpractice attorneys who represent injured patients believe it is.

Proposals for federal laws would enforce changes in the laws about suits for medical malpractice in every state. Several states have already changed such law, calling it "tort reform." A "tort," from an old French word, is a "wrong." In some states the reforms have been held to violate state constitutions. Almost every state constitution provides the individual harmed a right of access to the courts (a right to sue for damages).

Experts question whether the federal government has the power to change state tort law in this way. The 11th Amendment to the U.S. Constitution reserves to the states all powers not specifically granted to the federal government. The power to regulate state tort law is not specifically granted to the federal government.

Some provisions of proposed federal law are to limit (cap), the amount of noneconomic damages that a patient can recover for harm. Economic damages are expenses that were paid or owed to the doctor, hospital, and nursing care, as well as loss of wages. The other damages are non-economic. Plaintiff's lawyers use the term pain and suffering, for obvious reasons. California, for instance, currently limits noneconomic damages to $250,000, although state legislators are considering raising this cap.

Also proposed is a limit on the percentage of the award to the patient, which the attorney and patient agree to be the attorney's fee. This could limit poor people's ability to get into the legal system. Malpractice suits are expensive and risky for the plaintiff's attorneys. The attorney usually advances all expenses for the suit and gets nothing if the patient doesn't win.

Also proposed is a limit on the amount of punitive damages. These are damages awarded to punish the defendant for intentional, wanton, or reckless behavior. These damages are not usually awarded in malpractice cases. They require a high degree of culpable conduct. Also possible in reforms is increased funding for state licensing boards to increase practitioner discipline.

MODEST SUGGESTIONS

You know by now that there is no wonderful answer to all of these issues. You know by now also that paying indirectly for care, through insurance and other third party payments, does not make the system any better.

We could encourage direct pay as much as possible. Practitioners could give discounts for direct pay instead of insurance. The government could require Medicare recipients to prove economic need. The howls at that suggestion are heard even through my word processor. The government could give tax incentives for people who do not carry insurance, but who instead save the money for future illness care. This would be a kind of IRA, not for retirement but for possible illness. Several candidates for President and the President have endorsed this plan, called Medical Savings Accounts.

The government could tax people on the money their employer pays for insurance premiums as income. Workers would understand that insurance is not free, that it's paid for with their money that the employer now controls; we could provide "care stamps," vouchers for poor who can't pay for care, like food stamps, and save the 20% bureaucracy.

Changes are occuring rapidly. Dismantling the enormous industry that has been bloated by the indirect pay of government and insurance companies is cause dislocation; the economics of healthcare changes but the ethics do not.

STUDY QUESTIONS WITH ANSWERS

These are suggested answers. If you have something like these answers in your own words, consider yourself successful. If you have more (quality, not quantity) than these answers, consider yourself excellent.

1. Why are the ethical issues in the Share of Care chapter more important to you personally than any others in the course?

   Because the kind of system we have will affect your job, patients, family, and yourself as a patient in the future.

2. What is the problem with the existing system, assuming you think there's a problem?

   Write it down now, and see if your view changes after this chapter.

3. What is the percentage of illness care expense paid now by taxpayers through state, local, and federal governments?

42%

4. Which are the values most often mentioned when share of care is discussed?

- Social Justice, first.
- Autonomy, for patient and practitioner.
- And the one the whole thing is about, money, which is a substitute for work.

5. Which three specific things are protected from taking without due process of law under the 5th and 14th Amendments to the U.S. Constitution?

- Life.
- Liberty.
- Property.

6. These Amendments are examples of which value?

Justice.

7. What is the maxim or saying that best characterizes social justice?

The end justifies the means.

8. Which philosophy advocates the greatest good for the greatest number?

Utilitarianism.

9. Which is the value that keeps us from forcing people to do things we believe are good for them?

Autonomy.

10. What are the three parts to the economy of illness care?

- Demand.
- Supply.
- Cost.

- Just like the economy of anything else; in illness care we call the demand <u>share</u> (you'll see it wrongly called access); we call the supply "level of <u>technology</u>" (you'll see it wrongly called quality, though that's nearly impossible to measure); and we call cost<u>cos.t</u>

11. What happens to the cost when the demand for a service goes up and the supply stays the same?

    Cost goes up also.

12. What happens to the supply of technology in illness care if the demand or share of care goes up, and the government controls the price or cost at the same level?

    $\uparrow$ Demand + $\updownarrow$ Cost = $\downarrow$ Supply

13. What is the definition of GNP?

    - Gross National Product.
    - The total production of goods and services in a country.
    - Also called Gross Domestic Product.

14. What percent of a country's gross national product is too high a percentage to produce in illness care?

    - Your call—12%?
    - Experts guess it will go to 15% at least before any decrease.
    - It is going to go down!

15. Why do people confuse health care with health and life, and the absence of health care with illness and death?

    - Because logically it has the word "health" in it.
    - Then, health care is associated with health, then with life.
    - Logically following, health care means life, and lack of it, death.

16. How many people are uninsured for illness care in the U.S.?

    You're right (nobody knows).

17. What is the difference between "uninsured" and "unhealthy?"

    - Mention that they are not the same concepts.
    - Insurance does not produce health; lack of insurance does not produce illness.

- You might have also mentioned that as a group, uninsured people include people who can't get insurance for health reasons, so the group is likely to be "unhealthier" overall.

18. What is the difference between "uninsured" and "uncared-for?"

   - Mention again that they are not the same concepts.
   - People without insurance receive care, some pay for it out of their own pocket, and some do not.
   - Data show that people without insurance see the doctor and go to the hospital almost as often as people with insurance.

19. How does insurance work?

   - Many people pay premiums.
   - Only a few of the people paying premiums will need care.
   - Otherwise, the insurance company would go broke.

20. What are the values involved in refusing to pay for patients who have "self-inflicted" diseases?

   - Our value of beneficence, doing good, goes down the drain.
   - We sort of uphold autonomy; the patient has the choice, even when it's bad for her.
   - We elevate justice to a religion, especially the Old Testament idea of justice as "an eye for an eye".
   - We say the person deserved what she got.

21. Which philosophy allows us to force individuals to buy insurance they don't want if it is better for the society?

   Utilitarianism.

22. Illustrate the contract between patient and practitioner with a schematic.

   Patient Gives $$ Practitioner
   Practitioner Gives Care Patient

23. Illustrate the relationship when the payment is made indirectly, by a third party.

   Insurer (Private or Taxpayer)
     $$$$ $$$$

   Patient ◄——(Care)—— Practitioner

---

24. Why does indirect payment cause increased use of care?

   Because the care seems to be "free".

25. Why does increased money available for care stimulate increased use of technology?

   Industry has an incentive to develop more technology to improve potential profits.

26. Why is technology more likely to be paid for than other kinds of care?

   Technology is more visible, documentable, more easily quantified by a number than is some more subjective activity like patient teaching.

27. Why does increasing money available for care, or seemingly available through the "free" care attitude resulting from indirect payment, cause inflation in the industry?

   • Inflation results from unlimited resources and limited supply.
   • This is exactly the appearance when care is paid for indirectly.

28. What is the effect of indirect payment on malpractice suits?

   • Because the care seems "free," the standard of care is elevated to doing everything possible, not just what is necessary.
   • The patient's expectation is higher, so the suit is more likely to be filed in the first place.
   • And because the practitioner has had no input from the patient as to what limits to set, the practitioner is held to a higher standard so she is more likely not to meet that standard.

29. How have limits on illness care been set in the past and presently?

   Care is limited (not rationed, a much more formal system in which supply is fixed) by where you live, how much money you have, what your insurance will pay for, and what the government will pay for.

30. What are some "socially just" illness care systems already functioning in the U.S.?

   • The old (Medicare).

- Poor (Medicaid)
- Disabled (Medicare again)
- War veterans (VA)
- Native American Indians (Indian Health Service)
- And relatives of people in the military (CHAMPUS, Civilian Health and Medical Program of the Uniformed Services)

31. What are the intended consequences of the Medicaid program?

    To provide illness and illness prevention care for poor people who otherwise could not afford it

32. What are the unintended consequences of Congress' adding more requirements each year to the benefits under Medicaid?

    The states, in order to meet their limited budgets, add the required procedures and remove people from the program

33. What are the intended consequences of the Medicare program?

    To provide care for over-65 people

34. What is the unintended effect of the Diagnostic Related Group cap on reimbursement to hospitals for Medicare?

    The patients were discharged sicker quicker in order to meet costs to the hospital, and require care at home still at government expense

35. What is the good news about the VA?

    They are efficient, and they don't have the big overhead that private insurers do

36. What is the bad news about the VA?

    They are efficient at the cost of staffing, and limit care with waiting lists

37. What are the main differences between Hawaii and Massachusetts regarding employer-mandated insurance?

    - The economies are different, the people and their environment are different
    - Massachusetts is not an island

---

38. What are the three principles of the Oregon reform of Medicaid?

  I. Money for care (thus care) is limited
  II. More care does not always mean more health
  III. Care that results in less illness can be determined

39. What is the criterion for determining which care will be paid in Oregon?

  The care will be paid that results in longest life combined with best quality of life

40. What is the philosophy or ethic that underlies the Oregon plan?

  The most valued persons are those who will have the longest and healthiest lives

41. What are your feelings about the Oregon plan of Medicaid reform?

  • Whatever you feel is OK
  • Your feelings are probably based on how you view life, whether you value more the practical aspect of the plan or dislike the non-ideal aspect of it
  • Remember the process in Chapter Three—stop first, and feel what you feel; then you will have your bias in mind as you look for information; you're more likely to know when you're not being honest with yourself

42. How do your feelings about the plan relate to your philosophy of life?

  • I'd love to see what you said!
  • Did you say you were a utilitarian or a romantic? Or a dozen other things?

43. What is the definition of "monopsony?"

  • An economic term, meaning "only one buyer"
  • Like "monopoly" (which is the opposite) "one seller" can only exist with government force

44.	How does Canada hold down costs in its national health system?

	•	Limiting technology
	•	Using waiting lists for procedures
	•	Delaying capital improvements
	•	Avoiding the administrative costs of multiple private insurers by prohibiting private insurance contracts

45.	How do the European national health systems solve the problem of two levels of care?

	Most of them don't

46.	How does Great Britain hold down costs in the National Health Service?

	•	Limiting technology
	•	Waiting lists for procedures
	•	Denying some treatment to certain groups (e.g., people over 65)
	•	Removing procedures from lists of care that will be paid
	•	And as in Canada, by enforcing a monopsony, which cuts down on administrative costs

47.	What is the sequence of cost-shifting for nonpaying people's illness care?

	•	In the beginning . . . nonpaid care was added to the cost of care paid by other individuals
	•	As more individuals were covered by the government (Medicare) and private insurers, those two entities got the costs shifted to them
	•	They have tried to minimize this, and additional costs of nonpaid care are now being shifted onto the hospitals and independent practitioners
	•	The insurers have shifted their nonpaid care costs onto the people buying the policies, the employers

48.	What are the three groups most vocal in the request for national "health" insurance?

	•	Big businesses that already pay for employee insurance and are experiencing cost-shifting
	•	Hospitals and other providers now giving really free care and getting cost-shifted
	•	And insurance companies for obvious reasons

49. What are the three major proposals for illness care payment reform?

    - A national health system like Canada's and Great Britain's
    - A "play or pay" employer-paid insurance
    - Or tax credits for individuals to buy their own insurance

50. What are the major problems with a national health system?

    - Several are possible; the most glaring is its cost
    - Ethical issues of control, autonomy, government intervention, are present as well.

51. What is the major problem with a "play or pay" employer-paid health insurance system?

    - Some employers might fire workers to pay for the increased cost per worker, resulting in net job loss
    - The ethical objection is the violation of autonomy resulting from government force on the employer

52. What is the major problem with a tax credit for purchase of individual health insurance?

    - The "health" insurance industry already operates with a taxpayer-paid government subsidy; this would add to it
    - The philosophical or ethical problem is with autonomy, if individuals were forced to buy insurance; and with the autonomy of the taxpayer who is forced to pay more taxes in order to pay for the subsidy of the industry.

53. What is the difference between buying insurance and gambling in Las Vegas?

    In Las Vegas, the casinos guarantee to give some of the money back to the bettors.

54. What is the difference between a tax credit and a tax deduction?

    - A tax deduction of $1000 is worth $150 to you if your income is taxed at 15%.
    - A tax credit is worth $1000 to you, period.

55. What is the ethical question of malpractice insurance?

- If lawsuits were prohibited, the cost of all malpractice insurance could be given in more care, or in less cost of the care
- However, the legal and ethical questions of the individual's autonomy in suing, and the value of justice under the law in being compensated for harm, would arise

56. What are your reactions to the Modest Suggestions at the end of this chapter?

- Please mail to: Jacky Hall (or Michael Johnson), in care of CCHS
- No grade
  Thanks!

Unit Three Exam

HSM 510
Ethical Considerations in Health Care Delivery

SCANTRON FORM INSTRUCTIONS

Please follow these instructions for completing your Scantron form:

1. Use a #2 pencil **only.**

2. Enter the five-digit Test Number in the box marked **TEST No.** Shade in the corresponding boxes.

   The test number for this exam is: **51003**

3. Enter your Social Security Number in the box marked **SOCIAL SECURITY NUMBER.** Shade the corresponding boxes.

4. Enter your Course Code number in the box marked **COURSE CODE.** Shade in the corresponding boxes.

   The course code is: **510**

5. Print your name, address, and social security number on the lines provided.

6. Enter the estimated number of hours (to the nearest whole hour) you spent on this lesson (this is for our statistical purposes only). Fill in the appropriate boxes.

7. Be careful to darken the entire area within the boxes.

8. Do not make any marks outside the boxes. Completely erase all mistakes. **Do not use whiteout.**

9. Send the Scantron form to CCHS for grading. Your test results will be mailed to you.

If you have any questions regarding your exams or any other questions or comments, please write them on a **Request for Help** form and send it in to CCHS with the Scantron form. **DO NOT STAPLE** anything to the form. Be sure to write your name, SSN, phone number (optional), and Test Number on the **Request for Help** form. GOOD LUCK!!

UNIT THREE EXAM

MULTIPLE CHOICE

Select the *best* answer to each of the following questions. Mark your responses on the Scantron form.

1. What is <u>not</u> one of the reasons in the text that the ethical issues in the share of care unit are important?

    a. you will be a patient in a future system
    b. you will be a practitioner in a future system
    c. you will pay for a future system
    d. history will be affected by what we do

2. State the percentage of illness care expenses paid now by taxpayers through state, local, and federal governments.

    a. 24%
    b. 42%
    c. 100%
    d. 0%

3. Which of the list below is <u>not</u> one of the three specific rights that are protected from taking without due process of law under the 5th and 14th Amendments to the U.S. Constitution?

    a. privacy
    b. life
    c. liberty
    d. property

4. Identify the philosophy that advocates the greatest good for the greatest number.

    a. existentialism
    b. individualism
    c. utilitarianism
    d. materialism

5. Which is <u>not</u> one of the three parts to the economy of illness care?

    a. supply
    b. cost
    c. demand
    d. administration

6. People who are uninsured for illness care are _____.

    a. without health
    (b.) without insurance
    c. without care
    d. without concern

7. Identify the philosophy that allows us to force individuals to buy insurance they don't want if it is better for the society.

    (a.) utilitarianism
    b. individualism
    c. materialism
    d. existentialism

8. Identify the reason from the list below that is not a reason why technology is more likely to be paid for than other kinds of care.

    a. more visible
    b. more quantifiable
    (c.) more effective
    d. more easily documented

9. Which is not one effect of indirect payment on malpractice suits?

    a. increases the standard of care
    b. increases patient expectation of care
    c. causes practitioner to do more procedures
    (d.) causes more malpractice

10. Which is not an example of a "socially just" illness care system already functioning in the U.S?

    a. the Veteran's Administration
    (b.) private fee-for-service care
    c. the Indian Health Service
    d. patients cared for under Medicaid

11. Describe the unintended consequence of Congress' adding more requirements each year to the benefits under Medicaid.

    (a.) some poor people are denied any coverage under Medicaid
    b. some poor people get more coverage under Medicaid
    c. states are required to pay more money for Medicaid
    d. practitioners are reimbursed for more services under Medicaid

12. Describe the unintended effect of the Diagnostic Related Group cap on reimbursement to hospitals for Medicare.

    a. costs for Medicare decreased
    b. hospitals became more efficient
    c. patients required home illness care
    d. patients had shorter hospital stays

13. Which of the list below is not one of the three principles of the Oregon reform of Medicaid?

    a. money for illness care is limited
    b. more illness care is not the equivalent of more health
    c. the most effective illness care is that which gives the most people, the longest, healthiest lives
    d. people who most need care are the priority

14. Which is not the philosophy or ethic that underlies the Oregon plan?

    a. the healthiest get priority
    b. the most ill get the most care paid
    c. the people who will live longest are most valued
    d. younger and healthier people are more valuable than others

15. Which people get priority under the Oregon plan?

    a. the sicker
    b. the healthier
    c. the older
    d. the treacherous

16. In an economic system, a "monopsony" is _____.

    a. many potential buyers
    b. one enforced supplier
    c. one enforced buyer
    d. many potential suppliers

17. Which one of the list below is least vocal in the request for national "health" insurance?

    a. big employers
    b. insurance companies
    c. hospitals and other providers
    d. government bureaucrats

18. A subtraction from taxes (not income), is called a _____.

    a. tax deduction
    b. tax credit
    c. play or pay
    d. national health system

19. Which is not one of the three major proposals for illness care reform (it is the present system)?

    a. tax deduction
    b. tax credit
    c. play or pay
    d. national health system

20. Which group has not had costs for nonpaid care shifted to it as a result of indirect payment through insurers and government?

    a. providers
    b. employers
    c. all the people involved have had costs shifted to them
    d. uninsured people who self-pay

21. Social Justice is best characterized by which phrase?

    a. the end justifies the means
    b. the means justifies the ends
    c. people are means to an end
    d. the interests of society are justified

22. Health care is the same thing as health.

    a. True
    b. False

23. Indirect payment for care increases use of care because _____.

    a. more good technology is available to use
    b. people feel less healthy under such a system
    c. people need more care under a system of indirect payment
    d. there seems to be no cost for the care

24.	Which is <u>not</u> a difference between Massachusetts and Hawaii?

    a.	the people and environments differ.
    b.	Hawaii is "rich" while Massachusetts is "poor"
    c.	both states propose or mandate employer-paid health insurance
    d.	Massachusetts is not an island

25.	Which is <u>not</u> a way that Canada limits cost of illness care?

    a.	making its people healthier
    b.	creating waiting lists for care
    c.	limiting technology available
    d.	cutting administrative costs by prohibiting private insurers

26.	Without enforced cost controls, when the demand for a service goes up and the supply stays the same, the cost of the service goes up.

    a.	True
    b.	False

27.	If the demand or share of illness care goes up, and the government controls the price or cost at the same level, the supply will stay the same.

    a.	True
    b.	False

28.	The Gross National Product, GNP, is the total production of goods and services in a country and is also called Gross Domestic Product in some countries.

    a.	True
    b.	False

29.	The percent of a country's gross national product that is too high a percent when it consists of illness care is _____.

    a.	dependent on how much we value such care
    b.	12%
    c.	15%
    d.	6%

30.	The number of people <u>un</u>insured for illness care in the United States is _____.

    a.	47 million
    b.	37 million
    c.	31 million
    d.	since it's estimated, nobody knows

31. "Uninsured" is the same thing as "unhealthy."

    a. True
    b. False

32. "Uninsured" is the same thing as "uncared-for."

    a. True
    b. False

UNIT FOUR

CHAPTER FIVE
PROFESSIONALS AND EMPLOYEES

OBJECTIVES

Upon successful completion of this chapter, you will be able to:

1. Discuss why even self-employed practitioners have some of the same concerns as employed professionals.

2. Discuss the conflicts between professionals and employers.

3. List the earliest traditional professions.

4. Discuss the definition of "profession."

5. Identify the model occupation in illness care that other occupations have sought to emulate.

6. List the qualities of medicine that other illness care occupations seek to copy.

7. Describe the two ways of setting compensation for workers (professional or not).

8. Discuss the idea that professionals are more ethical than other people.

9. Identify the main difference between the ethics of the professional and the ethics of the nonprofessional.

10. List the values most discussed in codes of ethics in illness care occupations.

11. Discuss whether the violation of a code of ethics means the practitioner is unethical.

12. Differentiate the code of ethics from law.

13. List the values implicit in the codes' standards for competent care.

14. List the values implicit in the codes' standards for patient dignity and for participation in research.

16. List the value implicit in the codes' standards for patient advocacy and reporting of unsafe practices.

17. List the value implicit in the codes' standards for patient confidentiality.

18. List the value implicit in the codes' standards for work settings.

19. Discuss how codes of ethics address law.

20. Identify what should happen if the code of ethics of your profession required some action, but the law made the action illegal.

21. Identify the values implicit in the codes' standards that practitioners work to improve the public health.

22. Discuss the differences and similarities between licensure, and registration or certification.

23. Define the purpose of licensure and certification from the public's perspective.

24. Define the purpose of legal credentialing from the practitioner's interest or point of view.

25. Discuss potential problems with an administrative board's enforcement of licensure laws.

26. Discuss the other edge of the licensure sword.

27. List the factors other than licensure that protect the public from unsafe practitioners.

28. List the ethical values implicit in discussions about practitioner education.

29. Discuss the reason that education is used instead of competence as a standard for safety in a practitioners' practice.

30. Discuss the evidence that more schooling improves competence.

31. Describe the effect on the profession of increasing education .requirements for entry.

32. Describe the effect on the public of increasing education requirements for entry into professions.

33. Distinguish "standards" from "standardize" regarding education.

34. Discuss the intent of mandatory continuing education for practitioners.

35. List some factors that would change if practitioners attained increased competence in a mandatory CE state.

36. Discuss the measurable difference in states where practitioners are required to have CE for relicensure.

37. Identify the one essential factor of readiness for learning as reported by theorists in education.

38. State the value to be preferred when conflicts arise between cost saving and patient benefit.

39. State which value the jury will likely consider most important in a malpractice case.

40. Describe how payment for referral of Medicare patients became a crime.

41. Discuss why it is illegal for a physician to own a laboratory and refer patients to that lab for tests.

42. Describe the two purposes of Institutional Review Boards.

43. State the requisite for participation in unethical research such as the Nazis conducted.

44. Identify the values in the cell research and ownership issue.

45. State how research consent differs from therapeutic consent.

46. List which characteristics seem to make animals more valuable to us humans.

47. State the values in the taxol-breast cancer conflict.

48. Discuss the values that people hold who are in conflict about futility and a patient's demand for treatment.

49. Discuss the origin of the word "confidence" and relate it to the value of loyalty.

50. Describe a situation in which you would be ethically bound to reveal a patient's confidence.

51. Describe why the term "informed consent" has one word too many.

52. Identify the value in consent conflicts.

53. Discuss the two legal standards for consent.

54. Describe the exception to getting consent that is most difficult to prove in court if a malpractice case is filed.

55. Discuss two opposing points of view regarding Rust v. Sullivan.

56. List the values underlying conflicts like this.

57. List the policies in your institution that have the most ethical implications.

58. Identify the values in your agency's DNR policy.

59. Identify the interests of the parties discussed in the policy.

60. Discuss the implication of the enormous fear the public has of HIV infection on illness care practitioners.

61. Identify the value underlying a demand for patient testing if practitioners are required to be tested for HIV.

62. Name the two values in the whistle-blowing conflict.

63. Describe the benefit from having some possible penalty for whistle blowing.

64. Describe the lesson in the text which demonstrates that the worst damage from unethical behavior is to your own view and opinion of yourself.

65. Identify the two areas in which managers have ethical concerns.

66. Describe the advantages the manager has in ethical conflicts.

67. State a short maxim that reflects the manager's reconciliation of business with ethics.

68. State the purpose of most labor laws.

69. Discuss the "at-will" doctrine in employment law and the exceptions with ethical implications.

70. List the labor laws that would not have been necessary if all employers and employees would have acted ethically toward each other.

71. State the **rule** for legal and ethical behavior in illness care labor management.

STUDY QUESTIONS

This is not a test. Read the study questions before you begin the chapter. Answer them as you go along or after you finish the chapter. Then look at the suggested answers at the end of the chapter to see if you agree with the answers.

1. Why do even self-employed practitioners have some of the same concerns as employed professionals?

2. What are the conflicts between professionals and employers?

INTRODUCTION

Practitioners of illness care usually work as employees. Some physicians are entrepreneurs, sole proprietors or partners or own part of their corporation, but this accounts for a small percentage of all illness care practitioners.

The IRS and other laws interpret "employee" in specific ways. But as we speak about employees in this section, an employee can be an independent contractor, in a partnership, or in a corporation. Managers are employed, by someone, and only the entrepreneur is actually his own boss.

Even among self-employed people (doctors, therapists), there is a relationship between the practitioner and the insurance company or the government who is paying the bill. They are increasingly in an employee relationship with the payor (who is not the patient, but is the government or insurer).

In the old days, the practitioner was an employee (a contractor, a servant) of the patient. Now with payment of the bill by the insurers, either private or government, the practitioner is not directly responsible to the patient but to that anonymous "third-party-payor," or "3PP." Do recognize that the "third party" is us. Unfortunately there isn't any rich uncle out there, just us. (See the Unit Three "Share of Care" section for elaboration.)

The mythical 3PP (third-party-payor) is the boss -- the employer we will refer to during most of this section.

THE PATIENT–3PP–PRACTITIONER RELATIONSHIP

In any work setting, there will be some conflict of interest between what the employer wants and what the employee wants. Between practitioners and their employer, there is always a potential conflict. The usual difference of interests concern money, hours, conditions of work. Between practitioners and their employer are, in addition, considerations of ethics or standards of behavior.

This conflict is not unique to health care. Engineers have a standard other than that given by their employer to build safe buildings and cars. Lawyers who work as employees have a standard of professional responsibility not just to their employer but also to their clients. They even take exams in ethics (and pass them at very high rates).

Does the fact that they can take an examination and recognize the rules and know the answers according to the rules make them ethical? If you pass this course, will that make you ethical?

STUDY QUESTIONS

1. Which are the earliest traditional professions?

2. What is the definition of "profession?"

3. Which is the model occupation in illness care that other occupations have sought to emulate?

4. Which are the qualities of medicine that other illness care occupations seek to copy?

5. What are the two ways of setting compensation for workers, professional or not?

6. Are professionals are more ethical than other people?

7. What is the main difference between the ethics of the professional and the ethics of the nonprofessional?

PROFESSIONAL

What is a profession? The traditional professions of law, medicine, clergy, military, were first formalized in England as something for the younger sons to do. (The oldest son inherited the farm under a system called primogeniture.)

Sociologists have spent a lot of time and paper coming up with definitions and describing the characteristics of a profession. Some assert that historically there are three ideas involved in a profession: organization, learning, and a spirit of public service. Earning a livelihood is secondary in that interpretation. The idea of a profession is a concept, a construct. Its definition and meaning are subject to individual interpretation like so many ideas we have examined in this course.

Reference: Pound, R. The Lawyer from Antiquity to Modern Times. West, St. Paul, 1953.

People who work in occupations that don't fit the traditional or sociologist definitions have spent a lot of time trying to mold themselves to those definitions. Because? Being a member of a "profession" is valued. The people who are called "professionals" are seen as more educated, thoughtful, wise, wealthy, and trustworthy than the average person.

In illness care, the obvious professional role model was medicine. So the more "doctor-like" the occupation, the more "professional." Doctors are seen to have a long education. (Actually they didn't until about the turn of this century, after a man named Flexner reported that there were a lot of quacks calling themselves doctors). Then medicine started to lengthen and standardize its education.

This lengthening and standardization of education is still seen as the route to professionalism for most illness care occupations. (See below under "Education" for discussion.)

Independent or solo practitioner job structures are preferred for the same reason—independence from, leading to equality with, the physician. However, doctors increasingly work formally as employees.

All the occupations talk about teams, making themselves independent of and equal to and as professional as physicians. They all seek "autonomy" in their practice like physicians. But, doctors increasingly have

---

people looking over their shoulders in the form of quality review, payment review, peer review committees, state medical boards, and the ultimate review of malpractice suits.

(This review is not a new idea. The medical guild - union - in Florence in the late 1300's required that "bad cases" be reviewed by a committee of the Guild).

Wannabe professionals seek to increase the thinking part of their jobs. They seek to decrease the portion of their time they spend doing physical things, although physicians' jobs seem more now to be physical skills, passing catheters and various other tubes, and looking at machines and lab results.

These physical activities by physicians have been more highly valued than cognition, or thinking activity. The new payment system initiated by HCFA in 1992 promised to value more highly the "cognitive" work of medicine, but in reality will probably just pay all practitioners less.

Most sociologists' definitions of "profession" mention somewhere up among the most important the professional's characteristic of putting the patient or client first, before her own self-interest.

This does not occur in the way just described. What happens is that the practitioner puts her interest in being a good practitioner or professional first before her other interests of eating or going home early or making a lot of money.

Being defined as professional has not kept lawyers and physicians from making a lot of money. But merely being described as a profession will not make your occupation one that earns a lot of money. Teachers, clergy, military people are called professionals, but they do not make a lot of money.

What makes a lot of money for an occupation is not education. It is that people value what you do. You don't have to agree that they're right. You may not believe that doctors should be more valued than nurses. But somehow the patients do, as a whole group. Otherwise nurses would be paid more, in the fairly unrestricted market which still exists in this country. The people pay more for professional baseball and basketball players than they do for professional physicians. They don't pay the players for their education.

The alternative to this system is Plato's Republic, where all activity is valued and controlled by the state. They thought this was a good idea in the old Soviet Union, too. The problem is that some people are the state. Even in the old Soviet Union, the "state" people got to drive nice cars and shop at special stores. It sounds unfair to let the market determine price, but it does seem to be the only thing that finally works, if you measure what "works" as having food to buy in the stores.

ARE PROFESSIONALS MORE ETHICAL?

The idea that professionals have some "higher" ethical or moral sense than other people is simply not true. They do have an interest in benefitting their patients. They prioritize that self-interest before some other self-interests at times. That results in benefits for their patients. That is the value to the society of having such people around. They can be relied on to act in their professional interest, which is to say in their patient's interest.

Certain people derive pleasure from helping other people. They are attracted to occupations that have components of self-interest in helping people. The training or practice in helping occupations convinces some people they chose wrongly. They discover they would be happier doing jobs without such values as beneficence for patients. People self-select themselves into illness care, or out of it, depending on how highly they value the self-interest of helping other people.

Other occupations also have self-interests that are "higher," if you characterize other than immediate interest in gratification a "higher" interest. The factory worker also has some obligation or concern to her fellow woman to make products that are as safe as she knows how. This is the same obligation we have toward each other as people. "Do unto others" preexisted the concept of the "professions."

But in the occupations that call themselves professional, those obligations are formalized, somewhat agreed upon, written down, and taught. That's what you are learning in this course.

The assumption is the following: If the interest of the client/patient/ customer conflicts with another self-interest of the "professional," the "professional" will put his other self-interest second. The professional is putting a work, a "professional," interest first. That turns out to benefit the patient, but the professional still acts in his own interest.

Nicely, both professional and patient benefit. The patient's need for care is met. The professional's need to be a good practitioner (or help others or whatever his self-interest is in doing his job is also met).

Professionals do not put our interests ahead of theirs. They prioritize their own interests so that the work interest (the interest in doing a good job) comes first most of the time. It probably comes first more of the time than for other people. That is what is implied by "professional." Any other implication, that professionals are better or kinder more ethical than other people, is not true.

This ethical standard is probably more pronounced in illness care. The people the professional serves could be injured or die as a result of the professional's act or failure to act. But the airline mechanic too has such responsibility. We can hope she is a "professional" and puts our safety (her professional interest) before her interest in getting off work early.

Professions usually have a moral/ethical code of behavior. That should not imply that people who are not "professional" have a lower standard of behavior. Other occupations than those designated as "professional" do have ethics, but they may not be standardized, formalized, written—or written about.

STUDY QUESTIONS

1. Which are the values most discussed in codes of ethics in illness care occupations?

2. Does the violation of a code of ethics means the practitioner is unethical?

3. What is the difference between a code of ethics and law?

4. Which are the values implicit in the codes' standards for competent care?

5. Which are the values implicit in the codes' standards for patient dignity and for participation in research?

6. What is the value implicit in the codes' standards for patient advocacy and reporting of unsafe practices?

7. What is the value implicit in the codes' standards for patient confidentiality?

8. Which is the value implicit in the codes' standards for work settings?

9. How do these codes of ethics address law?

10. What should happen if the code of ethics of your profession required some action, but the law made the action illegal?

11. Which are the values implicit in the codes' standards that practitioners work to improve the public health?

CODE OF ETHICS

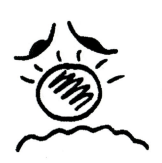

Most of the health care occupations have a written code of ethics, a series of statements about what behavior is expected of a person in that occupation. Such codes differ, but they have some things in common. They put beneficence and autonomy for the patient first. They discuss loyalty to the occupation, and improvement of the occupation, its autonomy. Through promises to maintain competence they speak to the value of nonmaleficence of the patient. They promise confidentiality and advocacy for the patient. They may hint at social justice, and underlying all as always is the conflict about money-work.

EXAMPLES

The code of ethics for pathologists is a different kind of code. It is a long list of courtesies and protections for other pathologists. It amounts largely to a list of promises not to invade another's economic turf—covenants not to compete.

WHO WRITES THEM?

Important point. Usually the association of the occupation's members writes the code of ethics. This means that the most politically active (not necessarily the most ethical) write the code. Even if "experts" in ethics write the code, it does not reflect what every member of the group thinks is ethical behavior. It is a compromise of what most of the group thinks are the most important ethical behaviors the people do.

A code of ethics by definition is not law. If it were mandated behavior, it would be written law, and practitioners would be forced to follow it. Instead, it is a guide, suggestions for action in situations that practitioners find themselves in. To violate the code (to behave differently from what the code recommends) doesn't mean that the practitioner behaves unethically necessarily. It means that the practitioner believes that the situation calls for another action. The practitioner in that situation either believes that action to be either ethical, or the only realistic choice for her in the situation.

THE RESPIRATORY THERAPY CODE—CONSIDERED AND COMPARED

The code of the American Association for Respiratory Care, the professional association for respiratory therapists, is examined in detail below and contrasted with the nurses' and physicians' codes. This analysis incorporates the ARRC Code prior to December 1995, when a new Code was adopted. Does a new "Code" mean the values of the profession changed, or merely the expression of the values?

PREAMBLES

AARC CODE OF ETHICS

Preamble
As health care professionals engaged in the performance of respiratory care, respiratory care practitioners must strive, both individually and collectively, to maintain the highest personal and professional standards.

The principles set forth in this document define the basic ethical and moral standards to which each member of the American Association for Respiratory Care should conform.

(American Association for Respiratory Care, 11030 Ables Lane, Dallas, TX 75229)

Notice that the respiratory therapists immediately claim "professional" status. They seek "individual and collective" highest standards. The first paragraph gives attention to personal as well as work behavior.

The second paragraph speaks to "ethical and moral," which to some mean the same thing. The word "should" is important. If "must" were used it would imply force of law, or at least removal from the organization for violation. The RT code consistently uses the word "shall," as does the physician code, which usually would imply force of law. These codes are not law.

The AMA Code of Ethics

The Preamble of the American Medical Association's Principles of Medical Ethics (1980) says some of the same things:

> **Preamble**
> *The medical profession has long subscribed to a body of ethical statements developed primarily for the benefit of the patient. As a member of this profession, a physician must recognize responsibility not only to patients, but also to society, to other health professionals, and to self. The following Principles adopted by the American Medical Association are not laws, but standards of conduct which define the essentials of honorable behavior for the physician.*

The Nurses' Code of Ethics

The nurses' code preamble never says that it is <u>not</u> law. It does not use either the word "should" or "shall." It implies that to be a nurse means that one just does these things. Does this mean that no deviation is likely, or tolerable?

COMPETENCE: AN ANALYSIS

The Respiratory Therapy Code of Ethics

> **Respiratory Therapy Code, Paragraph I:**
> *The respiratory care practitioner shall practice medically acceptable methods of treatment and shall not endeavor to extend his practice beyond his competence and the authority vested in him by the physician.*

Not to practice beyond one's competence is a basic requisite for beneficent or nonmaleficent care. The reference to the physician's authority makes clear that the Respiratory Therapist practices under the authority of the physician. There is a clear covenant not to compete with physicians here. The autonomy of the RT is derived from the autonomy of the doctor.

Physician and Nurse Codes

> **Medical Ethics: Principles**
> *I. A physician shall be dedicated to providing competent medical service with compassion and respect for human dignity.*

Nurses
Point 5. The nurse maintains competence in nursing.
Point 8. The nurse participates in the profession's efforts to implement and improve standards of nursing.

RT's
The respiratory care practitioner shall continually strive to increase and improve his knowledge and skill and render to each patient the full measure of his ability. All services shall be provided with respect for the dignity of the patient, unrestricted by considerations of social or economic status, personal attributes, or the nature of health problems.

The increase in knowledge and skill are for the benefit, beneficence, of the patient. The respect for the dignity of the patient indicates value of autonomy of the patient. An ethical conflict would arise here if a new system of illness care denies treatment for certain health problems, (for example DNR for people with AIDS), because the RT is to give care unrestricted by the nature of the problem.

Physicians
See Principle I above for dignity (the value expressed is autonomy)   Further, regarding competence and increase of standards through research:

V. A physician shall continue to study, apply and advance scientific knowledge, make relevant information available to patients, colleagues, and the public, obtain consultation, and use the talents of other health professionals when indicated.

Nurses
The above Points 5 and 8 speak to competence and increase of standards. Following is the component for research for nursing ethics.

Point 7. The nurse participates in activities that contribute to the ongoing development of the profession's body of knowledge.

Regarding dignity
Point 1. The nurse provides services with respect for human dignity and the uniqueness of the client unrestricted by considerations of social or economic status, personal attributes, or the nature of health problems.

This is identical to the second sentence of the RT's Code.

RT's
The respiratory care practitioner shall be responsible for the competent and efficient performance of his assigned duties and shall expose incompetence and illegal or unethical conduct of members of the profession.

The principle of fidelity to the employer can be seen here, in "competent and efficient performance," and also beneficence for the patient again. The "whistle-blowing" mandate expresses the values of veracity and non-maleficence to the patient, above fidelity to co-workers, co-professionals, or one's employer.

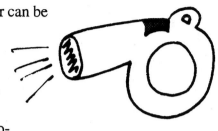

"Illegal" or "unethical" is a correctly stated expression; the words do not mean the same thing. It is not specifically stated that the RT has an ethical obligation to report bad conduct of members of other professions, though that could be implied.

Physicians
II. A physician shall deal honestly with patients and colleagues, and strive to expose those physicians deficient in character or competence or who engage in fraud or deception.

Nurses
Point 3. The nurse acts to safeguard the client and the public when health care and safety are affected by incompetent, unethical, or illegal practice of any person.

Confidentiality

RT'S
The respiratory care practitioner shall hold in strict confidence all privileged information concerning the patient and refer all inquires to the physician in charge of the patient's medical care.

This refers to the requirement of confidentiality, which expresses the value of fidelity to the patient. Confidentiality also indicates the values of beneficence and nonmaleficence. The reference to the physician again makes clear the relationship of this occupation to physicians.

Physicians
IV. A physician shall respect the rights of patient, of colleagues, and of other health professionals, and shall safeguard patient confidences within the constraints of the law.

Nurses
Point 2. The nurse safeguards the client's right to privacy by judiciously protecting information of a confidential nature.

Money and Practitioner Autonomy

RT'S
The respiratory care practitioner shall not accept gratuities for preferential consideration of the patient. He or she shall guard against conflicts of interest.

This section deals with economic matters that might cause the practitioner to put his own money interest before the patient's interests. The physicians' code is different. It speaks a lot more about autonomy for the physician.

Physician's
VI. A physician shall, in the provision of appropriate patient care, except in emergencies, be free to choose whom to serve, with whom to associate, and the environment in which to provide medical services.

This has been changed from earlier days when the code prohibited physicians from being employees.

Nurses
Point 9. The nurse participates in the profession's efforts to establish and maintain conditions of employment conducive to high quality nursing care.

Nurses recognize in their code of ethics that their economic interests are important. This section is often cited as the ethical foundation for collective bargaining.

Also related to the work setting of nurses is the following:

Point 4. The nurse assumes responsibility and accountability for individual nursing judgments and actions.

Point 5. The nurse exercises informed judgment and uses individual competence and qualifications as criteria in seeking consultation, accepting responsibilities, and delegating nursing activities to others.

This can be related to the physicians' V, which speaks to consultation and "use" of other professionals. Nurses have been advised to use these sections of the code of ethics when refusing or accepting delegation of responsibility from physicians. These sections also are used in delegating work to LPN's and nurse aides. Nurse leaders have been adamant that nursing be seen as an independent profession not under the supervision of doctors. Hence this emphasis in the code.

Dignity and Honor to The Profession

RT's
The respiratory care practitioner shall uphold the dignity and honor of the profession and abide by its ethical principles. He or she should be familiar with existing state and federal laws governing the practice of respiratory care and comply with those laws.

Upholding the dignity and honor of the profession is an example of fidelity to one's colleagues and occupation. But to have an ethical principle which says to uphold ethical principles is like saying that one of the 10 commandments is "to obey the 10 commandments." The promise to comply with the law seems to be aimed at practitioners who might practice without being licensed in states that require such license. See what the doctors do with this.

Physicians
III. A physician shall respect the law and also recognize a responsibility to seek changes in those requirements which are contrary to the best interests of the patient.

At issue here is not the doctor's interest, but the patient's. (Of course, one could say the patient benefits when the doctor benefits.)

Nurses
Point 10. The nurse participates in the profession's effort to protect the public from misinformation and misrepresentation and to maintain the integrity of nursing.

Mixing a little beneficence for the public with fidelity to the profession, this could be used to justify enforcing nurse licensure laws.

Promoting Community

RT'S

The respiratory care practitioner shall cooperate with other health care professionals and participate in activities to promote community and national efforts to meet the health needs of the public.

That's why the chapter on "Share of Care" is important. The docs and the nurses have similar concerns.

Physicians

VII. A physician shall recognize a responsibility to participate in activities contributing to an improved community.

Nurses

Point 11. The nurse collaborates with members of the health professionals and other citizens in promoting community and national efforts to meet the health needs of the public.

Sounds familiar.

Role Model Statement For Respiratory Care Practitioners

In addition, RT's have a role model statement which speaks to research, teaching, public education, and disease prevention programs. In particular, the Role Model Statement admonishes the RT not to use tobacco, and to hold himself up as a model. The Code of Ethics uses politically correct gender neutral language (he and she), while the Role Model is a male.

The physician code is gender neutral, (he and she avoided altogether), and so is the nurse's code. Both professions have many other pronouncements elaborating on ethical positions taken in their code. They have committees or divisions to address ongoing ethical problems that their practitioners face.

STUDY QUESTIONS

1. What are the differences and similarities between licensure and registration (or certification)?

2. What is the purpose of licensure and certification from the public's perspective?

3. What is the purpose of legal credentialing from the practitioner's interest or point of view?

4. What are some problems with an administrative board's enforcement of licensure laws?

5. What is the other edge of the licensure sword?

6. Which are the factors other than licensure that protect the public from unsafe practitioners?

LICENSURE

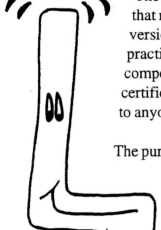

The euphemism for licensure and junior versions of that monopoly is "legal credentialing." Some junior versions of licensure exist. In laws that register or title practitioners, certain people with certain education or competence are designated as (predictably) registered, or certified. The practice of what they do is not prohibited to anyone else.

The purpose from the public's interest is to inform the public that this person has these qualifications. The purpose from the practitioner's interest is that this is the first step toward licensure. Such laws may be designated as permissive credentialing; one may be licensed. The other status is mandatory credentialing -- meaning one must be licensed to practice. No one else may maintain that practice other than the one licensed.

Licensure in some form is a status devoutly wished for and diligently sought by many occupational groups in states. Respiratory care has legal credentialing at some level in 33 states. Physicians and nurses have mandatory licensure in all 50 states. Licensure is granted by the state government.

Licensure is one of those powers reserved to the states in the 11th Amendment to the U.S. Constitution; not having been granted to the federal government, it is reserved to the states. Therefore, who is licensed, how, with what qualifications, and to do what, is determined by law in each state.

Licensure is a monopoly, a restriction on services, granted by the government. Economists assert that this is the only kind of monopoly that can persist. A "monopoly" in the private sector will be destroyed by competition sooner or later. But the state can use its police power, its force, to maintain the monopoly.

This is what happens with licensure. Suppose you start doing something, some illness care. You are competing with some other people also doing the care. If you don't have the required license (the monopoly permit from the government), the government will come in and stop you—physically, if necessary. The sheriff may put you in jail. Some licensing statutes carry misdemeanor or felony penalties for people who violate them. Conviction of either could mean jail time. The monopoly persists through the force of the state—enforcement of the statute.

The freedom of the practitioner to work is restricted, and the freedom of the patient to hire whom she wants is restricted.

There is a reason given for enforcing such a monopoly for the benefit of a few practitioners who are licensed. The reason given is that the safety, good, of the public is a greater benefit, higher value, than the freedom or autonomy of the practitioner—higher than the freedom and autonomy of the public to choose a practitioner, also. Paternalism is justified here, it is asserted.

The assumption is made that the public cannot know from the usual marketplace information whether or not the practitioner is safe. So the state government takes over that function for the individual. The state functions as the market, inquiring about the safety of the practitioner. The state then prohibits practice by any person not meeting the safety standard by not licensing that person to practice in the monopoly.

Ideally, then, the licensure law is to protect the public. It should establish minimum standards for practice and no more. In reality, the bureaucracy administering licensure laws behaves as all bureaucracies do, tending to more and greater power and people within an agency.

Boards then take it on themselves to be guardians of the profession, protecting practitioners from the public. At the same time they are charged to be watchdogs over the profession, protecting the public from bad practitioners. The latter is their actual role. As in all law enforcement, they cannot safeguard the public from all harm. Usually they can only act after harm has been done and remove from practice a person who has harmed the public.

The effect of any state-granted monopoly like licensure is to increase cost, decrease access, and obtain more money for practitioners. It should also increase the safety of the public.

The freedom of individuals to contract with each other is diminished. A citizen cannot hire a non-nurse to be his "nurse," a person he knows to be competent from his own experience, because the premise is that he is unable to judge her expertise in practice. And a person who is competent to do a job cannot contract to do a job because she lacks the proper pieces of paper.

STIFF AS BOARDS

Boards of licensure tend toward absolute power. Often, their decisions can be reviewed only with difficulty. The Boards' findings are given great weight on appeal, as the initial tribunal or court in most cases. This is because the Board has personally heard the witnesses and examined the evidence, while the appellate court can only examine the case from the paper record.

This weight to the Board's decisions is the same credence, or belief, given to trial courts by courts on appeal. It doesn't mean the court will always agree with the Board, but the Board starts with the advantage over the practitioner who is appealing the Board's decision.

Licensure boards almost always have the power to discipline (cut off the meal ticket) of licensees for unprofessional conduct. And this is conduct that is necessarily subjective in the eye of the beholder.

Boards may go beyond enforcing safe practice to enforcing "ethical behavior." In the Tuma case, an Idaho nurse believed she should discuss a therapy for her patient which the doctor had not discussed. She was disciplined by the Idaho nursing board for unprofessional conduct.

Her case is unusual in that we know about it; usually we don't. We know about it only because she appealed the Board's discipline of her license and won. That took several years, much money, and anguish and publicity. Thousands of other cases in which Boards find unprofessional conduct are never appealed.

A woman with terminal cancer, a hospice patient, dies in agony because her physician refuses to increase her dose of painkillers. Six nurses are so upset that they begin to hoard extra doses of narcotics, mostly morphine suppositories, donated by families of deceased patients. The nurses gave the morphine only after a doctor's order, but sometimes out of their illicit stockpile because there was no all-night pharmacy.

Sometimes the stockpile was used for patients without money; once for a patient who couldn't swallow liquid morphine. A nurse told the supervisor, who reported it to the Board of Nursing in Montana. The board placed the nurses on probation for unprofessional conduct for 3 to 5 years. In 1993, the case was appealed to the courts and the Board's discipline was reduced.

References: "Pain Control an Issue in Montana's 'Hospice Six' Case," *Medical Ethics Advisor*, November 1991, pp. 136–37. Tong, Rosemarie, "The Ethics of Medical Licensure," *Federation of State Medical Boards Bulletin*, 1991; 78:174-183.

THE DOUBLE-EDGED SWORD

The legislatures have seen an opportunity to solve some money problems by using the licensure laws. As noted in the section on "Share of Care," the increase in cost of illness care, since indirect payment through Medicare and insurance shifting is now being shifted to providers.

Legislators do this by tying mandatory free work to requirements for licensure. A Massachusetts law requires doctors to accept assignment (take a minimum fee and not bill the patient more) for Medicare patients. The same has been done with Medicaid in West Virginia and lately in Minnesota. These laws have been upheld in court as being reasonable actions on the part of legislatures.

That is the only test for that kind of law, not whether the requirement is related to the safety of practitioner. The court asks: Is the action of the lawmaker somehow related to the problem seen? If the answer is yes, the law stands.

A Massachusetts nurse objected to part of her license questionnaire that asked whether she'd paid her state taxes. The appellate court said that was a legitimate question to ask. Failing to pay taxes (or answer questions about them) is immoral, they said, and that's related to your licensure no matter how good a nurse you are.

The lawmakers know that they are granting a state-enforced monopoly when they license you. They are charging a price for it. With one edge of the licensure sword you as practitioner cut out the competition from "uneducated, unsafe practitioners." The other edge of the sword can cut you, the licensed.

The sword of licensure law enforcement allows the government to tie requirements to licensure. These requirements need have nothing—or very little—to do with the safety of the public or your competence to practice.

So much for the fundamental reason for licensure—to protect the safety of the public. The legislature knows it is also an economic tool to keep practitioners' competition down, to keep the supply low so demand stays high. If practitioners get the state-granted monopoly, they may pay for it.

INSTITUTIONAL LICENSURE

From time to time a solution to the proliferation and restrictive problems of licensure is offered. Economists and planners and some hospital management people advocate that the state not grant licenses from the government for each kind of occupation. Instead they recommend that institutions be licensed.

Who is qualified to do what would then be decided within the agency. This would keep the monopoly of licensure for agencies, and end the benefits of licensure (monopoly) for practitioners. Occupations that have or seek licensure oppose this. The power to decide who is a safe practitioner would rest with the employer. Practitioners fear that employers would not have the same interests of the patient (interest in quality of practice) that the practitioner does.

Some arguments for institutional licensure exist. Fear of malpractice would keep agency standards high, or at least safe. They do now. Pressures of competition would keep agencies employing qualified people with proper credentials. They do now.

Inspection by JCAHO would keep agencies employing people with specified credentials (they do now). Insurance companies would only pay for procedures done by qualified people (they do now). The loss would be to the occupations' "professional" status, to their power as licensed people.

Since all these benefits of agency control already exist, perhaps no institutional licensure is necessary. Perhaps abolishing existing licenses without additionally licensing hospitals to credential people formally would suffice.

Note that licensure is not necessary for everything. For example, physicians are not licensed specifically to do chest surgery. Those privileges are granted by the institutions and other groups of doctors. It's not a state power, but an informal group power. The market works, as it always has and always will.

If licensure were abolished altogether, the change wouldn't be great. The taxpayer would save some bureaucrat money and the practitioner would lose some hassle. The pressures of malpractice suits, loss of privileges, inability to get a job without competence and knowledge, would keep the status quo. The Latin is "status," or standing; "quo," the way it is.

References: Holzer, Henry Mark, "The Physician's License: An Achilles' Heel?" *Journal of Legal Medicine* 1991;12:201-20.

Kusserow, Richard P., et al., "An Overview of State Medical Discipline," *JAMA* 1987;257:820-23.

STUDY QUESTIONS

1. What are the ethical values implicit in discussions about practitioner education?

2. Why is education used instead of competence as a standard for safety in a practitioners' practice?

3. What evidence exists that more schooling improves competence?

4. What is the effect on the profession of increasing education requirements for entry?

5. What is the effect on the public of increasing education requirements for entry into professions?

6. What is the difference between "standards" and "standardize" regarding education?

7. What is the intent of mandatory continuing education for practitioners?

8. What are some factors that would change if practitioners attained increased competence in a mandatory CE state?

9. What is the measurable difference in states where practitioners are required to have CE for relicensure?

10. What is the one essential factor of readiness for learning as reported by theorists in education?

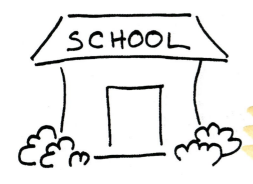

The reason we educate professionals is that we believe it will make them good at their practice. We want them to be good at their practice, for the good of their patients. The ethical value that underlies the requirement of competence of professionals is beneficence. The same value, good of the patient, underlies any attempt to ensure competence to enter the profession through education. The value of professional autonomy is here also—the increase in that autonomy created by more education. Money is the other value underlying education. More education yields more money, as the supply of practitioners is limited.

To be professional (more like the professional prototype of medicine) all the illness practitioner groups seek requirements for more education for new practitioners. Whether more education is necessary to do the job is not the issue; the goal is to "improve the profession."

The advantage of using education instead of competence or knowledge as the standard for practitioners, is that it can be measured easily. One can count easily the number of hours that have been spent sitting in chairs, listening to lectures. In essence, that is what degrees or hours of continuing education represent.

Harder to measure are competence and knowledge. It is easily understood why occupations use formal education as "standards" for entry into the practice, and seek to "standardize" (make specific) the way of entry. Formal education has the double advantage of being easy to measure, and having the effect of increasing the "professionalization" of the occupation.

"Standardizing" education is not the same as "setting standards" for practitioners. "Setting standards" means that all practitioners will have to prove they can achieve some standard, either in competence or knowledge. "Standardizing" is making specific the way that practitioners are taught, so that only people educated in the prescribed way can enter the occupation. This keeps out a lot of people, and cuts down the competition. It increases the demand and therefore the rewards for the practitioner. (See the "Share of Care" chapter for explanation of supply and demand.)

Professional groups (in some cases unions) seek more education as a requirement for new practitioners to join the guild, the monopoly of licensure. This is always said, and sincerely believed, to be required to improve the profession and thus the service to the patient.
Indeed, higher education requirements will improve the practitioner. Making her richer should be an improvement. More education required always results in decreased supply of people having the required education. Decreased supply results in increasing demand, thus higher pay for the fewer practitioners.

The second reason given for requiring more education for entry to practice is to improve service to the patient. Objective data that proves that people with more years of schooling give better service is very hard to come by in any occupation. Such proof is nonexistent in most. People with more formal schooling may give different kinds of service, as in management, or research, or teaching, but not better care. That is where the patient would see the difference if there were any.

A decreased supply of practitioners and higher cost of service both result from increasing the education requirement for entry into practice. Neither benefits the patient.

MANDATORY CONTINUING EDUCATION

Mandated continuing education is not a new issue. A guild of doctors in Florence required continuing education of their members in 1389!

Mandated continuing education of practitioners promises safe care and more quality care to the public. Whether requiring a certain number of hours per year in class will ensure competence is the question. Mandatory CE does force changes in behavior. It guarantees attendance at courses, or payment of money for correspondence courses. Since competence is hard to measure, that attendance is all that CE measures.

Continuing education promises the public competency of the practitioner. The premise is that more education results in a safer practitioner. This has not been proven. No increase in competency is documented in states with mandatory continuing education.

No decrease in malpractice case filings, settlements, or verdicts has been noted. No fewer disciplines by state boards have been reported. No objective outcome measurements can be documented to prove that requiring continuing education for relicensure accomplishes its purpose—to protect the public.

Since competence cannot be measured or demonstrated, the intent of mandatory CE laws may not be to protect the public. They may instead just lead the public to <u>believe</u> the practitioner is more competent. Misleading the public in this way is of questionable ethics; it counters the value of veracity to patients.

Another intended consequence of such a law may be to make the practitioner go to courses. Such behavior is seen as what good practitioners do, whether or not the outcomes of competent practice are met. The reasoning: Good nurses get CE. Therefore, CE caused the nurses to be good. Fallacy! The nurses were good <u>in the first place</u>. This value is seen in the codes of ethics emphasis on maintaining competence and improving standards.

The difficulty is that codes are voluntary, while licensure is law and mandatory. Should codes of ethics become written into the law? Should they be the minimum requirement for behavior, not the ideal?

Competency can be ensured by requiring all practitioners to repeat the licensing exam every year. That would ensure at least that the practitioner did not know <u>less</u> than when she entered practice. Licensure examinations are not perfect at measuring competence either, but they are all we have at present.

DISCLAIMER

Lest this analysis of <u>mandatory</u> continuing education seem negative about education as a whole, it must be stated: Voluntary continuing education is a good thing. People choose voluntarily to learn something they are interested in. They do learn, they are better people, and sometimes they are better practitioners too.

As theorists in education realize, it is essential that education be voluntary. Only with the condition of voluntariness are people able and ready to learn. People cannot be forced to learn something, which is quite apart from the question of whether it is ethical to try to make them.

STUDY QUESTIONS

1. Which value is to be preferred when conflicts arise between cost saving and patient benefit?

2. Which value will the jury likely consider most important in a malpractice case?

3. How did payment for referral of Medicare patients became a crime?

4. Why is it illegal for a physician to own a laboratory and refer patients to that lab for tests?

MoneyMoneyMoneyMoneyMoneyMoneyMoney

The money factor. The patient has an interest in good care. The employer/ HMO has an interest in saving money or in making more. The employee has an interest in more money, whether through increased or decreased treatment for the patient (increased in fee-for service, decreased in managed care).

A Government Accounting Office (GAO) report on a Florida Health Maintenance Organization (1992) charges that at least 35 Humana HMO doctors gave "poor quality care." For example, the report charges they failed to order appropriate medical tests or failed to follow up on abnormal test results. Did they withhold necessary medical care because it was in their financial interest to do so?

Practitioners are asked to serve two masters, patient and payer—either employer or insurer. Cost containment puts pressure on practitioners to hold costs down; but dedication to good care for their patients may require costly treatment. At least one "ethicist" believes that practitioners will have to change their ethics from doing the best for the patient, to doing the best that the payor will pay for.

References: Veatch, Robert M., "Professional Ethics vs. Cost Containment: The Inevitable Clash," *The Internist*, June 1991, pp. 9–11, 15.

Harris, T. Reginald, "Serving Two Masters: Conflicts in Practice," *The Internist*, June 1991, pp. 12–15.

Technology is easy to see and measure; that's why procedures have been better paid than diagnosis. The new Relative Value Resource Based Scale (RVRBS) used by Medicare to reimburse fee-for-service workers proposed to fix that. The criteria for payment do mention skill and thought. But also mentioned is time spent with the patient. Again, failure to measure quality of care results in measuring anything measurable.

On a related front, malpractice cases have arisen and are bound to increase when the failure to treat is seen as a result of the practitioner's financial interest. Juries are not sympathetic to practitioners who make more money when the patient is refused care, or to practitioners who make more money when inappropriate care is given.

When costs are held down by third parties, not the patient herself, is there a conflict with the patient's interest in care? Schemes that limit beneficial care will have to be accompanied by a limit or prevention of liability. They will have to a limit the injured's right to sue for injuries caused by the limited care.

Otherwise, the agency that manages the care, which causes too little or damaging care to be given, will be liable vicariously. They won't have done the damage directly like the practitioner, but as a result of being the employer of the practitioner. The Latin legal phrase is respondeat superior, "let the master respond," means the superior or boss pays for the damage. The rationale is that the boss wanted the thing done, it's for the boss's benefit, and (most important) the boss has the money to pay for the damage.

The managing agency might also be directly liable for setting up the system to encourage less-than-optimum care. Managed care conflicts have only just begun!

CREATING THE CRIME OF COST INCREASE

In July 1991, a big set of regulations came from the Health Care Financing Administration (HCFA). The Medicare law prohibits and punishes people who get "kickbacks" for increasing payments made by Medicare. These HCFA regulations establish safe harbors, business deals that are exempt from the law that "kickbacks" are a fraud on Medicare.

Real fraud is obtaining money by lying. Remember how we value veracity in our society. Real fraud is committed against Medicare when practitioners charge for procedures not done or do procedures that are not needed.

Most "kickbacks" charged under the law are not really fraud. Most of the procedures charged for are done, and are necessary in such cases. The law creates a crime of spending money. The government believes that increasing procedures, even if they are necessary, increases costs. They're right. The same activity, payment for referral, is legal in some businesses outside illness care, outside government subsidy. Those referrals constitute good business in those industries.

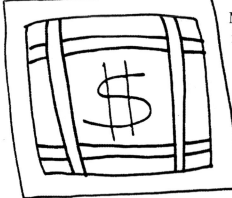

Most professions believe the conduct of paying for referral is unprofessional, therefore unethical. Some licensing boards discipline the practice because it is considered "unprofessional conduct."

Another conflict can arise—the issue of self-referral. A cardiologist does heart catheterizations. Is it ethical to refer all her patients to herself for catheterization? If she owns a lab, is it unethical for her to refer patients that need tests to the lab?

Laws now prohibit the latter. Not because the activity is unethical, necessarily, but because it is associated with increased costs in some instances. We are fast approaching a point at which just increasing cost will be considered unethical, unprofessional, and illegal, even if the patient needs the care.

The cardiologist is under a mandate to benefit her patient, not to cause harm. If the good of the patient requires a lab test, or a cath, what should she do?

Reference: Iglehart, John K. "Efforts to Address the Problem of Physician Self-Referral," *NEJ* 1991;325:1820-24.

STUDY QUESTIONS

1.   What are the two purposes of Institutional Review Boards?

2.   What is the requisite for participation in unethical research such as the Nazis conducted?

3.   Which are the values in the cell research and ownership issue?

4.   How does research consent differs from therapeutic consent?

5.   Which characteristics seem to make animals more valuable to us humans?

6.   Which are the values in the taxol-breast cancer conflict?

7.   Which are the values that people hold who are in conflict about futility and a patient's demand for treatment?

RESEARCH CONCERNS

Practitioners who are involved in research generally know that the interests of subjects have to be protected. This is under the value of beneficence, nonmaleficence, and veracity. Help, don't harm, tell the truth.

In a syphilis research study in the U.S., it was discovered in the '70's that some patients in the study had remained untreated for decades after penicillin was available. Now a federal law mandates that all experiments be reviewed by an Institutional Review Board.

The review boards look at the purpose of the research and the protection of the subjects, and balance those interests. Individual practitioners also have to balance interests. They must consider their own interest in participation in the research and their patient's interest in being protected from harm and in getting good care.

Excellent examples in such conflict come from the Nazi era. Such detail is beyond the space in this course but the practitioner should be aware that under the Nazi government, physicians and nurses and technicians freely participated in horrible experiments on people who had not consented.

It could never happen again if we continue to remember that it did happen, and that good people like us were the perpetrators. It will never happen again if we determine that we as individuals would never let such things occur in our own experience. The requisite for those experiments was only this: the research was more important than the subjects.

WHOSE GARBAGE IS IT, ANYWAY?

John Moore, surveyor on the Alaskan Pipeline, sought medical treatment for leukemia from an oncologist at UCLA. His spleen was removed (it had gone from 1/2 pound to 14 pounds). Moore got better. The doctor isolated and cultured a cell line from the spleen, which could produce several products. The cell line was patented in 1984.

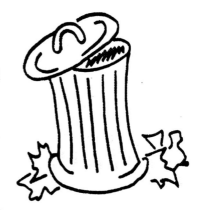

Was the removed spleen waste, garbage? Did it belong to

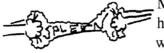

Moore. Did he have the right to the profits from his cells? What should the doctor get for the work, without which the spleen would have been worthless?

Controversy still exists over who owns the products of research. This important California case gave potential compensation and some interest in the profits to the man whose tissue was used in the research.

Reference: *Moore v. Regents of the Univ. of California, et al.*, 88 D.A.R. 9520 (Cal. Ct. App., 2d Dist., Div. 4, 1988).

CONSENT TO RESEARCH

Consent is always an issue in research. Yes, Mr. Moore had consented to research, but said he had checked the box granting ownership of the cells "no." The consent issues in research are generally the same as those related to treatment. They may be more involved because the research may involve procedures that are not therapeutically necessary.

Consent for research is more scrutinized than consent for therapy, usually. The research consent process will be reviewed in advance of the procedure by the Institutional Review Board. In contrast, consent for therapy may never be reviewed at all, unless a malpractice action is filed.

FINDERS KEEPERS

Another controversy is the payment of finders fees for residents or other practitioners who identify and refer patients to researchers. Such fees range from $50 to $350, and are justified by the difficulty of finding suitable patients, say researchers. Opponents believe the use of such fees will influence "finders" to persuade patients to enroll in research projects regardless of the value to the patient.

Reference: Interview with Stuart E. Lind, Harvard University Medical School, in August 15, 1991, *Chronicle of Higher Education.*

FLIPPER IN THE CONCENTRATION CAMP

The subject of research using animals is beyond the scope of this course. Practitioners should be aware that controversy exists in this area as well. Again the factors are different interests, and conflict among people (and animals) with different interests.

The interests are those of humans—in having the best drugs, techniques, and illness care. Also to consider are the interests of the animals themselves, in life and being free of pain. And the interests of people who are concerned with how we humans value (or don't value) animals, and our ability to dominate, as opposed to the rightness of doing so.

Research in animal behavior itself reveals more intelligence, more "feeling," than we previously suspected (or wanted to know). We humans clearly have the ability to impose our will on other living creatures. Because we have the power, do we have the right? Do we have a responsibility to other humans, to our species, to use whatever resources we have to promote our species' survival and well-being?

The more intelligent the animal, like the dolphin, the more they seem like humans. Does that "humanness" make our use of them worse? Is intelligence the condition we value—in animals or humans? Do we save baby seals because they're endangered, or because they're cute? Are cows less valued than veal calves, and why?

References: American Medical Association Council on Scientific Affairs, "Use of Animals in Medical Education," *JAMA*, 1991;266:836-37.

Pardes H., West A., Pincus H., "Physicians and the Animal-Rights Movement," *NEJM*, 1991;324:1640-43.

TAXOL OR TREES

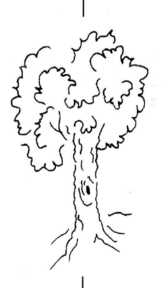

Further, practitioners should be aware of the ethical issues that arise when the environment is threatened in order to provide illness treatment. The most obvious example is the use of the bark of a rare species of yew tree to make an anti-cancer drug. Is the life of one woman with breast cancer worth killing all the yew trees? Should we preserve all the yew trees, even if it costs thousands of women's lives? Is there a compromise we can reach—X number of trees per life saved?

Be aware of the utilitarian argument implicit here, that it is OK to lose some individuals (trees or women) for the greater good. Do not fall for the "all-or-nothing" argument stated above; life is almost never like that. Science has developed an analog for the taxol so the trees ares safe already!

Health risk in the environment is a related issue. Is it ethical to impose on the autonomy of the individual, to prohibit all smoking, for instance, when smoking causes health risk to a relative few?

STUDY QUESTIONS

1. What is the origin of the word "confidence" and its relation to the value of loyalty?

2. Describe a situation in which you would be ethically bound to reveal a patient's confidence.

3. Why does the term "informed consent" have one word too many?

4. What is the value in consent conflicts?

5. What are the two legal standards for consent?

6. Which exception to the requirement for getting consent is most difficult to prove in court if a malpractice case is filed?

7. What are two opposing points of view regarding Rust v. Sullivan?

8. What are the values underlying conflicts like the above?

9. Which policies in your institution have the most ethical implications?

10. What are the values in the DNR policy in your agency?

11. What are the interests of the parties discussed in the policy?

PATIENT NEEDS, PATIENT DEMANDS

The value here is "professional autonomy" in conflict with the value of patient autonomy. It means the practitioner has the interest in doing what he sees as best, and in maintaining his integrity ("wholeness" is another word, not getting broken into pieces). It results in the position that you won't do just anything your employer asks you to do, because you're a professional.

What about doing just anything the patient asks you to do? Will you assist in removing a leg, because a patient wants to become a beggar and get more sympathy? In removing a breast, because a patient believes she might get breast cancer? If she has no relatives with cancer? If every woman in her family for centuries has developed cancer?

What about the patient who requests elective abortion? Sterilization? In vitro fertilization? Circumcision? A Cesarean section? These all are about patient's interests in having what they want. The classic and the slippery slope already stepped on is cosmetic surgery. The vast majority of these procedures are not medically necessary. They are socially driven and patient initiated and demanded.

And practitioners grant those wishes. If physical health is not the criterion for whether the practitioner acts, then can the practitioner resist the patient's wishes about CPR or antibiotics for viral infections? If the rationale for cosmetic surgery is psychological health, surely these other procedures are as important to psychological health as are cosmetic procedures.

Reference: Ross, Judith A. "Judgments of Futility: What Should Ethics Committees Be Thinking About," *Hospital Ethics Committee Forum*, 1991; vol. 3, no. 4, pp. 201-10.

CONFIDENTIALITY

A long-held ethical value of practitioners is to keep confidential information about the patient. This is part of the Hippocratic Oath and no doubt came before. It arises from the great power the practitioner has from information—information that the patient has not shared with any other "stranger" information that could harm the patient or embarrass her.

The first reason for the principle of confidentiality, which is based in the value of fidelity, is that the patient will give the practitioner all necessary information. If the patient thought the practitioner would not keep her confidence, she'd be less likely to confide information needed for diagnosis and treatment.

Second, it is in the practitioner's interest to keep confidences, even without laws to force this. If a practitioner tells secrets, people get to know the practitioner as an untrustworthy, unfaithful, infidel. ("Infidel" is also a word for "unfaithful," in the religious sense; compare "infidelity," and your dog "Fido," whose name in Latin is Faithful.)

The result of not keeping confidences is that the practitioner gets less information, makes worse diagnoses, kills patients, gets fewer patients. People stop using a practitioner who will reveal her patients' secrets.

We now have codes of ethics and laws to tell us what the market already told us—it's wrong to tell things about your patient that you know from your relationship.

TARASOFF

Sometimes there will be a reason to tell—when other people are threatened. A famous case in California, <u>Tarasoff</u>, held a psychiatrist's employer responsible for not telling the patient's friend that the patient had threatened to kill her. The patient killed her.

When you find out that your patient has HIV and hasn't told his sexual partner, you'll face a conflict between your patient's interest in privacy and his lover's interest in life. Your interest in professionalism, professional autonomy, will be in there too somewhere.

There may also be law that says you must tell things you learn—such as infections the legislature has determined must be reported, violence, neglect, and drug use by your colleague. Could such a law ever be unethical?

Reference: Tarasoff v. Regents of the University of California, 131 Cal. Rept. 14551, P. 2d 334 (1976)

CONSENT

Informed consent, like "best interest," has one word too many. In order to even be a consent, the patient must be informed of the procedure to be done and the attendant benefits and risks. To say "informed consent" is redundant; a valid consent is an informed consent.

All you need call it is consent. If a patient consents without information, she hasn't consented at all. If I "consent" to a colostomy and you haven't informed me of what the word means and my likely condition afterward, I haven't consented at all.

We use a variation of the veracity value when we ask the patient to tell us the truth. To get information about him that we need, we promise not to betray his confidence. Then he'll have confidence in us. He'll confide in us.

The other side of the veracity value is involved when we tell the truth to the patient. We have in turn an obligation to be truthful to him as he has been to us. That truthfulness is implied in consent. That's why it's not necessary to say "informed" consent.

If the patient has information or truth offered, and chooses not to take the information, that is his option. He has not been lied to, not had information withheld. That is the basis of the information part of consent—that lying by omission is lying all the same.

The courts (juries and then judges) have said that failing to tell someone of a possible risk, that any reasonable person would consider important, or a reason to decide against a procedure, means that the person did not consent. Doing something to someone (just touching them, actually), is a battery and can result in liability in a lawsuit.

In the old days, the standard for consent was whether a reasonable doctor would tell a patient. Reasonable doctors often withheld information that reasonable people would use to decide, the juries and judges have held. Now the standard has been changed in many jurisdictions.

In those jurisdictions, it's no longer a reasonable practitioner's standard. It's a reasonable patient's standard now.

Exceptions to consent are in the laws. The exceptions come out of what is originally ethical behavior. One exception to getting consent is an emergency situation. To wait for the consent would be to let patient die, and we value life. We excuse consent by implication. We "imply" that we would want it done for us. We would have people do unto us as we will now do for another. Express consent is the opposite, the expressing of consent in writing or verbally.

Consent can be waived if the patient indicates he will give up the information voluntarily. In that case we value the patient's interest in choosing, his autonomy and freedom. When the patient is unable to consent, we get another to give consent for him. We say this is the patient's surrogate, stand-in, representative. She is someone else who "is" the patient for purposes of consent.

Nowhere do you see the practitioner deciding for the patient, unless the patient waives his right to give consent. This can be tricky to decide in retrospect. The practitioner sued for failure to obtain consent would testify that "the patient said he didn't want to know."

The patient who is now plaintiff would testify, "I never said that." People can consent verbally as well as in writing. The writing is not magic, but it is easier and stronger evidence to introduce in court.

New concerns have arisen about confidentiality from new technology in record-keeping. With computer access we can do research on patient outcomes. This will allow comparison of individual practitioners' records and hospitals' outcomes. Will they be discoverable in malpractice cases?

As a practitioner, your sensitivity to patient confidentiality should extend to new technology, also including facsimile transmissions of patient records that could be misdirected. The principles of protecting your patient confidence are the same, there are just new applications of that value of loyalty.

PROFESSIONAL EMPLOYEE: DUTY TO INFORM

The Supreme Court upheld a regulation prohibiting practitioners from advising patients in federally funded family planning clinics about abortion. (See discussion in Chapter Three, "A Time to Be Born," Rust v. Sullivan.) Though the regulation was later rescinded, the case says the government can order practitioners to advise or not advise patients.

To some writers, this is an unthinkable invasion into the practitioner-patient relationship. To others, it is a reasonable authority of an employer to require certain attitudes and policies on the part of employees. Since the government does not have to pay for family planning at all, when it does it may choose to subsidize and encourage certain kinds of family planning and not others.

Other examples of required speech on the part of practitioners abound, including informed consent statutes that require practitioners to tell patients about such treatments as electroconvulsive shock therapy, sterilization, breast cancer therapies, and now abortion.

The opponent of such intervention into the practitioner-patient relationship would cite regulations that provide for informed consent for AIDS testing. These laws in some cases regulate counseling that would promote, directly or indirectly, homosexual activity or intravenous drug use.

In addition, there is some concern that failing to inform a patient, even if required to do so by law, could result in a malpractice suit for lack of informed consent.

The values of patient autonomy, practitioner autonomy, patient beneficence, and loyalties to the patient, group of practitioners, and employer can all be seen here.

In March of 1992, the Bush Administration changed the rule regarding doctors, so that physicians may advise patients about abortions. Other practitioners still could not. What are the ethical implications of that differentiation between professionals?

As noted above, the rule was rescinded in 1993 by the Clinton Administration. What if a rule <u>required</u> info about abortion be given? About the "right" to suicide?

References: Sugarman, Jeremy, and Powers, Madison, "How the Doctor Got Gagged: The Disintegrating Right of Privacy in the Physician-Patient Relationship," *JAMA*, 1991;266:3323-27.

                   Physician's Financial News, January 15, 1992, pp. 15-16.

The Professional Employee And Agency Policy

Related to the conflicts involving regulations, some employers have policies on a number of ethical issues. For example, your employer probably has regulations regarding living wills and other advance directives, no-code orders, reporting child and elder abuse, gunshot wounds, organ donations, required pre-op pregnancy checks, ICU selection, determination of death, and code blue policies. There are more, no doubt.

Any and all of these policies have ethical implications. Some of them were probably made with the help of the ethics committee at your institution. Discussion of their specifics is impossible, but you should be aware of them and know their content generally. After this course you should be able to analyze the values expressed in the policy. In addition, you should be able to identify the interests of the people likely to be affected in a given situation.

Employer policies are not laws. As you may see when you examine the policies, they may not even be ethical by your standards. Conflicts may arise, and the choice is yours whether you as an employee follow them, or whether you as a professional adhere to what you believe is the right, ethical, behavior.

Study Questions

1.   What is one implication of the enormous fear the public has of HIV infection on illness care practitioners?

2.   What value underlies a demand for patient testing if practitioners are required to be tested for HIV?

AIDS And The Professional Employee

People panic about being infected by their practitioners with HIV (Human Immunodeficiency Virus) or AIDS (AutoImmune Deficiency Syndrome). People have been carefully taught to be afraid of HIV. The fear results from a deliberate campaign by a group of people at risk for AIDS.

The people at risk for AIDS have an interest in frightening the larger group of non-IV drug users and heterosexuals. If the larger group believes that it too is at risk for the disease, they will feel sympathy for and vote money to research and care.

The fear is coming to roost, particularly on the illness care sector.

The fear of AIDS by nonpromiscuous, non-IV Drugusers (the majority of the population) is not justified. Transmission by nonanal intercourse is very difficult. Only 17% of women who are heterosexual partners of HIV-infected hemophiliacs, having regular unprotected sex over a period of years, have tested positive for the virus.

Most of the women who are now testing positive for HIV are in lower socioeconomic groups, having gotten HIV from heterosexual (sometimes anal) intercourse with bisexual males or IV drug users.

The epidemic of heterosexual AIDS in Africa cannot be generalized to the American population for a number of reasons. Africans use unsterilized needles for administering many different medications, freely available in bars and other places. The multiplicity of sexual partners among the population is a different order of magnitude than in this country.

Transmission between intravenous drug users is rising the fastest now. Some intrauterine transmission from such users to their infants occurs. Little transmission from contaminated blood products occurs. There is little risk to nonpromiscuous, non-IV drug using, Americans of any color or either sex. The infection is increasing fastest in people who engage in high risk behavior; many of those people are in groups classed as African American or Hispanic.

References: Johnson, Anne M., "Heterosexual Transmission of Human Immunodeficiency Virus,"*British Medical Journal*, 1988;296:1017-20.

Padian, Nancy S., et al, "Female-to-Male Transmission of Human Immunodeficiency Virus,"*JAMA*, 1991;266:1664-67.

If AIDS becomes a fatal disease that affects almost only groups considered minorities, the ethical conflicts about its control and treatment would intensify. The proposed Oregon Medicaid system discussed in Chapter Four, Share of Care, limits care for AIDS infected people since their longevity is short. What sounds like a class conflict could develop; indeed, a sizeable minority of black (African-American, people of color) people in America now believe that AIDS is an attempt at genocide.

The campaign to convince the general public that they are at risk for AIDS has worked. The average American is terrified of AIDS. One group they can politically safely target, to relieve a little fear and anger, is practitioners of illness care.

The interest of the patient is not to get HIV infected as a result of his care. The risk is very small, but the infection has deathly results. People want to know that they will not have any risk. At this writing, only one instance of a practitioner infecting patients has been documented and thought to have been deliberately done.

The practitioner has an interest in not contracting the virus from his infected patients; a still small risk but much more likely than transmission from practitioner to patient. Practitioners have a much higher likelihood of infection from (and to) patients with the hepatitis B virus, than HIV.

Universal Precautions (gloves, masks, eye shields, and gowns—depending on the degree of danger) have been instituted for all practitioners with possibility of contact with body fluids carrying the virus, which is just about all body fluids usually encountered from patients, except urine without blood in it.

The risk of transmission from patient to practitioner has prompted demands that patients be tested, so that practitioners can take appropriate precautions. Because that testing violates the privacy and possibly the confidentiality of HIV-infected patients, Universal Precautions must be used on all patients to protect against the few that might be HIV-infected. This cost, which all pay for in their care, must be weighed against the privacy interests of the few that are infected.

The practitioners also have an interest in privacy. This great fear of HIV by the public (which now believes that it can contract HIV from practitioners) has prompted a campaign to require testing and disclosure for all practitioners of their HIV status. HIV-positive practitioners' confidences have been violated, they have lost their jobs, and been denied privileges to practice. This is a result of the unreasonable fear of the many, fostered by a few people at risk for AIDS.

HIV-positive practitioners are protected by the Americans with Disabilities Act. Note the words here. It is now politically correct to say a person <u>with</u> a condition, such as a person with developmental disabilities. It is not politically correct to say a developmentally disabled person. The nice reason given is that we should consider the person first, and her disability second.

HIV-positive practitioners are considered handicapped under that law. The law requires that such persons can't be discriminated against in their work, unless they present a substantial risk of transmitting the disease. The population largely is not at <u>any</u> risk from the disease, but they have been convinced they are. People so fear the disease, that their legal system has converted, through judicial decisions, the words "substantial risk" to "<u>any</u> risk," of transmission. That limits the protection of the ADA law, and HIV-infected practitioners lose.

If practitioners are tested, then fairness would require that patients be tested as well. Time will tell just how far this fear campaign has carried us.

The Center for Disease Control (CDC) has backed off its blanket requirement that all HIV-positive practitioners stop invasive procedures, regardless of circumstances. The CDC now recommends that a committee in the practitioner's institution address the specifics of where and how and what procedures an HIV-infected practitioner should perform. The Occupational Safety and Health Administration (OSHA) has issued regulations extending Universal Precaution requirements to all employers of ten or more people. We may see ethics committees for HIV infected practitioners established in physician's offices, too.

STUDY QUESTIONS

1. What are the two values in the whistle-blowing conflict?

2. What is the benefit from having some possible penalty for whistle blowing?

3. What is the lesson in the text which demonstrates that the worst damage from unethical behavior is to your own view and opinion of yourself?

WHISTLE BLOWING

This is a cute new term for an old action—telling the truth. The values are veracity and truthfulness. People with those values may have a conflict with feelings of fidelity (loyalty) to the employer. Or the value might be fidelity to self (money interest) or to a friend, as when one refuses to report drug use or other harmful behavior of the friend. Another value involved is beneficence, doing good for someone. Usually this is seen as good for the patient or the group of patients, the public.

You have a mandate --a duty under the law-- to report a colleague who uses drugs on duty. If you don't you may be disciplined yourself. Your obligation to her conflicts with your obligation to yourself and to her patients (the public).

You may feel a fidelity to your patient and a professional obligation to keep confidential your patient's diagnosis. But what if his HIV test is positive, and the state law requires that you report what if there's no law, and the patient tells you he will not tell his wife of his diagnosis, and threatens to sue if you tell?

A negative side of this concept or truth-telling is the ability to stay anonymous and hide behind the qualified privilege of protecting another. This can be used to mount a character attack, or to tell personal things that are not justified. For example, it was important for Anita Hill not to stay anonymous, to come forward and be examined on her statements about Clarence Thomas.

This danger is why the Sixth Amendment to the U.S. Constitution gives you the right to confront witnesses against you in a criminal proceeding. In earlier times, other places, people could whisper an anonymous attack. And without the deterrence of knowing they'd be challenged by the accused, accusers were free to attack at will.

Several codes of ethics require that practitioners act in their patients' interest or advocacy, to the point of telling truth that might cost the practitioner her job. Some statutes protect people who tell. State laws may, through cases, encourage people to tell the truth when the public interest is at stake. An example is the Toxic Substances Control Act.

But there always has been and probably always will be some danger in telling truth that other people, especially employers, don't want to hear, even the comparatively small penalty that we suffered in school—"Tattle-tale, Tattle-tale."

That telling all is not completely free of retribution, however small, is not a bad thing. We have the bad example of Nazi Germany when children were encouraged to report their parents. Lately the examples are in the Eastern Bloc (formerly <u>East</u> Germany) where a high percentage of the population was reporting on their neighbors, family, and friends to the secret police.

Practitioners have to weigh the harm to patients if they don't report against the harm to themselves and the institution if they do. They have to remember the harm to their own view of themselves if they don't tell the truth in some cases.

The best ethics lesson I ever had was in law school, not in the long semester of the "professional responsibility" course, but in the response of my civil procedure professor to a student. The student asked, "if I do this (bad thing), who'll know?" "<u>You'll</u> know," Professor Ross answered.

He didn't add it, but we all knew who would be hurt most by unethical behavior. Not the patient, not the institution, but the practitioner.

Another lawyer, the Mayor of Springfield, Missouri, was really teaching ethics while teaching bankruptcy to neophyte lawyers: "You'll catch yourself lying. Everybody does sometimes. Just stop it." No preaching, no guilt, no assumption that you'll never do something you're ashamed of—but when you notice that you are, **just stop it**.

Reference: Bok, Sisela. "Whistleblowing and Professional Responsibilities," *Ethics Teaching in Higher Education*, Callahan, Daniel, Ed. The Hastings Center, 1980, Hastings-on-Hudson, New York.

STUDY QUESTIONS

1. In which two broad areas do managers have ethical concerns?

2. What are the advantages the manager has in ethical conflicts?

3. What is a short maxim that reflects the manager's reconciliation of business with ethics?

4. What is the purpose of most labor laws?

5. What is the "at-will" doctrine in employment law and which are the exceptions with ethical implications?

6. Which labor laws would not have been necessary if all employers and employees would have acted ethically toward each other?

7. What is the **rule** for legal and ethical behavior in illness care labor management?

MANAGEMENT ETHICS

Back when I was a labor organizer, I would say this was a contradiction in terms—management can't be ethical. That is the worst kind of tactic, to make the statement or assumption that your disagreement is with a person without ethics. That is the same as saying that he is without humanity, that he is not a person like you.

Managers have ethical concerns in at least two broad areas; one is their interests vis-a-vis (French for "face to face") their employees. (See below under specific labor laws.) The other is their own (or their institution's) interests regarding the patients of the facility.

In the patient situation, managers are usually concerned from a distance greater than the practitioners. The values of beneficence and nonmaleficence or autonomy are as obvious to the manager as those values are for the practitioner at the bedside.

The manager's interest relative to the patient's usually involves justice, the distribution or access to care. Sometimes fidelity to the institution or community, or veracity, telling the community the truth, is involved also.

STAFFING

Managers may have ethical conflicts regarding staffing, in particular. Staffing, as practitioners know instantly, directly affects the amount and kind of care that patients receive. The numbers and scheduling of staff matter often in the control of the managers and affect the employees' work and the patients' very lives. This is far more than juggling numbers; it's a big responsibility with ethical implications.

Managers may feel helpless to make any difference (everybody has bosses), and may be tempted to go home at five and forget it. Practitioners are, too.

But managers even more than practitioners can work to change what needs changing, and can make differences that are within their power. Using the process described in Chapter Three—Stop, Look, Listen, and Stop Again—can help, even if it can't give perfect answers. Sometimes there is no answer that everyone likes.

All bosses have bosses, and professional managers have the same interests and conflicts with their bosses about ethical problems that practitioners and employees do. In some cases, they have more conflicts, since the managers in illness care may be practitioners who've been promoted to management.

Managers may have access to information that lets them see the bigger picture—how more staffing or more services to patients will end up in bad financial statements and eventually even losing the hospital altogether. Managers have to walk the line. The line is between what's good for the individuals, patient, and employee; what's good for the institution, and what's good for the community. And somewhere in there has to come consideration of what's good for the manager. Saints are in short supply, even saints have self-interest in being saintly.

Some managers say good business decisions make good ethical decisions and vice versa. They say that a short-term, unethical decision will come back to haunt you, both ethically and financially; consider the implications of these examples: sweeping a malpractice incident under the carpet, instead of identifying, making amends, and working to correct the underlying problem; or accepting a patient for long-term care who cannot pay, when no other place will take her; or laying off 100 of a staff of 600 in a small town. Here managers have to consider their type of hospital, (public, private, or county), whether it's church affiliated, what the mission statement says, and the philosophy of the hospital.

"Administrative Ethics in the 1990's: CEOs Confront Payment, Access Dilemmas," *Hospitals*, January 5, 1992, pp. 20-28.

LABOR

The second conflict that managers have involving ethics is with their employees. The topic may look totally legal, not belonging in a discussion of ethics, but laws are based on ethics. These in particular are designed to enforce right behavior among people, in this case, between employees and employers. If all managers had acted "right" by their employees, there would have been no need for these laws.

You may have been an employee and are now a manager or going to be one in future. These laws and the ethics they represent do, and will continue, to affect your life considerably.

THE AT WILL DOCTRINE IN LABOR LAW—IS IT LEGAL? IS IT RIGHT?

"I have a written contract that says I can only be terminated for just cause. The hospital can't fire me for any other reason." WRONG.

"I have to uphold nursing standards; if I tell JCAHO inspectors about violations I can't be fired for that." WRONG.

These two cases illustrate the strength of the "at will" doctrine in labor law. What is this "at will" doctrine? The question is whether an employer can fire an employee "at will," or whether the employer must have a good, or just, cause to fire the employee.

In some states the answer is this:

> [I]n the absence of a contract of employment for a definite term or a contrary statutory provision, an employer may discharge an employee at any time, without cause or reason, or for any reason and in such cases no action can be obtained for wrongful discharge. Amaan v. City of Eureka, 615 S.W.2d 414 (Mo. Banc 1981), cert. denied 454 U.S. 1084, 102 S.Ct. 642 (1981).

This answer has been much discussed in legal articles. Some states' courts have different rules. For example, in Illinois an employee can charge that she relied on the employer's promises, even though not in a contract, to her detriment. And in Wisconsin and California, some fired employees have won cases that establish a requirement of good faith or fair dealing on the employer's part. Sound like ethics?

EXPLANATION OF CASES

CASE I

When is a contract not a contract? A nurse has sued her former employer, alleging that the nurse was fired without cause though a written agreement with the employer said the nurse could be terminated only "with just cause."

The court of appeals said the contract had no ending date, and therefore was a contract "in perpetuity, condemned in [early cases]." So the nurse was really an employee "at will" and the hospital had the right to discharge without cause. The idea of upholding contracts is related to the ethical value of keeping promises, of fidelity. <u>Main v. Skaggs Community Hospital</u>, MLW No. DS5-117, (Mo. App. 1991).

CASE II

Can you be fired for refusing to falsify documents? Generally you can't be fired for refusing to violate a statute, or legal rule. You can't be fired for exercising a statutorily created right, or for performance of a statutory duty. For example, you have a duty to report another practitioner's drug use. You can't be fired for "whistleblowing" if you report the violation of a statute that is to protect the public.

So why didn't this nurse have a case? The nurse claimed that she reported violations to JCAHO inspectors and was subsequently fired. There are other legal problems with the case, but one reason cited by the court in finding against her was that JCAHO requirements are not law. It's important to know what's law and what's not! The court stated:

> To be sustainable as an actionable claim for wrongful discharge, an employee suing under the public policy exception to the employment at will doctrine must allege and prove that conduct required of him by the employer would have amounted to a violation of a statute, constitutional provision or regulation adopted

pursuant to a statute, and also that his discharge was attributable to a refusal to perform the unlawful act or his performance of a mandated lawful act contrary to the directions of his employer.

The ethical value that this exception of whistle blowing upholds is veracity, and beneficence for the patient. If the facts alleged in this case are true, it put the practitioner in a squeeze between her value of veracity (not to lie on the report) and her need for the job (money value). She chose the veracity. Crockett v. Mid-America Health Services, 780 S.W.2d 656, (Mo. App. 1989).

Further cases have found employers liable or firing nurses when they uphold their nurse practice act (law).

The "at will" doctrine is upheld by some states' courts because it is the courts' job to interpret law, not make it. If a change is desired in this policy, the people through the legislature can make new law.

ADVICE TO YOUR EMPLOYEES

If you write a contract with your employer, be sure it's a real contract for a specified time. Anything else is sort of a glorified personnel policy. Yes, that means the contract might not be renewed when it expires, but if you want the protection you must take the risk. The contract that's upheld promotes the value of fidelity. If there's no contract, there's no promise.

The public policy exception to that doctrine only applies to violation of **law**. The exception values the idea of veracity and beneficence. If you think you're fired because you obeyed the law, talk to a lawyer about it. And if you don't know law when you see it, analyze by whether it's written, and made by people with authority to make law. Law is always in the form of a statute, a regulation, or a court case.

Sometimes the promises in employee handbooks (personnel policies) plus verbal promises made by managers are enough to create a contract. The ethics, and the law, of that for managers is to treat others as you'd like to be treated. Don't promise what you can't keep. Especially don't promise what you don't know or know to be untrue.

There are laws (statutes) that specify several reasons that people can't be fired or otherwise discriminated against. You can't fire or discriminate in employment because of a person's age, sex, race, ethnicity, handicap, or veteran status. All those laws have ethical bases.

Don't promise to be your employees' mother and father. You care about their interests, because that's who does the work. And they may be your friends. But they are employees; they are important to the **work**. It's not fair to them to think they're in a family when they are not. Employment is not supposed to be family; it can't be. Employers who say this are trying to make children of their employees.

And you are going to be sorry when you have to fire someone.

We can be friends, we can work for each other's self-interest, but we can't go back into the womb at work and assume that Big Daddy will always be there for us. We have to do good work, expect fair pay, plan to take care of ourselves and have skills to transfer.

IS IT LAW OR IS IT ETHICS OR IS IT BOTH?

The Americans with Disabilities Act, passed in 1990, went into effect gradually in 1992 and beyond. It mandates that people with disabilities be integrated into the mainstream of the work force. (We are changing the words again from "handicapped." Let's hope it works). The law mandates (forces) what we thought was an American ideal all along. That ideal is that all of us should have an equal chance at a job if we can do the work with a little accommodation. The ethical principle of justice should be apparent here—not social distributive justice, but real justice, justice of equal chance.

Title VII of the 1964 Civil Rights Act protects people from being discriminated on the job for reasons of race, color, national origin, sex (this went in as a joke, believe it or not), and religion. Religion can be tricky where Sunday work is concerned. As an aside, have you noticed people are not black and white? We're sort of tan and pink. I think we should change the words, call ourselves tanney and pinky. That would be a nice change, maybe change our attitudes toward tan and pink people.

Agencies of the federal government go further. They say: This program or activity will be conducted on a nondiscriminatory basis without regard to race, color, religion, national origin, age, sex, marital status, or disability. You can still discriminate against people because they have blue eyes (though if it's because of their Swedish origin you may be in trouble).

But why do you want to? Keep the value of justice and work (getting the most done) firmly in mind. You will be doing all the right things without knowing a single thing about these statutes.

The 1991 Civil Rights Act clarifies the standard of proof necessary for a person to prove that she's been discriminated against. Employer groups believe it is now easier for people to sue employers.

The burden of proof has shifted back to the employer. The employer whose work force is not in the same proportion of pink and tan people as the community will have a burden. She'll have to prove that a work force that is not racially reflective of the community was not gained as a result of discrimination.

Regardless of that, if you will do the right thing by people you will 1) probably not get sued, and 2) if you do, the person suing you will probably not win. I did not say certainly, I said probably. The certainty is that if you do the right thing by people that work with/for you, you will sleep at night and be content with yourself.

Doing the right thing by people does not mean letting them take advantage of you; if you do that you are being unfair (unjust) to the other people who work for you. This is the argument against affirmative action -- the immorality of paying for past sins, forcing payment to the child for past actions toward his ancestors.

Federal law forbids discriminating against people because they're pregnant. It applies to women only, at present. (See discussion in Chapter Three, "A Time to Be Born," for fears that men may take that away from us.) An important case in this area of employment is the Johnson Controls case. In that case women won the right to work in areas the company had considered to be dangerous to their babies (should they become pregnant). Employers said they felt trapped between possible liability to a child born damaged from such work, and the requirement under the federal law to allow women to do such work. That is a self-interest argument, avoiding liability, when the more appealing ethical argument would have been based on beneficence, protecting potential babies.

In the health care setting, the law may make it difficult to be beneficent if a woman wants to work in an area formerly considered dangerous to pregnant women, such as anesthesia or radiology. But the argument can be made that beneficence for the child is a shield hiding paternalism, which keeps women out of higher paying jobs. Examine motives carefully, including your own.

The Age Discrimination in Employment Act prohibits discrimination in jobs against people 40 to 70, solely because of their age. Again, if you really try to do the right thing, you will interview people and look at their qualifications and what job you need done. If you don't worry about their age, you don't need to worry about the law. Good ethics is good law.

Related to age is the law about pensions, the Employee Retirement Income Security Act. This law requires companies to do the right thing about pensions. The law is quite complex and causes many employers to have experts run their pension plans, because bureaucrats tend to go overboard and require such detail that the substance is lost.

The substance was, again, to get people to do the right thing. Some very wrong things that were done before included firing people the day before they qualified for pensions. The cure is unpleasant. Doing the right thing would have been cheaper and easier in the first place.

The National Labor Relations Act governs collective bargaining between employee groups and their managers. Not-for-profit health care institutions have been covered since 1974. Note that they are not called "nonprofit." The first demand for the law was back in the 30's when people (strikers and owners) were shooting at each other over labor disputes.

People organized into unions for a long time before that. Employers have opposed that strength in their employees. The process was not always peaceful, but some resolution of differences always came. The intent of the NLRA, first passed in 1935, was to promote peaceful collective bargaining. This was another attempt to get people to do the right thing by one another.

One provision of the law, not allowed in "right-to-work" states, allows union and management to force mandatory union membership or payment of fees to the union. This payment is enforced by the law. The person who does not pay loses her job and has no remedy. Does this violate the individual's autonomy, freedom? Is the resulting union strength, the collective good, worth the loss to the individual?

Whether the law has succeeded is debatable depending on whether you're union or management. People in labor disputes don't shoot each other; maybe they wouldn't without the law.

One easy thing to remember, instead of learning all the separate laws governing employees and their employers, is this: "Be ethical." The **rule**, is to treat other people the way you'd want to be treated. You'd want to be treated fairly, but with no special favors. You'd want to be rewarded when you do a good job, to pay the penalty prescribed when you don't. You'd want to be laid off without bias against you, if a layoff were necessary.

Reference: Luke 6:31.

STUDY QUESTIONS AND ANSWERS

These are suggested answers. If you have something like these answers in your own words, consider yourself successful. If you have more (quality, not quantity) than these answers, consider yourself excellent.

1.   Why do even self-employed practitioners have some of the same concerns as employed professionals?

     Increasingly, third party payors control their practice in the same ways that employers control employed professionals' practices

2.   What are the conflicts between professionals and employers?

     •   The usual conflicts about pay, conditions of work are present
     •   In addition, potential conflicts exist about ethics or standards of behavior that involve the professional's duty to her patient

3.   Which are the earliest traditional professions?

     •   Law
     •   Medicine
     •   Military
     •   Clergy

4.   What is the definition of "profession?"

     Like other constructs, it is an idea whose meaning depends on what people believe it is at any given time

5.   Which is the model occupation in illness care that other occupations have sought to emulate?

     Medicine

6. Which are the qualities of medicine that other illness care occupations seek to copy?

    •   Lengthy or longer education
    •   Independent employment status
    •   Independence or autonomy in practice
    •   More thinking and less sweat in their jobs
    •   More money

7. What are the two ways of setting compensation for workers, (professional and not?)

    •   The market
    •   The government

8. Are professionals more ethical than other people?

    •   A professional puts his own work interest before his other self-interests
    •   His work interest is to benefit his patient's interest
    •   It comes out that the patient's interest comes before the professional's lesser interests, before his interest in having lunch, for example
    •   He does not have <u>more</u> ethics than another person
    •   He has a different ethic, and it is written

9. What is the main difference between the ethics of the professional and the ethics of the nonprofessional?

    The ethics of the professional about his job are discussed, standardized, written and written about

10. Which are the values most discussed in codes of ethics in illness care occupations?

    •   Beneficence
    •   Nonmaleficence
    •   Autonomy (professional and patient)
    •   Money-work
    •   Social justice
    •   (Not life?)

11. Does the violation of a code of ethics means the practitioner is unethical?

   - The code is an agreed-upon guide for behavior
   - Each individual uses it as a guide, but it is not a law that must be adhered to at all times
   - To violate the occupation's code is not necessarily unethical
   - To violate one's own ethical code is unethical

12. What is the difference between a code of ethics and law?

   The codes are written usually in terms of should. Since they are made by associations and not lawmakers, they do not have the force of law

13. Which are the values implicit in the codes' standards for competent care?

   Beneficence and nonmaleficence of the patient

14. Which are the values implicit in the codes' standards for patient dignity and for participation in research?

   - Patient dignity is a "code" [sorry] word for patient autonomy -- (you know you do a lot of undignified things to patients)
   - The research component has two values:
       1) the good or beneficence of the patient, and
       2) the profession's autonomy
   - Professions are by definition supposed to advance human knowledge in their area

15. What is the value implicit in the codes' standards for patient advocacy and reporting of unsafe practices?

   Beneficence and nonmaleficence for the patient, and some side effect of autonomy for the profession from other professions and from the employer

16. What is the value implicit in the codes' standards for patient confidentiality?

   As discussed in Chapter Three, "Values," confidentiality is a variation of loyalty to the patient

17. Which is the value implicit in the codes' standards for work settings?

    - Moneymoneymoneymonymoney
    - The codes speak openly and explicitly about the economic interests and conflicts that practitioners have
    - Money-work is a value always present in ethical conflict
    - It is appropriate and honest that it be referred to in codes of ethics
    - Autonomy is another value present

18. How do these codes of ethics address law?

    - They sometimes admonish the practitioner to uphold the law
    - Sometimes they suggest that the practitioner work to change the law

19. What should happen if the code of ethics of your profession required some action, but the law made the action illegal?

    - Depends on whether you think ethics is more important than law (Lawyers always say "it depends")

20. Which are the values implicit in the codes' standards that practitioners work to improve the public health?

    Beneficence, not just for one patient but for the society

21. What are the differences and similarities between licensure and registration or certification?

    - The words may vary from state to state
    - They are all a form of "legal credentialing" and all tend to protect the public from unsafe practitioners and inform them
    - They restrict competition for the practitioner
    - Licensure is mandatory, no one can practice except one licensed
    - Other forms of registration, certification, or titling indicate that only certain persons can use the title bestowed by the state

22. What is the purpose of licensure and certification from the public's perspective?

    - To protect the public
    - To provide a minimum safe level of practitioner
    - To inform the public of who such practitioners are

23. What is the purpose of legal credentialing from the practitioner's interest or point of view?

To advance the public safety (the professional self-interest), but primarily to enforce a monopoly or limit the numbers of competing practitioners, thereby increasing the demand and price for her services

24. What are some problems with an administrative board's enforcement of licensure laws?

- The boards have almost absolute power, because review of their actions is expensive, lengthy, and difficult to overturn
- Boards have a roving commission to judge personal behavior under sections of state laws that say licensees should not be "unprofessional"

25. What is the other edge of the licensure sword?

Legislatures can tie licensure to requirements of practitioners that have nothing to do with competence to practice or safety of the public

26. Which are the factors other than licensure that protect the public from unsafe practitioners?

- Malpractice suit fears
- Institutional requirements for the job
- Outside agencies like JCAHO standards for certification
- Insurance company standards for payment
- Requirements for privileges in institutions

27. What are the ethical values implicit in discussions about practitioner education?

- The value of beneficence, doing good for the patient through requiring education to produce a competent and safe practitioner
- The value of autonomy for the professional and her occupation
- The value of money which accrues to the professional in an occupation with numbers of practitioners limited by educational requirements

28. Why is education used instead of competence as a standard for safety in a practitioners' practice?

    It is easier to count hours spent in class or degrees conferred than to measure competence

29. What evidence exists that more schooling improves competence?

    As noted, competence is very hard to measure, so such evidence is lacking

30. What is the effect on the profession of increasing education requirements for entry?

    • The profession's status is enhanced
    • Practitioners gain economically from limited competition

31. What is the effect on the public of increasing education requirements for entry into professions?

    • The public gets fewer practitioners that can qualify, thus less care
    • The care costs more because the supply of practitioners is limited

32. What is the difference between "standards" and "standardize" regarding education?

    • "Standards" are a set of criteria for competence or knowledge
    • To "standardize" is to make the path of education the same for all, so that no variation exists

33. What is the intent of mandatory continuing education for practitioners?

    The intent is to protect the patient through practitioners with increased competence

34. What are some factors that would change if practitioners attained increased competence in a mandatory CE state?

    • Malpractice actions should decrease
    • Disciplines by state boards decrease
    • Patients should be healthier, faster, and cheaper
    • Patients should be happier with their care

35. What is the measurable difference in states where practitioners are required to have CE for relicensure?

More people go to more courses

36. What is the one essential factor of readiness for learning as reported by theorists in education?

The learner must seek the education voluntarily

37. Which value is to be preferred when conflicts arise between cost saving and patient benefit?

- Neither can be a priori stated to be most important in every case
- That question is what much of this course is about

38. Which value will the jury likely consider most important in a malpractice case?

The value of beneficence, good of the patient

39. How did payment for referral of Medicare patients became a crime?

- Congress made it a crime in the Medicare statute, in an effort to reduce cost
- Not because payment for referral is generally a crime in the private sector, but because we want to save public money

40. Why is it illegal for a physician to own a laboratory and refer patients to that lab for tests?

- Because a statute says it is
- Allowing that practice cost the government more money in some cases

41. What are the two purposes of Institutional Review Boards?

To promote the purpose of the research while protecting the subjects of the research

42. What is the requisite for participation in unethical research such as the Nazis conducted?

The research is more important than the subject

43. Which are the values in the cell research and ownership issue?

   - Patient autonomy
   - Veracity (informed consent)
   - Money for the researcher who does the work and for the subject whose "property" the tissue is

44. How does research consent differs from therapeutic consent?

   - The consent process used in research is reviewed by a committee that is supposed to protect the subjects
   - Therapeutic consent may never be examined at all unless it is the subject of a malpractice action

45. Which characteristics seem to make animals more valuable to us humans?

   - Intelligence (dolphins, apes, dogs)
   - Cuteness (baby seals, kitty cats)
   - Rarity (snail darters, spotted owls)
   - Age (young calves, not old cows)

46. Which are the values in the taxol-breast cancer conflict?

   - Real life for the patient with breast cancer
   - Ideally better life for the society with a better environment
   - Any life for the tree

47. Which are the values that people hold who are in conflict about futility and a patient's demand for treatment?

   - The practitioner has an autonomy value
   - The patient does, also

48. What is the origin of the word "confidence" and it's relation to the value of loyalty?

   The base of the word is "fid," fidelity, loyalty

49. Describe a situation in which you would be ethically bound to reveal a patient's confidence.

   - You probably can think of several from your experience
   - Examples include reportable diseases, child or elder abuse, or when in your judgment the patient would be harmed by your not revealing; when the patient tells you of a symptom and tells you not to tell the doctor

50. Why does the term "informed consent" have one word too many?

    • Because "informed" is implied in valid consent
    • To have consent be real, the patient must be informed

51. What is the value in consent conflicts?

    Truthfulness (veracity)

52. What are the two legal standards for consent?

    • The older standard is that consent is valid if the practitioner told the patient what a reasonable practitioner would tell a patient
    • The newer standard is that consent is valid if the practitioner told the patient what a reasonable patient would believe important and would use to decide against a procedure

53. Which exception to the requirement for getting consent is most difficult to prove in court if a malpractice case is filed?

    The waiver of consent, when the practitioner says "the patient didn't want to know."

54. What are two opposing points of view regarding Rust v. Sullivan?

    • It is an invasion of the practitioner-patient relationship
    • Or, it is a reasonable expression of an employer's preference which employees adhere to as usual

55. What are the values underlying conflicts like the above?

    • Autonomy, for patient and practitioner
    • Beneficence to the patient
    • loyalty to the patient, practitioner group, or employer

56. Which policies in your institution have the most ethical implications?

    Find them in handbooks, policy and procedure manuals, from the nursing or administration office, or from ethics committee staff

57. What are the values in the DNR policy in your agency?

    • The value of life
    • Beneficence to keep the patient comfortable
    • Nonmaleficence to prevent harm from an unwanted code
    • The value of autonomy should be seen in some provision for consultation with patient or family

- The autonomy of the practitioner in not giving useless care
- I missed the money-work—where is that?

58. What are the interests of the parties discussed in the policy?

- The hospital, in not being sued
- The practitioner, in giving appropriate care
- The patient, in peaceful life and avoiding harmful unwanted care
- Does anyone or anything have a money interest?

59. What is one implication of the enormous fear that the public has of HIV infection on illness care practitioners?

The patient is afraid he'll get HIV from his caregiver

60. What value underlies a demand for patient testing if practitioners are required to be tested for HIV?

Justice

61. What are the two values in the whistle-blowing conflict?

- Truthfulness (veracity) and loyalty (fidelity)
- Another value that might be here is beneficence to the patient or group of patients, the same people who benefit from the fidelity
- Fidelity to the employer might be here also
- Again, money is missing, or is it? Might you keep quiet about an employer's illegal action for fear you'd lose your job (your money)?

62. What is the benefit from having some possible penalty for whistle blowing?

- We don't want to live in a Nazi-like state, where everyone is reporting everyone else all the time
- And we don't want to encourage irresponsible or malicious tale-telling

63. What is the lesson in the text that demonstrates that the worst damage from unethical behavior is to your own view of and opinion of yourself?

- Who'll know?
- You'll know

64. In which two broad areas do managers have ethical concerns?

    In the area dealing with their employees, and in the area dealing with the institution's patients and public

65. What are the advantages the manager has in ethical conflicts?

    - The manager may have more information to see the effects of his actions, a bigger picture
    - The manager should have greater power or flexibility to effect change or maneuver toward a better outcome

66. What is a short maxim that reflects the manager's reconciliation of business with ethics?

    Good ethical decisions are good business decisions, and vice versa

67. What is the purpose of most labor laws?

    To enforce ethical or "right" behavior between employer and employee

68. What is the "at-will" doctrine in employment law and which exceptions have ethical implications?

    - The at-will doctrine means that the employee relationship exists at the will of both
    - The employer doesn't have to keep them employed if she doesn't "will"
    - The exceptions are many
    - One exception with ethical implications is contract, in which a promise is made; the ethical value of fidelity is implicit in that
    - Another exception is whistle blowing, in which the values of veracity and beneficence are encouraged to protect patients or public
    - The statutes prohibiting discrimination are other exceptions with the values of justice implicit

69. Which labor laws would not have been necessary if all employers and employees would have acted ethically toward each other?

    - The Americans with Disabilities Act
    - Title VII of the 1964 Civil Rights Act
    - The 1991 Civil Rights Act
    - The Pregnancy Discrimination Act
    - The Age Discrimination in Employment Act

- The Equality in Retirement Income Security Act
- The National Labor Relations Act

70.   What is the **rule** for legal and ethical behavior in illness care labor management?

Treat other people the way you'd want to be treated

UNIT FOUR EXAM

HSM 510
Ethical Considerations in Health Care Delivery

SCANTRON FORM INSTRUCTIONS

Please follow these instructions for completing your Scantron form:

1. Use a #2 pencil **only.**

2. Enter the five-digit Test Number in the box marked **TEST No.** Shade in the corresponding boxes.

   The test number for this exam is: **51004**

3. Enter your Social Security Number in the box marked **SOCIAL SECURITY NUMBER.** Shade the corresponding boxes.

4. Enter your Course Code number in the box marked **COURSE CODE.** Shade in the corresponding boxes.

   The course code is: **510**

5. Print your name, address, and social security number on the lines provided.

6. Enter the estimated number of hours (to the nearest whole hour) you spent on this lesson (this is for our statistical purposes only). Fill in the appropriate boxes.

7. Be careful to darken the entire area within the boxes.

8. Do not make any marks outside the boxes. Completely erase all mistakes. **Do not use whiteout.**

9. Send the Scantron form to CCHS for grading. Your test results will be mailed to you.

If you have any questions regarding your exams or any other questions or comments, please write them on a **Request for Help** form and send it in to CCHS with the Scantron form. **DO NOT STAPLE** anything to the form. Be sure to write your name, SSN, phone number (optional), and Test Number on the **Request for Help** form. GOOD LUCK!!

UNIT FOUR EXAM

MULTIPLE CHOICE

Select the *best* answer to each of the following questions. Mark your responses on the Scantron form.

1. Which conflict is unique to employment between professionals and employers?

   a. duty to the patient
   b. working conditions
   c. pay
   d. hours of work

2. Which is <u>not</u> considered among the earliest traditional professions?

   a. medicine
   b. nursing
   c. law
   d. clergy

3. Which is <u>not</u> a quality of the medical profession that other illness care occupations seek to enjoy?

   a. autonomy in practice
   b. longer education
   c. low pay
   d. cognitive instead of physical work

4. Identify the main difference between the ethics of the professional and the ethics of the nonprofessional.

   a. continues her education
   b. cares about her client or customer
   c. seeks to do excellent work
   d. has a written Code of Ethics

5. Professionals are more ethical than other people.

   a. True
   b. False

6. Which value in the list is <u>not</u> implicit in the usual code of ethics' standard for competent care?

    a. beneficence for the patient
    b. autonomy for the patient
    c. nonmaleficence for the patient
    d. physicians always are the best equipped to judge ethics

7. List the most important value implicit in the codes' standards for work settings.

    a. beneficence
    b. nonmaleficence
    c. money
    d. fidelity

8. The most restrictive legal credential, thus most desired by the occupation, is _____.

    a. credentialing
    b. titling
    c. permissive registration
    d. mandatory licensure

9. What is the primary purpose of legal credentialing (listed in the text) from the practitioner's interest or point of view?

    a. to make care less expensive
    b. to improve the profession
    c. to benefit the patient
    d. to limit competition

10. Which is <u>not</u> a factor that protects the public from unsafe practitioners?

    a. agency hiring requirements
    b. malpractice fears
    c. registration or titling only
    d. indirect payer requirements

11. The main reason education is used instead of competence to determine practitioner safety is because education _____.

    a. makes a better practitioner
    b. can be measured more easily
    c. advances the profession
    d. benefits the practitioner

12. Which is <u>not</u> an effect on the profession of increasing education requirements for entry?

    a. lower pay
    b. more status
    c. less competition
    d. fewer practitioners

13. To set standards for practitioners does not mean the same thing as to standardize education for practitioners.

    a. True
    b. False

14. What is the measurable difference in states where practitioners are required to have CE for relicensure?

    a. fewer malpractice suits
    b. more attendance at more programs
    c. fewer disciplinary actions by state licensure boards
    d. better outcomes in patient care

15. State the requisite for participation in unethical research such as the Nazis conducted.

    a. the subjects are more important than the research
    b. the researchers are unethical scientists
    c. the research is more important than the subjects
    d. the participants are forced to participate

16. Which characteristic does <u>not</u> seem to make certain animals more valuable to us humans?

    a. life span
    b. intelligence
    c. cuteness
    d. rarity

17. Identify the most important value in consent conflicts.

    a. beneficence, good of the patient
    b. nonmaleficence, no harm to the patient
    c. fidelity, loyalty to the patient
    d. veracity (truthfulness) to the patient and autonomy

18. Which is not a legal standard for consent?

    a. what a reasonable doctor would have told her patient
    b. what a reasonable hospital would have allowed to be done to its patient
    c. what a reasonable patient would have thought important
    d. what information a reasonable patient would have used to decide against a procedure

19. Identify the major value underlying a demand for patient testing if practitioners are required to be tested for HIV.

    a. beneficence, goodness
    b. veracity, truthfulness
    c. justice, fairness
    d. money, work

20. Describe the lesson in the text that demonstrates that the worst damage from unethical behavior is to your own view of and opinion of your self.

    a. Nobody will ever know
    b. If it's not a crime, it's not unethical
    c. I have to uphold my image
    d. Who'll know? You'll know

21. State a short maxim that reflects the manager's reconciliation of business with ethics.

    a. good ethics is good business
    b. good business is good ethics
    c. good ethics is good law
    d. answers A and B are both right

22. State the purpose of most labor laws.

    a. to hassle the employer
    b. to enforce minimum ethical behavior
    c. to give employees special favors
    d. to set ideal standards for labor relations

23. Which is not one exception with ethical implications to the "at-will" doctrine in employment law?

    a. statutes prohibiting discrimination; fairness done, value is justice
    b. whistle blowing; truth told, value is veracity
    c. firing for good cause; fairness done, value is justice
    d. contract; promise kept, value is fidelity

24. Which law is <u>not</u> among those that would have been unnecessary if all employers and employees had acted ethically toward each other?

    a. Americans with Disabilities Act
    b. Age Discrimination in Employment Act
    c. Attorney's Full Employment Act
    d. Pregnancy Discrimination Act

25. State the **rule** for legal and ethical behavior in illness care labor management.

    a. treat other people as you would have them treat you
    b. don't fire anybody if you think they would sue you
    c. don't hire anybody if you think they would sue you
    d. treat your employees as though they were children

26. Self-employed practitioners have some of the same concerns as employed professionals, because increasingly third party payors control their practice in the same ways that employers control employed professionals' practices.

    a. True
    b. False

27. Which is the model occupation in illness care that other occupations have sought to emulate?

    a. nursing
    b. medicine
    c. health service managers
    d. respiratory therapy

28. The two ways of setting compensation for workers (professional or not) are through the free market or through government control.

    a. True
    b. False

29. Violating her <u>profession's</u> code of ethics always means the practitioner is unethical.

    a. True
    b. False

30. Which statement is <u>not</u> true about codes of ethics and law?

    a. codes are written usually in terms of "should"
    b. codes do not have the force of law
    c. law is written in terms of "must"
    d. law is permissive, not mandatory

31. Which is <u>not</u> an intended purpose of licensure and certification from the public's perspective?

    a. to protect the public
    b. to provide a minimum safe level of practitioner
    c. to decrease the numbers of practitioners
    d. to inform the public which practitioners are qualified

32. The <u>intended</u> consequence of mandatory continuing education for practitioners is to protect the patient by increasing the competence of practitioners.

    a. True
    b. False

IMPORTANT

Have you checked your answers for accuracy? Your score on this exam will be used in calculating your course grade.

UNIT FIVE

CHAPTER SIX
A TIME TO DIE

OBJECTIVES

Upon successful completion of this chapter, you will be able to:

1. Discuss the error in the idea that to get old is to have failed.

2. Define "end-of-life."

3. Define "longevity."

4. Indicate how life expectancy is computed, and give a synonym.

5. Identify one factor that affects life expectancy numbers.

6. Identify correctly that more people are living to be old now, not that people are living to be older.

7. State your her own personal risk of heart attack if you are in a group whose risk (class probability), of heart attack is 30%.

8. List the values encountered in ethical conflicts around the time to die.

9. Identify a complicating factor in our relationships with patients that affects our work as practitioners.

10. Discuss what you observed on your visit to a nursing home, and whether you would rather live there as a patient or be dead.

11. Repeat the definition of insanity given by the physician in the text.

12. Identify the greatest fear the competent have of becoming incompetent.

13. Differentiate between people who are incompetent and people who are incapacitated.

14. Define "competency" as decisional capacity.

15. Recognize that the determination of competence is legal and also informally made by the practitioner.

16. List the three components of decisional capacity.

17. Describe a patient who seems to have capacity but fails the third part of the test, the knowledge of consequences of his decision.

18. Discuss why the practitioner's standard for decisional capacity or competence must be a personal one.

19. Define "guardian" and "ward."

20. Define "advance directives."

21. Discuss the effect of advance directives if the patient is competent.

22. Differentiate living will from durable power of attorney.

23. Discuss verbal living wills.

24. Identify the relationship we now have with patients which has in part caused the increased use of advance directives.

25. Speculate on why people don't write living wills or durable powers of attorney.

26. Indicate what the attitude of the practitioner should be toward advance directives that seem inappropriate under the circumstances.

27. Speculate on why most people seem not to want their advance directives followed rigidly.

28. Discuss why some people think a written advance directive is preferable to a verbal one.

29. Discuss the validity of a verbal advance directive compared to a written one.

30. Discuss the ethics of ignoring the directives in a living will or durable power of attorney.

31. Discuss one ethical concern that has been raised about advance directives.

32. State the main requirement of the Danforth Amendment to the Medicare law (the Patient Self-Determination Act).

33. Speculate on the purpose of that law.

34. Discuss the terms: withhold versus withdraw, active versus passive, and treating versus limiting treatment.

35. Identify the mental condition of the patients that most ethical conflicts are about.

36. Discuss two of the myths about terminating life support that are false.

37. Indicate what value is highest in the American Thoracic Society's guidelines for terminating futile treatment.

38. Identify the values in the futility issue—specifically in the Helga Wanglie case.

39. Discuss whether the doctors could have handled this case differently, or whether they may have wanted to go to court.

40. Discuss examples of practitioner acquiescence to patient demands which may make it harder for practitioners to assert their autonomy to decide when treatment is futile.

41. Identify the primary purpose of any "tool" or measurement of health or illness or quality of life.

42. Cite evidence that courts are not often involved in decisions to limit treatment.

43. Speculate on what an opposite decision would have meant in the Wanglie case.

44. Differentiate the use of the terms "substituted judgment" and "best interest."

45. Discuss the reason that family or people close to the patient are named as decision makers.

46. List the three standards of evidence used in American law, and give examples where each is used.

47. Discuss why the Cruzan case is so significant in American bioethics.

48. Indicate one reason the courts might want to impose a standard of clear and convincing evidence before terminating treatment.

49. Identify another source of rights, remedy, or relief for persons who want treatment terminated, other than the U.S. Constitution's right to refuse treatment under the 14th Amendment liberty interest.

50. Define "Persistent Vegetative State."

51. Define "death."

52. List the consequences of declaring PVS patients to be dead.

53. Identify an earlier disease in which the patient diagnosed as such was declared to be dead.

54. Differentiate "artificial" from "natural" feeding.

55. Identify the year that closed chest massage at a fast rate was first reported.

56. List the conditions for which CPR was first considered effective.

57. Identify the conditions under which CPR is done in the hospital or nursing home setting now.

58. Describe the only condition under which CPR is <u>not</u> performed in most institutions.

59. Discuss the ethical problem facing the Emergency Medical Technician when called to a hospice patient.

60. Describe the discrimination evident in DNR orders.

61. Discuss futility and the DNR order.

62. Discuss your opinion of whether DNR orders should be suspended in the OR.

63. Discuss the CPR policy recommended in the text.

64. Define "euthanasia."

65. Identify the Nazi assumption that allowed killing of millions of people.

66. List the three pairs of conditions applied to euthanasia.

67. Distinguish "active" from "passive euthanasia."

68. Distinguish "voluntary" from "involuntary euthanasia."

69. Distinguish "direct" from "indirect" euthanasia.

70. Define "suicide."

71. Define "assisted suicide."

72. Disagree with the statement that euthanasia, or assisted suicide is a relatively new ethical conflict.

73. Provide examples of attempts to pass laws allowing assisted suicide in the U.S.

74. Explain the position of the Catholic Church on pain control and death.

75. Express your opinion on whether Nancy Cruzan's death was euthanasia and whether it was caused directly or indirectly, actively or passively, voluntarily or involuntarily.

76. Identify some of the values present in an assisted suicide conflict.

77. Explain why societies either make suicide illegal or discourage dead.

78. List some examples of the preoccupation about death.

79. Discuss reasons some give in support of practitioners assisting suicide.

80. Discuss reasons some give in support of practitioners not assisting suicide.

81. Discuss the statement that euthanasia is not illegal in Holland.

82. Explain why you think the Dutch process should or should not be adopted in this country.

STUDY QUESTIONS

This is not a test. Read the study questions before you begin the chapter. Answer them as you go along or after you finish the chapter. Then look at the suggested answers at the end of the chapter to see if you agree with the answers.

1. What is the error in the idea that to get old is to have failed?

2. What is the definition of "end-of-life?"

3. What is the definition of "longevity?"

4. Explain how life expectancy is computed, and give a synonym.

5. What is one factor that affects life expectancy numbers?

6. Which is the correct statement? People are living to be older now. More people are living to be old now.

7. What is your own personal risk of heart attack if you are in a group whose risk (class probability) of heart attack is 30%?

8. What are the values encountered in ethical conflicts around the time to die?

9. What is a complicating factor in our relationships with patients that affects our work as practitioners?

INTRODUCTION

Aging, illness, and death are realities, but you might never know it to look at television. They are not the ideal in our pretty, ideal, TV world. The old go "away" to nursing homes, it is believed, out of sight out of mind. The dying go to hospitals. And the great majority of us die in the hospital or nursing home, not at home. The undertaker takes us away in the night; maybe we're cremated and people never have to confront the dead body.

Practitioners are different. We work with them, the old, the ill, the dying. If we have any insight at all, we know that we will be one of them—aging, dying, dead. Sometimes we can get a skewed view, and it looks like all old people are sick, or all sick people are old; neither is true. I used to be very negative about back surgery, because the patients I remembered (and saw a lot) on our orthopedic ward were people whose surgeries had failed. I "forgot," because I wasn't confronted with them, the ones that succeeded.

We "forget" that old people are not all sick, and the population "forgets" that they are not all in nursing homes. Actually, they've moved to Florida; go down there and drive around. They're not sick, they're not in homes. They're out driving around with you. Slowly.

Aging is not a disease. Old people don't get old by being sick, by being unsuccessful. The advertisers would have you believe that if people would just take care of themselves (buy Oil of Olay) they wouldn't get old. It seems that old people did something wrong to end up old like that—when the opposite is true. They did something very right, a lot of right, or they were very lucky. They people who don't get old are dead.

Reference: Williams, T. Franklin, "Aging or Disease," *Clinical Pharmacological Therapy*, December 1987, pp. 663–64.

We surely don't want to talk about death. That's our goal as practitioners, isn't it, to "defeat" death? Isn't there a "war" on various diseases, on death? Are we "losers" when our patient dies? Not if we realize that everybody dies; we're in a losing game in the first place.

But it seems we cannot bear even to speak of death; now we're talking about "end-of-life" decisions, instead of dying. We care for "end-of-life" people instead of people about to die. It's everywhere.

LIFE EXPECTANCY

Related to aging, and death, and important in many ethical discussions, is the concept of life expectancy. The term is often misunderstood.

How do we know how long a baby born this year will live? Conditions will change in the next century. Life expectancy doesn't really mean how long a baby born this year can expect to live. It should be called "average age at death." It's determined by writing down all the ages of all the people who died **last** year.

For example, say only four people died last year. One was 97, and three others were one year old. Add: 97 + 1 (one baby), + 1 (second baby), + 1 (third baby) equals 100. Divide by the number of people who died, 4. 100 divided by 4 equals 25. The life expectancy for a baby born this year is 25. Actually, it's the average age at death of all the people who died last year.

Life expectancy numbers depend on how many babies die. If we counted the 1.5 million abortions each year as "infant deaths," our life expectancy would be a very low number of years. In 1900, the "life expectancy" was 50 or so because many infants died. Their low ages at death, averaged in, brought the number, the average age at death, down. But most people who survived infancy lived far beyond 50. Look at a graveyard of that time, and notice the ages on the tombstones.

The actual lifespan of people who survive infancy has increased only about two years since 1900.

Fewer babies die now because of better public health, including diet, housing, sanitation, and water. Very little of the small increase in life expectancy is due to "health care." But we are pretty good at taking care of illness and making sick people better, and making better the years people do live.

Because fewer babies die at infancy, now more people do live to be old. Not older than they did before, but more of them get to be old. But they didn't die at 50 in 1900, they either died as infants or as old people and it got **averaged** to 50. Many people, politicians, medical experts, and about half the medical texts make this error. Now you won't. Sometimes you read the headline, "Elderly Increasing at Rapid Rate." You'd think they were breeding and having old babies.

(Yin, Peter, and Shine, Marsha, "Misinterpretation of Increases in Life Expectancy in Gerontology Textbooks," *THE GERONTOLOGIST*, 1985; 25: 78-81.)

Another number concept that is used a lot when ethical conflicts arise, especially conflicts about which group or "disease" should get money, is risk probability. Those numbers are about "populations," a term used by epidemiologists about large groups, and have little relevance to individuals.

For example, say you are in a population with a 50% risk of having breast cancer during your lifetime. You, the individual, do not have a 50% risk. The population's risk, (called the class probability), is that 50 of 100 women will have breast cancer during their lives. But you will either be one of the 50 that does get it, or one of the 50 that doesn't. Your own probability is not 50%; it is either zero or 100%.

The group of 100 can have a percentage of risk, a class probability, because the 100 can be split into pieces. A group, a concept, of 100 can have 50% cancer. But you are not a group. You are just one person. You cannot be split into a percentage of yourself that will have cancer, and a percentage that will not.

Your own probability of breast cancer can only be 100%, that is, you have it; or 0%, you do not. All you do when you "reduce your risk" is join a different group with a different probability for the group. This is not to be fatalistic, nor to say you shouldn't try to get in a lower risk group. Taking actions to reduce your "risk" will help keep you healthy.
Think of the analogy to the weather forecast. The man says "There's a 50% chance of rain today." That doesn't mean that where you are, it will rain 50% of the time. He got that number from a computer that told him about past situations with the same conditions of temperature, humidity, etc. About half the time, it rained that day somewhere in the area. That's all it means. It will either rain where you are, or it will not. If you want to have less risk of rain, move to Arizona. But on any given day, it still will either rain in Arizona, or it will not.

This is important. We won't know what your own personal "risk" was, meaning what actually happened to you, until you die—either having had breast cancer during your life, 100%, or not, 0%. You need to think about that before you have a prophylactic mastectomy for a "50% risk of breast cancer."

VALUES OR PRINCIPLES ABOUT DEATH

The values most talked about concerning death are the values of sanctity of life, and autonomy, and beneficence and nonmaleficence. That is, we want to preserve life, all else being equal. What may not be equal is the autonomy of the patient. We want to do good (beneficence) and to do no harm (nonmaleficence). Sometimes we can agree on the right action. If the patient is competent and doesn't want treatment (autonomy), if treatment will do no good (no beneficence), if it will actually prolong pain (maleficence), we will agree that she can refuse treatment.

What we haven't agreed on is what to do if she is incompetent. Or if she's in a coma ("vegetative"). Or if the treatment will keep her alive, but not return her to the function she had before. Or if the treatment is very expensive.

In the old days we still had to worry about whether to treat, especially when treating meant a drain on resources. The drain was more personal, not abstracted to a figure like dollars per day for the ICU bed, or percentage of GNP. The drain was whether the family could spend its time and money (work) on someone who was not going to recover, or be a functioning member of the family if she did.

Physically and technically, we couldn't treat people in some of the ways we can now. We couldn't use ventilators to prolong breathing if people just stopped breathing. We couldn't use tube feedings to prolong nutrition if people just stopped eating. Now we can. The conflict is over whether we should.

STRANGERS

We have now turned the treatment over to strangers, literally. We the strangers don't know all about the patient that the family did in former times. We don't always know that our patient was a happy, busy grandfather until his stroke two days ago. We don't always know that our patient has been lying in a nursing home without family, without cognition, for months before his stroke two days ago.

We don't have all the information. Because of that, we tend to treat all the patients the same, or nearly the same. It's as near as we can come to justice. But that means treating all patients as aggressively as possible, since we as strangers we can't distinguish the quality of life for another stranger. We treat them all as extensively as possible.

STUDY QUESTIONS

1. What did you observe on your visit to a nursing home, and would you rather be there as a patient or be dead?

2. What is the definition of "insanity" given by the physician in the text?

3. What is the greatest fear the competent have of becoming incompetent?

4. What is the difference between people who are incompetent and people who are incapacitated?

5. Another two-word term for "competency" is _____.

6. Is the determination of competence a legal process only?

7. What are the three components of decisional capacity?

8. Describe a patient who seems to have capacity but fails the third part of the test, the knowledge of consequences of his decision.

9. Why is the practitioner's standard for decisional capacity or competence always a personal one at first?

NOT A PROBLEM FOR COMPETENTS

The conflict here is not usually about competent people. (definitions below). We almost always honor the wishes, the autonomy, of a competent person. We assume the person is acting in his own best interest. Plato questioned whether one could act in any other fashion. Most people want as much treatment as possible, if they believe the treatment will return them to their life as it was before their illness.

What they fear is the worst case scenario. They say they fear becoming incompetent and being treated aggressively and lingering on as a "vegetable" for years. Because the people doing the treating don't know their wishes, they are strangers. This fear is not based on a common occurrence.

Only 5% of people over 65 years old are in nursing homes. Of those in nursing homes, most have some meaningful life experience. Only about 2% of that tiny minority of people in a nursing home are "vegetative." Go and visit if you don't already work in one. Try to leave your "young person" bias at home. Remember when you were 20, you thought that it would be living death to be, say, 50 years old.

There are different qualities of life, and we must be careful when we look at others' lives from our vantage point of seeing, walking, talking, thinking. It's very easy to believe that we "wouldn't want to live like that." Some healthy young people believe they wouldn't want to live if they were 90 and needed a wheelchair to get around. The Nazis believed they were doing the Jews a favor. The Nazis believed they wouldn't want to have lived like that, being a Jew.

AUTONOMY AGAIN

Autonomy was defined back in Chapter Three but we will discuss it more here. Autonomy is not an absolute; that is, we do not base everything on autonomy. We limit autonomy in driving a car; you're not free to drive as fast as you want. You're not autonomous, free, to physically touch other people when and wherever you want, or even to say whatever you want to or about them (at least not without threat of a lawsuit or penalty).

You can't even do just what you want with your own body. You may not go to the doctor and order her to cut off your hand, even if you're obeying a Biblical injunction and it has offended thee. In some states, if you neglect your health to the point that you are "dangerous" to yourself (self-neglectful) you may be taken into custody and forced to get medical treatment.

You can't take just any drug you want, you can't drink alcohol to intoxication and walk on the street (much less drive). We limit autonomy pretty severely sometimes.

DEFINING INSANITY

But we value it nonetheless. All things being equal, we will in this society of paramount individual rights, honor the autonomy of the patient in health care decisions (as long as they decide the "right" thing). A physician told me of his patient who refused to consent to a procedure. The doctor said the man was clearly out of his mind. "How do you know that?" "Because, he refused to consent to the procedure." He'd have been sane had he consented.

Some of the other words used in deciding whether people actually have autonomy, whether they can act for themselves, are "competence," and "incapacity." These are also legal terms too. As you understand by now, legal terms are also words and have to be defined in the context of our experience, just as "ethical" words do.

COMPETENCE OR INCAPACITY

If you are not competent, in most states you can be made a ward, either of the court or some private individual. That means you cannot make decisions for yourself about anything, literally. The other person, usually termed a "guardian," becomes you for all purposes.

Interjection: The word "incompetent," not surprisingly, has come to have a stigma about it. First, we use it to characterize someone who cannot carry out his business or tasks with ability—as in "the TV repairman is incompetent." And at the legal level, it not only implies but expressly states that the person so designated is unable to carry out his business or take care of himself at all.

Incompetence is the ultimate loss of control over the most basic activities of life—where he lives, what he wears, what he chooses to eat. No wonder people fear this! It is this loss of control (not continued treatment) that people hope to ward off by the silver cross (signing of living wills and durable powers of attorney).

Of course, the signing won't prevent the loss of control. Or perhaps the idea is that one would rather die than to live as an incompetent person. This is precisely the assumption underlying Cruzan and other cases like that. People who are not functioning as they did before, or as we function now, would rather die. And their families, and many of us, would rather they died than live "like that."

The stigma about incompetency has been dissolved some say by changing the word to "incapacitated." We dissolved the stigma, in another case, by changing "graveyard" to "cemetery" to "memorial park." There are still dead people buried there. We solved the stigma of "venereal disease" by changing it to "sexually transmitted disease." Presto, no stigma, everyone is proud to have an STD now.

Now that we start to call these people "incapacitated," will people think of them differently than if they were "incompetent?" Missouri law since 1817 has provided for a procedure to deal with, or for, people with what was then called "unsound mind." Not a bad term again.

"Incapacitated" will work to reduce the stigma, just because we're not used to it. For a while the word does not immediately not refer to the thing we mean, the person who used to be incompetent. For a while, we're not sure what the word does refer to. Maybe the "thing" we are referring to changed, since the word changed. (See the discussion about word-referent-thing in Chapter Two.)

YOU DECIDE COMPETENCE

Short of a legal proceeding, many times you will have to decide if your patient is competent. A common situation is when the patient is asked to give consent, usually to a surgery or procedure. If you believe the patient is not able to give consent, you probably have made a decision that she is not competent.

DECISIONAL CAPACITY

Another phrase for "competent" is "decisional," or "decisionmaking capacity." Note the use of the word "capacity" as a preferred term for "competent." There are formal steps to determine this but they come down to some common-sense questions:

1. Is the patient able to receive and understand information about his condition and treatment necessary to a decision?

2. Is he able to think (cogitate, reason) about the information, make a decision and communicate the decision?

3. Does he know the consequences of his decision?

If Mrs. Jones can't even understand what you are telling her (the first criterion), she isn't competent. If she can't think about it and decide and tell you some way, she isn't competent. If she doesn't know what will happen as a result of her decision, she isn't competent. For example, if she won't eat but says she won't die as a result, she hasn't met the third criterion.

If there's a question about the consequences of the decision, it's a little tricky. Sometimes you or other practitioners are sure that she'll die if she doesn't have some treatment. It's better to assess whether she understands that she might die. You probably can't be sure that any decision will cause any other specific result, except that refusing food and water will cause death. At least it always has until now.

CONSENT = COMPETENCE?

It's fascinating to see that we assume patients are competent when they consent to treatment that we believe they need, or that we would consent to in their place. We are much more critical and look harder at patients who make what we consider irrational decisions. Thus, the definition of an irrational decision is "different from what we'd decide."

YOUR STANDARD

In reality, the only standard we have for assessment is ourselves, our own experience. It's not wrong to use that as an initial standard, and it's not wrong to at least look for incompetence in people who choose something that will cause their death or detriment.

We do assume that rational, competent, capacitated people want the best for themselves. When they make a decision that will result in harm to themselves, we rightly examine whether they are able to understand that the decision will have that effect. (Refer to "Process" in Chapter Three.)

STUDY QUESTIONS

1. A person who has been adjudged incompetent in a court proceeding is called the _____; the person who is appointed to make decisions for her is the _____.

2. What is the definition of advance directives?

3. What is the effect of advance directives if the patient is competent?

4. What is the difference between a living will and a durable (springing) power of attorney?

5. Are verbal living wills of any use?

6. What relationship do we now have with patients which has in part caused the increased use of advance directives?

7. Why don't people write living wills or durable powers of attorney?

8. What should be the attitude of the practitioner toward advance directives that seem inappropriate under the circumstances?

9. Why do most people seem not to want their advance directives followed rigidly?

10. Why do people think a written advance directive is preferable to a verbal one?

11. What is the validity of a verbal advance directive compared to a written one?

12. What are the ethics of ignoring the directives in a living will or durable (springing) power of attorney?

13. What is one ethical concern that has been raised about advance directives?

14. What is the main requirement of the Danforth Amendment to the Medicare law or (the Patient Self-Determination Act)?

15. What do you believe is the purpose of the law?

"WHEN SOMEONE ELSE DECIDES"

GUARDIANSHIP

The most obvious incompetent patient is one you don't have to assess. She comes in with a paper that says she has been "adjudged," by a judge or jury in a court of law to be incompetent. She has someone else to make all decisions for her. She has become a "ward," a dependent. Someone has been appointed by the court to be her "guardian," to guard her and look after her best interests.

In this case you treat her guardian as the person who makes decisions. You have no ethical problem, merely a legal one as to who has been named the guardian. Right? See below on safeguarding your patient.

If your patient does not have a guardian but seems incompetent to you, you may have an ethical or even legal responsibility. You may have a duty to seek to have her declared incompetent and a guardian appointed. Some states have laws that mandate that practitioners report instances of adult abuse or self-neglect that might require court intervention.

ADVANCE DIRECTIVES

Another place you will have to consider competence is when a surrogate decision maker asserts herself, or when you believe one is needed. In the familiar ward–guardian situation, the patient will have been declared incompetent by a court. The guardian has been appointed as the surrogate decision maker. A surrogate literally stands in the place of the patient.

"Advance directives" is a recent term for a group of "tools," written or verbal. People use them to direct, as in the word "directive," what is going to happen to them in case they become incompetent and unable to decide about their illness care.

They do this directing in "advance" of incompetency, hence "advance directive." An ordinary will is an advance directive, as is a note to your son telling him to put dinner in the microwave at 6 p.m. since you won't be there. Used in this context, they refer usually to living wills, durable powers of attorney, or just statements made to indicate what people want to happen in case of incompetence and illness.

WE VALUE THE AUTONOMY OF THE COMPETENT PERSON

That concept is primary. Understand that an "advance directive" is made in advance of a person's becoming incompetent. She must be competent when she makes the directive. And the directive is only used when she becomes incompetent. Competent before and incompetent after are the only time advance directives are needed or used. If the person is still competent, the advance directive is still unneeded; the person herself can decide now.

If the person is already incompetent, she can't now make an "advance directive." She's not making it in advance of becoming incompetent, she's already incompetent! We only allow these "directives" to work because we believe they were made by people who had the capacity to consider what their best interest was. The incompetent person does not have that capacity now, so she can't make an advance directive.

The term "living will" means an instruction on what the person wants to happen to his body while he's living, at a time he can't decide for himself.

Within the last 15 years, most of the states have written formal laws to recognize these living wills, which were already written informally by individuals. Some states specify a form to use to write the will. Some specify exactly who may witness or notarize the will.

Some laws state when the will is to be honored, in terminal illness or coma, for example. Some statutes provide who shall decide when the will is to be effective, certain doctors, for example. Some of these restrictions in state law are probably unconstitutional now, after the Cruzan decision, as we shall see. See Cruzan both in Chapter Three, "A Time to Be Born," and in this chapter under "Withdrawing and Withholding."

The term "living will" was proposed by the Euthanasia Society (now called the Society for the Right to Die) used in 1969 in the *Indiana Law Journal*. In 1976, California passed the Natural Death Act, which like other statutes provided that the will would operate only if the person was terminally ill. Usually state living will statutes say that water and food cannot be withheld, no surrogate is named 'M the will, and no penalty provided for not honoring the directive. But in Missouri, the practitioner can be charged with "unprofessional conduct," which could result in loss of license.

A living will statute in Ohio says that treatment can be withheld if one is diagnosed as a Permanently Unconscious Person or will die within 12 months, and on permission of certain family and a probate court. Another law in Illinois is similar, but without necessity of a court decision. Any restriction on advance directives by a competent person is probably going to be unconstitutional after Cruzan, if tested in court.

A living will tells anyone reading it, what the writer wanted done with himself after becoming incompetent. A durable power of attorney is different; it tells someone reading it, who is to make decisions after incompetency. A living will speaks to all potential providers. A durable power of attorney speaks to one person, saying, "Decide for me when I can't."

Some forms used by patients for living wills are now quite specific, providing that people do or do not want dialysis, IV's, intubation, CPR, antibiotics, etc. In addition, they may conflict with other advance directives about organ donation. For example, what should you do if the patient's living will says **do** resuscitate but **do not** intubate or use a respirator? What if they want organs donated but do not want CPR or life support? The body must be maintained on life support until organs to be donated are removed (being a farm girl, I cannot say "harvested" about this process).

What if the living will says **do** dialyze but no IV's? No antibiotics? **Do** antibiotics but no IV's? More about this later in "**But** . . . ."

There is another more informal advance directive, used in many cases that have come to court, and they have been upheld as valid (true); that is an informal, spoken living will. In most cases that have come to court, the informal, spoken expressions of the incompetent person have been honored. This is so in the <u>Cruzan</u> case also, as we shall see below. In that case, Nancy Cruzan's feeding tube was pulled because she had said to a friend about another similar situation, "I wouldn't want to live like that."

Evidence is available that living wills are being used to limit the patient's treatment without her consent even when she is competent, not terminal, and has a good prognosis. Some nurses and doctors assume that a living will on the chart means the patient would prefer to be DNR if she arrests. Further, it means to many that the patient doesn't want any treatment even if her prognosis is good.

If everyone should have a living will (the intent of the Patient Self-Termination Act--oops, Determination act), and if all with a living will are assumed to want a DNR (Do Not Resuscitate) order, and if all who are DNR are assumed to want food and water withheld—we stand to save a lot of money on illness care.

People who advise patients on advance directives should be aware that those instruments are being used to justify an automatic limiting of treatment by doctors, nurses, and hospitals. The person advising the patient may be legally as well as ethically responsible for fully informing her of such potential consequences of executing an advance directive, analogous to the medical informed consent.

When used by illness care providers who are under pressure to save money by limiting care, a living will could become a "living won't." You won't live long with a such a document on your chart.

DURABLE (SPRINGING) POWER OF ATTORNEY

All states have had a durable power of attorney specified in law. This document allows a person (the principal) to choose another to manage his money now, and to continue (the durable part) after he becomes incompetent.

The relatively new arrangement in the law is a durable power of attorney for health care (a surrogate, an agent, an attorney in fact, a proxy). All those words mean a person who manages your body if you become incompetent.

The use of the word "durable" is inappropriate here, since the analogy to the financial durable power of attorney is flawed. In the money-management durable power of attorney, the power is granted to the agent immediately, and continues, is durable, even when the principal becomes incompetent. In the illness care power of attorney, it is not durable because it only first comes into being at the time the person becomes incompetent.

Other instances of this concept in the law, for example property law interests, use the term springing. It means to spring up into existence when a certain event happens. That is the case here. The power doesn't endure (stay durable) from competence through incompetence. Instead, only at incompetence does it spring into being. You are not giving power to someone to manage your body care on the day you write the power of attorney. You are providing for a power of attorney that will spring into effect only later, if and when you become incompetent.

These laws have been enacted in many states and all in some way provide for another person to take over and make decisions for your patient **without** the need for a court to make a decision of incompetence as is done when a person is declared incompetent and a guardian appointed.

Who makes the decision that the patient is incompetent and that the agent has power to make decisions? Statutes differ, usually it is the physician. Nonphysician practitioners will need to furnish information to whomever is to make the decision and maybe initiate the process (being the closest to the patient).

For years, without formal documents or law, we have been turning to surrogate decision makers, in the persons of parents, children, spouses, and siblings. All that is new is that the procedure is formalized, because there is more that we can do for/to patients that they might not want, and we are more strangers to each other than before.

BUT . . .

Living will statutes have been in evidence for more than 15 years, living wills themselves longer than that, and most states have had a statute for longer than 5 years. Yet only 8-15% of Americans have filled out some kind of advance directive, so the question must be asked whether this is a need all people feel.

As indicated above, the forms for living wills and durable (springing) powers of attorney are as lengthy and complex as people care to make them. They must be requested from each patient, copied and on the patient's chart, and some state laws will penalize you if they're not followed. How are you going to follow something that contradicts itself? Of course you're not. Just as has always been done with directives for funerals that the family can't stand, directives to bury people in their cars or with their pets, the directives in the living will or durable power of attorney will be contradicted when they don't make sense.

Studies indicate that many people don't want their advance directives followed, even if they're written. In a study of dialysis patients, people varied greatly in their grant of authority to change their directives to practitioners and surrogates. The study revealed that 39% wanted the directives followed strictly, 19% granted a little leeway, 11% a lot, and 31% say the directives need not be followed at all!

Patients varied also in how much they wanted practitioners to consider things such as pain or suffering, quality of life, new treatment possibility, indignity, financial problems, and religion. Most of them wanted these things considered when carrying out their advance directives. A few wanted the directive followed without consideration of any other factor.

Only 20% of these patients had a written advance directive, but 43% had a spoken advance directive. Interjection: the use of word "spoken" and the word "oral" can be easily remembered as the difference between oral and spoken sex. Oral = mouth; spoken = words.

After 30 minutes of interview about advance directives, at a follow-up at least 4 weeks later, few additional patients (4 of 150) had a written directive. Nine more had made verbal advance directives.

The authors' conclusion was that practitioners should talk to patients about whether to apply advance directives and whether to modify them. This advice means that having written directives is not a substitute for communication. Patients and practitioners and families must talk about treatment wishes.

Reference: Sehgal, Ashwini, et al, "How Strictly Do Dialysis Patients Want Their Advance Directives Followed?" *JAMA*, 1992;267:59-63.

The preference for written advance directives is an artifact of the legal process. It is easier and more persuasive to produce a document with writing on it than for a witness to testify what you said and when and under what circumstances. But spoken directives are just as valid, as they should be.

At Nancy Cruzan's first hearing on removing her feeding tube, her friends testified that she didn't want to live if she couldn't be "At least halfway normal." That did not meet the Missouri standard of clear and convincing evidence of what she'd want. At the second hearing, the testimony of another friend that she'd said "I wouldn't want to live like that," did meet the standard according to the judge.

People do not have to write an advance directive; it can be spoken. The form specified by the state does not have to be used, even if the statute says it does. There is no perfect document that will satisfy everyone, and the search for one is futile.

Reference: King, Nancy M. P., "Dying Made Legal: New Challenges for Advance Directives," *Health Ethics Committee Forum*, 1991;3:187-99.

There is evidence that about one-fourth of the time, treatment of the patient is different in actual practice than living wills request. Most of the time, less treatment was given than the living will requested.

Even when asked to imagine themselves with a poor prognosis and desperately ill, 30% of people would choose life sustaining treatment.

Reference: Davis, M. et al, "A Prospective Study of Advance Directives for Life-Sustaining Care," *NEJM*, 1991;324: 882-88.

Some state laws forbid insurance companies from requiring applicants to make an advance directive refusing treatment in order to qualify for insurance. Those laws seek to protect people from pressure to make a living will in return for cheap insurance. They also interfere with the ability of the person to make a contract with the insurance company which might given them cheaper insurance that they want.

Not all states have such "protective" laws. What if insurance companies didn't require it, but gave discounts to people who wrote advance directives? That would save the insurance companies big bucks, which they could pass on to customers.

Watch out for this: Some attorneys are thoughtfully attaching a revocation form to the living will or durable (springing) power of attorney itself. People who are competent can revoke the document, change their minds and change the document, or change the agent they appoint to be their "attorney in fact."

Unfortunately, some people and their witnesses have signed all the documents the attorney has attached, including the revocation, at the same time. They effectively establish and then revoke the instrument.

An "attorney in fact" is different from but related to the term "attorney at law." The word "attorney" comes from old French, based on turn, to arrange, to distribute. An attorney in fact need not be a lawyer.

An ethical problem is seen by one authority. Competent persons make advance directives to feel in control of their future. Their wishes now, however, may conflict with their actual interest later when they are incompetent patients. The use of advance directives fails to recognize that people have different interests at different stages of their lives.

We are really unable to predict our interests as well as the directives would assume we can. An unimaginable existence to a 20 year old may be tolerable when he actually is 90 and ill, or at least may be preferable to death. The advance directive also could remove responsibility from and give license to the practitioner who has no ethical standards. Such a person would carry out the directive as written no matter what the circumstances. "It's not my job, man, she wanted it this way."

When you write an advance directive and then become incompetent, you may lose your right to change your mind. Some would argue that have no mind to change, at that point.

Reference: Robertson, John A., "Second Thoughts on Living Wills," *HCR*, November-December 1991; pp. 6-9.

A case is documented of a patient dehydrated and starved in a Florida nursing home though she asked for food. The court said she was not competent to revoke the power of attorney she gave her brother.

WHY YOU MAY GET INVOLVED

A word about protecting the patient. Most codes of ethics of professionals (See Chapter Five, "Professionals and Employees") speak to the mandate that the professional has to act in the best interest of the patient. The practitioner protects the patient, or in some way acts on behalf of the patient. You will have a patient with a surrogate decision maker, such as a doctor, family member, court-appointed guardian, or agent appointed by the durable (springing) power of attorney acting according to a living will.

If that person is not acting in the patient's best interest, what will you do? You may have a legal duty to act under a statute that requires report of abuse or neglect, or case law that imposes liability for negligence of your duty of care.

Aside from consideration of the law, you may have an ethical duty to assist another human being—beneficence and nonmaleficence. Your ethical mandate is reinforced by your profession's code of ethics. Your action is because you believe it is right, not just because your "profession" believes it is right. Codes of ethics are properly used not as clubs but as reminders.

In the Florida nursing home case it was a nurse's aide who blew the whistle.

DANFORTH—OBRA '90—PSDA

The Medicare law is amended every year at least You'll see OBRA '89, OBRA '91, '92, and so on. . One amendment that concerns ethical issues around death was passed on November 5, 1990: The Omnibus Budget Reform Act (OBRA) '90. It went into effect in late 1991.

The Danforth Amendment (Patient Self-Determination Act) is that Medicare law amendment. It requires agencies that deal with patients to inform them of their rights under state law to accept or refuse medical or surgical treatment, and to inform their patients of their right to formulate advance directives.

The law requires the agency to ask the patient if she has an advance directive and to indicate that on the chart. Surveys say that only 4% of hospitals asked this of patients prior to Danforth. The law requires the agencies to follow state law regarding advance directives. The state laws would have required this themselves, but by requiring it in the federal law, what is the effect? See below. The law requires agencies to formulate written policies about all this, and to educate their staffs and communities.

In states where assisted suicide became legal (see below), patients would have to be notified they could kill themselves with help.

Always ask, especially when dealing with law, what's the penalty if I don't? Who'll know? What'll they do to me? In this case, the potential penalty is not jail or fine or civil liability in a malpractice case. The potential penalty for violation is loss of funding from Medicare. It's unlikely that violating this section would by itself cause an agency to lose funds, unless the violation were flagrant and continuous.

The question remains: What is the purpose of this law? Is it merely in reaction to the <u>Cruzan</u> initial decision, which appeared to leave Nancy alive against her wishes? Is it to prevent other Nancys from this fate? An article was written by a staffer to Senator Danforth, who sponsored the bill. In the article, a memo from Danforth prior to writing of the law is quoted. The Senator asked about economics, quality of life, artificial extension of life, and whether a lesser degree of care to the comatose was possible. Economics was mentioned and denied as a motivator.

Reference: McClosky, E., "Between Isolation and Intrusion: The Patient Self-Determination Act," *Law, Medicine and Health Care*, 1991;19:1-2, pp. 80-82.

Another author, after discussing the costs of Permanent Unconscious Persons (PUPs) maintenance, said that economics was not the primary purpose of the law. He did say the law would have the fortuitous side effect of reducing cost. He believes there is a state and federal interest in ensuring that PUPs do not receive long-term care they would not have wanted.

A poll of nursing home residents which asked them to imagine that they were PUPs showed 16% of them <u>would</u> want tube feedings. How will we know which 16 of 100 want to be PUPs, and which 84 want to die? Perhaps a reverse living will could be required, saying they **do** want care. Otherwise we must assume we know which ones would want feeding. Perhaps we would not feed them even if they wished it, because it's too expensive.

Reference: Greco, Peter, et al, "The PSDA and the Future of Advance Directives," *Annals of Internal Medicine*, 1991;115:639–43.

Perhaps an unspoken motive for the Danforth Amendment was to counter what some believe is the practitioner motive for maintaining Permanently Unconscious Persons.

A frank discussion about maintaining PUPs like Nancy Cruzan will sometimes reveal a cynical attitude on the part of nonpractitioners, and some practitioners. That attitude assumes that practitioners want to "protect" patients like Cruzan for selfish reasons. It is believed that the practitioners have an economic interest in keeping the patient alive to keep their jobs. These are the same people who think medicine has a cure for cancer that they are hiding, because practitioners will lose money.

The people who objected first to the removal of Nancy Cruzan's feeding tube were her nurses at the state hospital at Mt. Vernon, Missouri. That was a vile deed, if you believe Cruzan existed in a horrible state, and that the nurses who wanted to keep her in that life did so out of sheer greed. Psychologists tell us that imagining someone else's motive may be projection of our own. You are free to project what you think their motives were.

Practitioners do have self-interest. In their nature and training their self-interest is served, by helping people and in particular by protecting their patients. We cannot know the motivation of the nurses at Mt. Vernon, nor the motive of other practitioners in other cases who intervene in their patient's care. We can project onto them what our motive would be in a similar situation.

Practitioners often disagree with decisions made that prolong patients' dying. A study of nursing home nurses revealed that they disagreed with their patients' aggressive treatment. Since aggressive treatment kept the patients alive longer, that study should be some small evidence against the assumption that greedy practitioners want to keep their patients alive, no matter what their condition.

Reference: Wolff, Michael L., Smolen, Susan, and Ferrara, Linda, "Treatment Decisions in a Skilled-Nursing Facility: Discordance with Nurses' Preferences," *Journal of the American Geriatrics Society*, 1985;33:440–445.

STUDY QUESTIONS

1. What is the meaning of the terms "withhold" and "withdraw," "active" and "passive?" Contrast these terms with "to treat" versus "limit" treatment.

2. What is the mental condition of the patients that most ethical conflicts are about?

3. What are two of the myths about terminating life support that are false?

4. What value is highest in the American Thoracic Society's guidelines for terminating futile treatment?

5. What are the values in the futility issue—specifically, in the Helga Wanglie case?

6. Could the doctors have handled this case differently, or might they have wanted to go to court?

7. What would an opposite decision have meant regarding futility of treatment?

8. What are examples of practitioner acquiescence to patient demands, which may make it harder for practitioners to assert their autonomy to decide when treatment is futile?

9. What is the primary purpose of any "tool" or measurement of health or illness or quality of life?

10. What is evidence that courts are not often involved in decisions to limit treatment?

11. What is the difference in the use of the terms "substituted judgment" and "best interest?"

12. Why are family or other people close to the patient named as decision makers?

"Withholding" vs. "Withdrawing;" "Treating" vs. "Limiting Treatment"

Most of us die in a hospital or nursing home, and 70% of those deaths are as a result of a decision to limit treatment (defined as dyong with 3 DNR order). Withholding or withdrawing, giving or limiting treatment, is an issue that concerns every practitioner and potential patient. You are both.

There is no difference, in theory, between withholding treatment in the first place, and withdrawing treatment later. To withhold the first tube feeding is the same as withholding the next tube feeding and the next, after it is started. To remove the ventilator and allow a patient to breathe on her own is the same as not aiding that breath in the first place. This is the fact, in _theory_; in practice it feels very different.

There is no theoretical difference in the law, despite what you may read. There may be some practical difference, since a case about withdrawing has time to go to court. The patient will be maintained on the ventilator or tube feeding while the case is decided. A case about withholding, on the other hand may not have time for court action, since the patient may die before a court can act if the treatment is withheld in the first place.

Practitioners have the technology. You have seen dramatic results from its use. You tend to treat first and withdraw later if the results are not forthcoming. That is not a bad plan of action. Despite fears, you really can withdraw treatment later if it is not helping.

This nondistinction is the same nonissue as passive and active, killing versus letting die. Withdrawing treatment sounds as though it's passive, like letting die. But putting your hand down and pulling on a respirator plug, or shutting it down (turning the dial) is the same kind of _act_ as starting the machine. It's not passive; it's active, an action. "Passive" and "active" are not helpful distinctions.

The distinction is not between "withdraw" and "withhold," nor "active" and "passive." The question is whether to _treat_ or to _limit_ treatment. The practitioners taking this course could never condone "not treating" if that meant not positioning, turning, cleaning, giving pain medication. Surely total absence of treatment would have to include lethal injection to prevent suffering.

Hippocrates wrote that medicine included to "refuse to treat those who are overmastered by their diseases, realizing that in such cases medicine is powerless." Other professions are not powerless in such situations; indeed, professionals like nurses have even more of a role in the care of people "overmastered by their disease."

Reference: Hippocrates. *The Art.* Jones, W. H., ed., Vol. 2. Harvard Univ. Press, Cambridge, 1923: pp. 193, 203.

There is usually no issue about treating competent people; we treat when they want it and when it's medically indicated. Can you imagine discontinuing a ventilator from a competent patient who wanted it, and who couldn't breathe without it?

There may be issues about what is medically indicated. Some authorities believe that the practitioner's participation in cosmetic surgery has removed any objection that medicine could have against doing what is not "medically indicated." Little cosmetic surgery is medically necessary. The patient gets what the patient wants.

The problem with limiting treatment is with incompetent patients. As you've noticed by now, many (if not most) of our ethical conflicts are about incompetent patients. A competent patient decides for herself. We decide for an incompetent patient. How do we decide?

First, unlearn the myths about terminating life support.

1.   Myth: Whatever the law or authority does not specifically permit is prohibited. Not so. It is a strange idea of the law which would have us all carry immense volumes of law books permitting all the specific things we do. (It would look like a personnel meeting at the VA.) The opposite is true. Whatever is not prohibited is permitted. It's easier to get forgiveness than permission.

2.   Myth: Terminating life support is either murder or suicide. Not so. It's usually just death. People will die, if they are dying, whether we treat or not.

3.   Myth: A patient must be terminally ill to terminate life support. Wrong. That's the specification in some living will statutes, but many of those are unconstitutional after Cruzan. However, the patient must want the support discontinued.

4. Myth: It's acceptable to terminate extraordinary, but not ordinary, treatment. That misconcept is from Catholic terminology. "Extraordinary" is that treatment in which the burden outweighs the benefit (cost-benefit analysis). There is no requirement to treat under that circumstance.

5. Myth: Withholding is OK, but not withdrawing. See above for discussion. Since they are theoretically the same, if one is ok so is the other. If one is not, neither is the other. With drawing feels worse than withholding though.

6. Myth: Tube feedings are different legally. Even the Supreme Court has said they're not. Controversy exists over the _ethics_ of removing tube feedings in non-dying patients.

7. Myth: To terminate life support, a court order is necessary. Not. That's the whole point of living wills, powers of attorney, all advance directives.

Reference: Meisel, Alan, "Legal Myths about Terminating Life Support," *AIM*, 1991;151:1497–502.

The guidelines of the American Thoracic Society provide that autonomy is the paramount value in those guidelines. Competent patients decide on their own treatment. Or, the competent patient decides through his advance directive in a living will or by naming a surrogate. A surrogate can decide for an incapacitated or incompetent patient. Life support can be terminated without consent of the patient _or_ surrogate when treatment is "futile". See discussion of this concept below; remember the values of beneficence versus nonmaleficence here. The society advocates that institutions should promote ethical decisions about life support therapy through use of the ethicists.

Reference: American Thoracic Society, "Withholding and Withdrawing Life Support Therapy," *AIM*, 1991;115:478–85.

FUTILITY

This brings us to futility as a concept. That a treatment is futile means different things to different people. Is it futile merely to keep the patient alive. Is the treatment futile if it merely returns the patient to consciousness. Is treatment futile if it doesn't return the patient to a meaningful "quality of life" (and in whose judgment). Is treatment futile if it doesn't return the patient to the life she had before?

A recent case raising this issue was In re Helga Wanglie, 4th Judicial District, (District Court, Probate Division) PX 91-283, Minnesota, Hennepin County. The physicians requested the court to protect them from liability for discontinuing a ventilator on Helga Wanglie, an 84-year-old PUP. The physicians would have not brought the case to court, unless there were a conflict. The conflict was with the patient's prior expressed wishes (her advance directive that she wanted such treatment). And the doctor's conflict was with her husband (who wanted the treatment continued).

The doctors said the treatment was not in her best interest. They said the treatment was futile, though it would keep her alive. Their definition of futile was treatment that would not restore her to consciousness. She had not been conscious before being put on the ventilator, either.

Analyzing the interests here: The patient expressed her wishes before her incompetence and expressed them through her appointed guardian, her husband. The wish was to stay alive in any way possible, with any treatment including the ventilator. She had no interest in decreased pain, since she was unconscious before and during the treatment.

The doctors' interests were in treating her appropriately. They asserted a "professional interest" in not giving a patient an inappropriate treatment.

The hospital's interest could have been in having the bed for other patients. This was not stated and occupancy is not usually that tight these days. The hospital's bill was being paid by Wanglie's private insurance so the hospital had no economic interest in terminating the case. It could be asserted the hospital had an economic interest in continuing the treatment. And the nurses?

The insurance company had a contract with the Wanglies to pay her bills if she got sick. In return, the Wanglies paid premiums while she was not sick. Did the other people who pay premiums to the insurance company have an interest in not having their money "wasted?" There is no standing (no acknowledged legal interest) for them in a case of this kind. Perhaps they too would want as much for their money as possible should such a case arise for them.

Given the above interests, there can be little surprise that the judge chose to follow the family's wishes in this case. The value of autonomy of the patient, as expressed through the surrogate here, allowed treatment to continue. Three days after the decision, Helga Wanglie died on the ventilator.

There is an economic, money-work interest in all these cases. It may not be openly stated, but someone will sooner or later come around to "all the money it's costing," or "it's not fair to spend all this money on these old people, when we could spend it on prenatal care for the babies," or "no wonder our health insurance premiums are going up," or "look at the bill for the hospital/taxpayer in this case." To consider the money-work value in such cases is perfectly appropriate, but we must be sure to confront it openly and not hide it under other considerations of "futility," "practitioner autonomy," or "best interest of the patient."

Whether the patient's autonomy is respected by the practitioner should not depend on whether the patient agrees with the practitioner. Unfortunately, the Wanglie case could be thus characterized: If you agree with me that your treatment is futile, I respect your autonomy. If you don't agree with me, I don't respect your autonomy and I'll discontinue the ventilator or feeding tube anyway. I'll ask the court to ok it so you can't sue me.

FEEDING TUBE FUTILITY

In cases about removing feeding tubes, practitioners have not asserted their own autonomy as practitioners. They have hidden behind the patient's autonomy, saying that the patient or her surrogate wanted treatment limited.

Practitioners are not likely to be able to take that practitioner autonomy back now, and say that they can decide when treatment is futile. The patients are not going to let them.

Some physicians' assertions of futility, and limiting treatment to medical necessity, is severely compromised by actions on the part of other physicians. Doctors who perform and practitioners who assist with cosmetic surgery, abortion, sterilization, fertilization, and Cesarean sections have to consider this issue.

These are treatments in which the patient may initiate the request and the practitioner complies regardless of determination of the patient's physical need. All such compliance on the part of the practitioner erodes the ability of practitioners to assert their professional autonomy, to say they won't provide treatment they don't believe is good for the patient.

What about patients who have high risk of breast cancer, who mistake class probability (or risk) for case probability (or risk)—what if they want prophylactic mastectomies? What if they have large breasts and want them larger? Not very large breasts and want smaller? What if her nose already looks great? What if he's transsexual? What if he is impotent and could be

NOTES

treated medically, but wants a prosthesis? What if he could be saved with CPR after a lightning bolt, but has a living will that says "no CPR?" Does the practitioner have any say here? "The customer is always right" has a price.

There is a 13th Amendment to the Constitution that prohibits slavery. So it must be that practitioners are doing these things willingly. It is then hard to assert that the treatment the patient or family wants is futile and not medically justified. This is especially true if treatment the patient wants will preserve her life . Other practitioners applied no such standard when the patient demanded a prettier nose.

FUTILITY FOR INCOMPETENTS

It is easier to assert futility if the patient is incompetent and the family is not asserting anything. Then the practitioner will decide, but not solely on medical grounds. Then it is a value judgment, a quality of life decision made by the practitioner for another person.

The decision about real futility is one the practitioner should make. The decision is subjective depending on the definition of futility used. Practitioners have started to, and will increase, the use of "quality of life" criteria to justify their decisions about futility. That term is shorthand for a decision not to treat, made for a variety of reasons.

To make subjective quality of life assessments appear to be objective and numerical, several "tools" have been developed. The APACHE, Acute Physical Assessment and Chronic Health Evaluation, used in ICU's, was developed at George Washington University in 1985. APACHE predicts the rate of survival after intensive care.

Could treatment be classed as futile if the score gets too close to zero probability of survival? Should it? Is the scale perfect? Is the computer objective? Does the practitioner have any ethical obligation if the numbers say "quit?"

The practitioner must always use such numbers the way they are created, as probabilities for a class of patients. The numbers are determined by past experience with patients different from yours. The individual (your patient) is not a class. He is a case, and his probability of living to leave the ICU is either zero or 100%, no matter what the other 70-year-olds in the class did.

Reference: Knaus, S. A., et al: "APACHE II, A Severity of Disease
Classification System,"*Critical Care Medicine*,
1985;13:818-829.

You may see other "tools," the SIP (Sickness Impact Profile), PGWB
(Psychological General Well Being), the PQOL (Perceived Quality of Life).
All may be useful, and all must be used with caution and not as substitutes
for individual practitioner responsibility.

Reference: The Hastings Center; *Guidelines on the Termination of Life-
Sustaining Treatment*, Briarcliff Manor, NY: THC, 1987.

Academy of Critical Care Physicians/Society of Critical
Care Medicine Consensus Panel, "Ethical and Moral
Guidelines for the Initiation, Continuation and Withdrawal
of Intensive Care," *Chest*, 1990;97:949.

President's Commission for the Study of Ethical Problems in
Medicine and Biomedical and Behavioral Research;
Decisions to Forego Life-Sustaining Treatment, Government
Printing Office, Washington D. C.: 1983, pp. 236-239.

FEAR OF COURTING, PART II

Some 60 cases on the "right to withdraw treatment" have been recorded at
the appellate level in this country. A case doesn't get reported unless and
until it is decided by a lower trial court, appealed to the next higher court,
then that decision is reported. At that point it becomes law.

The American Hospital Association says that 1.3 million people die yearly
as a result of limiting treatment since few patients ordered "DNR" would
survive resuscitation, this figure includes all DNRs, not exactly the same as
removing a ventilator or feeding tube. Since the 1976 Quinlan case (see
below), 20 million people died after treatment was limited. Very few
decisions to limit treatment go to court.

The few cases that go to court are not always result of a conflict. Some,
including to some extent the Wanglie case above, are in fear of suit or fear
of responsibility. As another example, the Cruzan family could have taken
their daughter home years ago, and quietly let her die there.

Some doctors, hospital attorneys, guardians, and families, seek official paternal court sanction rather than accept responsibility for what they believe is right. That so few cases are seen is a tribute that most practitioners are acting responsibly.

Several court cases deserve specific mention for their lessons and their notoriety. The first was Karen Ann Quinlan, In Re Quinlan, 70 N.J. 20, 355 A. 2d 647 (NJ 1976). With a 22-year-old in a coma as a result of presumed alcohol and drug ingestion, the court used a substituted judgment test to remove her from advanced life support (a ventilator). She breathed on her own, and lived 10 more years with a feeding tube which her mother said she would never have requested be removed.

BEST INTEREST—SUBSTITUTED JUDGEMENT

Many legal and ethical cases make a distinction between "best interest" of the patient and the patient's "substituted judgment." We only worry about this if the patient is incapacitated or incompetent.

If the patient can say, she decides what she judges to be in her best interest. There's no difference between best interest and substituted judgment of the competent patient. If the patient is not competent, a substituted judgment is needed. The substitute makes a judgment as though he were the patient. He chooses or judges what the patient would judge. The patient would, if she could, judge or choose the treatment that is in her best interest. So substituted judgment is at the same time judgment of the best interest of the patient. There is no difference in the two concepts.

The next question: who gets to make this substituted judgment or best interest decision? Who decides is only important if we assume that the decision maker is influenced by his personal values. That is what we assume; otherwise we'd feed all this into a computer and get a printout.

We want someone who knows the patient, who most nearly can judge the way she would judge. We prefer her husband, or parents, kids, sibling, lover. The trend in recent court cases as we see in Cruzan and Wanglie is to let the family decide. They know her and, the assumption still is, love her.

STUDY QUESTIONS

1. What are the three standards of evidence used in American law? Give examples where each is used.

2. Why is the Cruzan case is so significant in American bioethics?

3. What is one reason the courts might want to impose a standard of clear and convincing evidence before terminating treatment?

4. What is another source of rights, remedy, or relief for persons who want treatment terminated, other than the U.S. Constitution's right to refuse treatment under the 14th Amendment liberty interest?

CRUZAN, CRUZAN, CRUZAN

The case is the most important bioethical case in American history; it is the first and only one ever to reach the U.S. Supreme Court, which is why we devote so much time to it in this course. (Another big case is coming: Is there a right to help in self-killing?).

Nancy Cruzan had a car wreck in 1980. EMT's and practitioners worked to save her life. A feeding tube was put in. She was diagnosed as PVS (see below) in 1988. Years later, her family wished the feeding tube to be removed. The nurses and the institution objected. Conflict arose, with recourse to the courts. (If no recourse to the court is possible, the family has absolute decision about treatment.)

The Rule: In Missouri (and New York, New Jersey, and Maryland), before treatment can be discontinued, you need clear and convincing evidence that the patient while competent would not have wanted treatment. It's not a best interest–substituted judgment test, as in Quinlan. The family does not decide. It's really an expression of absolute autonomy of the patient. The patient decides.

STANDARDS OF EVIDENCE

About clear and convincing evidence: There are three levels, or standards, of evidence in court cases. (Administrative agency hearings use the standard of "clear and convincing to a reasonable certainty," but we are concerned here with standards applied in courtroom proceedings.)

BEYOND A REASONABLE DOUBT

The highest standard of evidence, the most difficult to attain or prove, is evidence that convinces beyond a reasonable doubt. This is the standard used in criminal trials. That standard of evidence must exist before we take away a person's life or liberty.

CLEAR AND CONVINCING EVIDENCE

The second standard, clear and convincing, is the standard used in Missouri and several other states. This level of proof must exist before a person's life support (food and water) can be withheld, if there's a conflict about the withholding.

If there is no clear and convincing evidence that the patient would refuse, there is no refusal. If no refusal by the patient, no termination of treatment.

PREPONDERANCE OF THE EVIDENCE

The lowest standard to meet is preponderance of the evidence. That's the level used in civil court cases. For example, that standard of evidence must exist to establish liability in a malpractice lawsuit. Say you testify that the bedrails were up. The patient testifies they were down. If there is just a little bit more evidence for you, for example you <u>charted it</u> too, then that's a preponderance. Anything over 50%, and you win if the case is appealed.

The Supreme Court in <u>Cruzan</u> found that Missouri could use the clear and convincing standard, or a lower standard if it wished. The people of Missouri also could by statute establish some other standard of evidence in such cases. The Court held some very other important things in this case. (See the "Rights" discussion in Chapter Three, "A Time to Be Born.")

THE 14TH AMENDMENT TO THE U. S. CONSTITUTION GUARANTEES THE RIGHT TO REFUSE TREATMENT

There is a constitutional right to refuse treatment, based on the 14th Amendment to the U.S. Constitution. That Amendment says that no state can deny life, liberty, or property without due process of law. The liberty interest, the freedom, the autonomy value that is so dear in this country and this Constitution, protects individuals from state courts, legislatures, and majorities that would limit their right to consent or not to consent to treatment.

This is the first time we've acknowledged a constitutional right in this area. Before <u>Cruzan</u> we had "merely" a right established by judge-made law (common law) state by state.

The following quote is from New York case law, adopted in all other states in some form: "Every human being of adult years and sound mind has a right to determine what shall be done with his own body . . . ." Justice Cardozo in *Schloendorff v. Society of New York Hospital*, 105 N.E. 92, 93 (NY 1914).

Schloendorff established the right to sue for battery when unauthorized surgery was performed despite permission only for a pelvic exam.

As long as the right to refuse treatment was a common law right established by state judge-made or legislature-made law, states could interfere with and restrict it as they chose. They so chose in many "advance directive" laws which only operate when patients are terminally ill, and don't allow patients to refuse food and water in their advance directives. Now that the Supreme Court in <u>Cruzan</u> has recognized a constitutional right, states may not restrict the right of competent patients to refuse treatment through advance directives.

FEEDING TUBES ARE NO DIFFERENT FROM VENTILATORS

The court did not differentiate between basic treatment and advanced treatment. Food and water can be withheld if the advanced directive requires it. And the Court indicated that advance directives would constitute clear and convincing evidence in a case such as <u>Cruzan</u>. Remember, the advance directives can be spoken.

Later in the <u>Cruzan</u> case, witnesses were found that testified that Cruzan had told them (or didn't disagree when the statement was made), "I wouldn't want to live like that." The same trial court judge who originally ordered the tube out, found this spoken expression to be clear and convincing evidence of Nancy's wishes and ordered the tube out again. This time the institution (the state of Missouri) did not appeal his decision. Nancy Cruzan's gastrostomy tube was removed and she died. Was killed. Starved. Pick your ending.

NOTES

References: Cruzan v. Director, Missouri Department of Health, 110 S.Ct. 2972 (1990).

Numerous references collected under Fairman, R. Paul, "Commentary: Withdrawing Life-Sustaining Treatment— Lessons from Nancy Cruzan," *Archives of Internal Medicine*, Vol. 152, January 1992, pp. 25-27.

INCOMPETENT PATIENT, NO ADVANCE DIRECTIVE

A later Missouri case involved Christine Busalacchi, similar to Nancy Cruzan except that she had not expressed any earlier statement about her treatment in the event of such an event. In this case, there was contradictory evidence of her diagnosis as Persistent Vegetative State (see below for discussion). Busalacchi's father wanted to move her to Minnesota for diagnosis of PVS by neurologist Dr. Ronald Cranford (and subsequent removal of her feeding tube), (according to court evidence). In 1993, the Court dismissed the case when the new Missouri Attorney General refused to contest the father's request. Christine was "allowed" to die by dehydration.

In New York, In re O'Connor, 53 N.E. 2d 607 (NY, 1988) involved a woman with senile dementia. The court ruled that she keep the nasogastric feeding tube in the absence of clear and convincing evidence of the patient's wishes.

WHY IS ALL THIS CLEAR AND CONVINCING?

We can't be sure it's not reversible. A 45-year-old woman, comatose with severe brain damage since October 1989, after surgery for a brain aneurism, woke up. Completely. This case got less much publicity. Such examples confuse our understanding that such PUPs want to and should be put "out of their misery."

Reference: "Comatose Woman's Wakening a 'Miracle,'" *St. Louis Post-Dispatch*, December 22, 1991.

A policeman in PVS for eight years, awoke in 1996, *Newsweek*, February 26, 1996. p. 56

COMPETENT PATIENT, CURRENT DIRECTIVE

Elizabeth Bouvia, a young woman with cerebral palsy and quadriplegia, sought the right to refuse food and water and to be allowed to die with hospital care, though not terminally ill. She was granted that right by a court, but now lives on a liquid diet in another hospital after being given control of her morphine administration.

STATE CONSTITUTIONAL RIGHT OF PRIVACY

The court in Cruzan found the right to refuse treatment in the liberty interest of the 14th Amendment. They did not discuss the case under an "unwritten right of privacy" in the U.S. Constitution. Many state constitutions do have such a right. Individuals may find relief there from state laws requiring feeding tubes.

Florida's living will law prompted regulators to rule that nursing home residents who don't eat, get a feeding tube or be discharged. That state's constitutional right of privacy allowed a resident's guardian to authorize feeding tube removal.

Reference: In re Guardianship of Browning, (State v. Herbert) No. 74, 174) Fla. Sep. 13, 1990).

Check your state's constitution for a written right of privacy. Look at the front of the set of state statute books, found in every branch library. You may be surprised.

STATE REQUIRES OMBUDSMAN

Claire Conroy, 84, was a nursing home patient with senile dementia. (That's what people used to have before we discovered Alzheimer's.) The court decided that the substituted judgment or best interest standard should be used to decide if her tube should be removed. The court also ordered a state ombudsman, plus a guardian, be appointed to decide the fate of such people.

Reference: In the matter of Claire C. Conroy, 486 A.2d 1209 (NJ 1985).

WITHDRAWING CARE IS NOT MURDER

The worst fears of physicians was realized in the next case. Care was withdrawn from a comatose patient, according to the family's wishes. A murder charge was filed and later withdrawn, but not before testimony revealed that the family was not so clearly committed to the patient's death as the doctor had thought/wished. **Lesson:** Know the patient and family well enough to ascertain their wishes, even if a delay in terminating treatment is necessary.

Reference: Lo, Bernard, "The Death of Clarence Herbert: Withdrawing Care Is Not Murder," <u>Annals of Internal Med.</u>, 1984;101:248–51.

STUDY QUESTIONS

1. What is the definition of "Persistent Vegetative State?"

2. What is the definition of "death?"

3. What are the consequences of declaring PVS patients to be dead?

4. In the middle ages, which disease caused the patient so diagnosed to be declared dead?

5. What is the difference between "artificial" and "natural" feeding?

PERSISTENT VEGETATIVE STATE: THE RADISH SYNDROME

Nancy Cruzan was diagnosed in PVS, Persistent Vegetative State. Persistent vegetative state as a diagnosis was first described in 1972 in an English medical journal. It is not a specific disease, but a collection of symptoms. It is variously described as wakefulness without awareness; patient is unaware of self or surrounding environment; no voluntary movement, emotion, or cognition. Some patients gag or cough, or their eyes move.

The condition may be reversible and cannot be diagnosed permanently with certainty.

The diagnosis is not in standard lists of mental health diagnoses like the Diagnostic Statistical Manual of Mental Disorders, DSM III R. Nor is it listed in Jablonski's Dictionary of Syndromes and Eponymic Diseases. Nor is it a diagnosis listed in the International Classification of Diseases, 9th Revision, Clinical Modification (ICD 9 CM). Nor is it in the Dictionary of Medical Syndromes. The latter are lists of standard diagnoses, conditions, syndromes, and diseases.

This is said to be a new disease. It is said to have come about as a result of the technologies: IV or enteral feeding, IV antibiotics for infections, and good systematic nursing care which lets these patients survive various insults which in former times would have killed their bodies.

There is no published set of accepted criteria for diagnosis of this "disease." This is, therefore, unlike the Ad Hoc Standards from the Ad Hoc Committee of Harvard Medical School to diagnose brain death. No lab tests will diagnose it and no diagnosis may be made from x-ray; though x-rays may show damage to the central cortex. A proponent of the idea that persons in the PVS are "dead" and should be killed is Ronald E. Cranford, neurologist at Hennepin County Medical Center, Minneapolis.

Reference: Cranford, Ronald, "The Persistent Vegetative State: The Medical Reality," *Hastings Center Report*, 1988; 27–32.

Causes of the condition are said to be variable, mechanical, not understood. The symptoms overlap with other neurological symptoms, such as coma, dementia, irreversible coma, and "locked-in" syndrome. Experts use the term "permanently unconscious" as a synonym. They variously describe loss of all possible components of mental life—thought, feeling, sensation, desire, emotion, awareness of self or environment. The patients have not suffered brain stem death, therefore they are not brain dead according to the Harvard definition. (President's Commission (1983) p. 173.)

To simplify and clarify, we will use the term Permanently Unconscious Patients, or PUPs, for people considered to be in a permanent vegetative state, since it pleases us better than thinking of people as radishes.

A recent study has shed some light. The PUPs are capable of prolonged survival with good care. There are an estimated 5,000–10,000 of them in the country. They are either fairly young, in which they have had a brain injury with cerebral anoxia (Cruzan, Quinlan). Or they are old, with cardiovascular accident or dementia etiology (Conroy, O'Connor, others).

Of 1611 nursing home patients examined in the study, 62 were identified by staff to be PUPs, or about 3%. And 11 of the 62 were subsequently determined by the investigators not to be PUPs. That is, they had some awareness, volitional movement, and two of those had improved since admission.

Of those diagnosed as PUPs, 53% had CPR status ordered (see below). Of those 53%, do not resuscitate (DNR) was ordered for 93%. Those numbers are about the same for general hospital patients. All PUPs were on daily meds. 78% have pressure sores. 27% were on antipsychotic medications, though behavior should not be a problem for such patients. During the course of the study, 60% were hospitalized for some reason, usually acute infection. 29% had surgery for some reason, such as fracture, pacemaker replacement.

Reference: Tresch, Donald D., et al, "Clinical Characteristics of Patients in the Persistent Vegetative State," *AIM*, 1991;151:930–32.

PVS is not a terminal illness. If these people are not to live, it will be because we terminate treatment, specifically food and water. If we decide for a class of persons (humans, vegetables) that their lives are not worth living, we may do so. But we must be clear that the judgment is not the person's, but ours. We must be clear that we value a certain quality or style of life. We will have to be clear that we are deciding for other people that they shouldn't live, because they can't live as we do.

BRAIN DEATH

This is not a new issue; as we said, we've always had to decide whether to care for dying or injured people, and when to stop. But as we have gotten better at treating dying or ill or unconscious people, and as their treatment has been removed from the family and given to strangers, it's more difficult to decide when to quit treating.

We can surely stop treating people when they're dead. The definition of death used to be when the heart stopped beating (usually secondary to respiration ceasing). With respirators, we can keep bodies going for a few hours or days <u>only</u> after the brain is dead. You noted in Chapter Two that one of the earlier bioethical conflicts was over brain death. The primary benefit of declaring a patient "brain-dead" is that the body can be cut and organs removed for transplant without practitioners feeling they have killed the patient.

Some people at Harvard developed a definition of brain death several years ago. Subsequently, several state legislatures agonized over that and adopted it pretty much as law. So practitioners can all agree and can diagnose total brain death now.

WRONG

Practitioners can diagnose irreversible brain stem death with a high degree of certainty, but not an extremely high degree. There is still confusion over determination of brain death for organ retrieval. A study indicates that experts <u>can</u> identify patients with a permanent loss of all brain function. However three-fourths of a group of practitioners and one-third of a group of experts did not agree that this meant the patient was dead.

This evidence of disagreement over the definition of death as loss of total brain function comes as we hear requests to re-define death to a still more "alive" level. Proposals are to define death as loss not of the total brain, as at present. New definitions of death would be loss of function in the higher levels of thinking and awareness. These are the people described above, the PUPs. Mentioned as a beneficial outcome would be organ retrieval from potential donors among the permanently unconscious.

Reference: Wikler, D., and Weisbard, Alan, "Appropriate Confusion over Brain Death," *JAMA*, 1989;261:2246.

In Japan the person is more part of a tribe, so death of an individual is not an excuse to declare him dead and take organs.

Reference: "Obstacles to Brain Death and Organ Transplantation in Japan," *The Lancet*, 1991;388:1063-64.

Serious consideration is being given to labelling PUPs as dead. An organism with no ability to communicate, no awareness of self or others, that will remain forever so is a corpse, said one writer. In the same article, examples of two PUPs were given who had recovered thinking ability. One was characterized as paralyzed, emotionally disturbed, and dependent on others. The second recovered PUP was only able to respond by blinking. The implication is that these two would be better off dead.

Reference: Thalblum, Donna, "PVS's and Immortality: If This Is Technically Life, the Legal Definition of Death Should Change," *UMKC Law Rev*, 1991;59:2:439-67.

ARE THEY DEAD?

Calls have been made for a change in the definition of death to include PUPs. This would classify a group of people as dead because they are not conscious. The obvious conclusion is that their "lives" have no value, lives not worth living.

Some writers believe we are lying when we wish to give families the right to "decide" to refuse treatment for their loved one in PVS. We would do away with the clear and convincing evidence standard only in PVS cases. In those cases even a little evidence is enough to prove the patient wanted to die. We only give families this right to decide when they will decide to terminate treatment for PVS patients, not in other cases.

For example, when nonPVS children are the subject, we do not let families decide their beloved child's fate. There have been several prosecutions of Christian Scientist parents when their children were harmed by lack of medical treatment. We did not, in those nonPVS, nonhandicapped kids cases, let the parents make decisions for the children. We only do that with PVS patients and handicapped kids, and only when the parents decide what we want them to.

One writer asks that we not leave decisions about PUPs to their families. He believes we should be honest and declare them dead.

Reference: Baron, Charles, "Why Withdrawal of Life Support of PVS Patients Is Not a Family Decision," *Law, Medicine and Health Care* 1991;19:1-2, 73–75.

The diagnosis of PVS would have important consequences. One wonders why use the word "vegetable." It may be easier to deal with vegetables, easier to decide such diagnosed people are not really people at all. To call someone "human" is not helpful, if being human does not confer any rights.

We are not doing anything new, declaring diseased people to be dead. In the 1200s, persons diagnosed with leprosy were officially declared dead in a ceremony. They lost rights as citizens (for example, to inherit or bequeath property). .

The leper was brought from her home to the church, mass was read and extreme unction given as though she had died. She was warned never to go to church, market, tavern or bathhouse, never to work bare handed, drink from a well, touch anything bare handed, and must warn all she met of her condition. She was then taken to the cemetery and laid in an open grave where the priest three times threw earth on her; lastly, she was taken to the leprosarium where she stayed.

Reference: Riesman, David, "Medieval Diseases and Epidemics; Leprosy," in *The Story of Medicine in the Middle Ages*, Hoeber, New York: 1935, pp. 233-40.

We're a kinder, gentler people now.

What if the PVS patients are declared dead? Then we not only can but must discontinue treatment and kill their bodies. To declare them dead is a more honest and compassionate solution than inventing the fiction that they would refuse treatment if they could. After the PVS diagnosis is done and feeding is stopped, some lethal injection would be administered. We don't even kill rats by starving them to death.

It would seem the bodies could serve some useful purposes for experimentation, as the aborted fetuses might. (See discussion in Chapter Three, "A Time to Be Born.")

If we don't lethally inject the diagnosed PVS patients, but merely withdraw artificial feeding, a problem might arise. Some diagnosed with PVS will still eat "naturally." Artificial nutrition was thought to be a good technology, an advance in medicine when developed. It still has some good uses, but the connotation is that it is evil.

If the PVS-diagnosed will eat "naturally," are they still dead? Perhaps they are being force fed, still treated "artificially." Forced feeding is being defined as putting food in the mouth of another who can't use her hands to do so. If the patient chews and swallows the food, she is still force fed. The distinction between "artificial" and "natural" nutrition may work in some cases. For example, "artificial" may refer to tube feeding of a person who can't or won't swallow.

Putting food in the mouth is considered forced feeding and is classified as artificially feeding. This gets very far back on a distinction of artificial versus natural. What shall happen to babies and toddlers who can't feed themselves? To the quadriplegic? Theoretically, eating with a spoon is "artificial."

NOTES

STUDY QUESTIONS

1. What is the year that closed chest massage at a fast rate was first reported?

2. What are the conditions under which CPR was first considered effective?

3. Under which conditions is CPR done in the hospital or nursing home setting?

4. Which is presently the only condition under which CPR is not performed in most institutions?

5. What is the ethical problem facing the Emergency Medical Technician on a call to a hospice patient?

6. What discrimination is evident in DNR orders?

7. What is the connection between futility and the DNR order?

8. What is your opinion of whether DNR orders should be suspended in the OR?

9. What CPR policy is recommended in the text?

CPR–DNR

"Call the code." The intern's words, the same words that a few minutes earlier had gathered these technicians, now froze them. A vignette of strong, competent pink youth surrounded the bed of a nude waxen white-haired 90 year old doll. The pumping, pounding, probing, and shocking ceased with the intern's call as suddenly as they began. The lady was as dead as when the nurse who shouted those first "code" words found her. Her body was a lot worse for wear, the staff's time and skill were diverted from other patients, and the hospital bill was a lot higher. She was still dead.

HISTORY

Over 100 years ago, a German surgeon, Friedrich Maass, first did external cardiac massage that succeeded. That was in 1891. In 1827, a Frenchman, Leroy-d'Etoilles, attempted to ventilate the lungs. In 1858, Silvester instituted artificial ventilation which was used for a century. Remember the arms above the head for inspiration, arms back onto chest with pressure for expiration? You're too young.

The airway obstruction was handled by pulling the tongue forward to open the airway. In 1858, a Hungarian surgeon, Janos Balassa, treated a pharyngeal obstruction with tracheostomy and resuscitation. Using earlier anesthesias sometimes resulted in "chloroform syncope." A sudden circulatory collapse resulted from anesthesia. Professor Franz Koenig of Gottingen, Germany, outlined chest massage in his 1883 text of surgery. Before, chest compressions were to be done at the rate of respiration, 12-20 per minute.

Maass's improvement was to recommend compressions at the rate of a fast pulse, 120 per minute. Maass published two cases of surgery collapse and recovery in 1891. 69 years later, William Kouwenhoven "rediscovered" external chest compression for heart massage. Lately, recommendation for modification of standard practice is to increase chest massage to the "new" rate of 120 per minute!

Reference: Gaw, Richard L., Jr., "Historical Note: Dr. Friedrich Maass: 100th Anniversary of 'New' CPR," *Clinical Cardiology,* 1991;14:1000–02.

CPR was known in the 1900s, but not used until the 1950s. The event was considered a surgical problem. Collapse outside the hospital was usually due to drowning and respiratory problems.

CPR—THE ANSWER TO EVERYTHING

CPR was such a great idea, being able to bring people back to life. It was first suggested that it be used for witnessed arrests, young people, drowning, and arrests of known etiology like anesthesia. Instead . . .

The policy of almost all hospitals <u>and</u> nursing homes in this country is that cardiopulmonary resuscitation (CPR, a "code") be done on <u>all</u> patients who die—for any reason, of any age, with any condition. Only specific orders written to the contrary stop automatic CPR.

The damage done by attempts at CPR are well known to practitioners who have performed it. (Of course if it works, it may be worth it.) The problem is that nonpractitioners do not understand that the patient is dead when CPR starts. Patients who are resuscitated are definitely better off than they were when CPR started.

When CPR started the patient was dead. The comment by a lawyer for the Task Force on Life and the Law in New York, that the patient is more debilitated after CPR than at the start, shows that the public does not understand what is happening. If the patient survives CPR, she's gone from dead to alive. (September 1991, *Medical Ethics Advisor*, p. 119.)

In a very few patients, CPR can possibly save life. In others, it will only run up the hospital bill, either for the heirs, the taxpayer, or the hospital to absorb. Cost for CPR varies from hospital to hospital, but will run to thousands of dollars.

Reported data confirm that CPR performed in a large VA hospital on patients aged over 70, or patients ill with sepsis (blood infection) or with cancer was seldom successful. Not one person resuscitated survived long enough to leave the hospital.

More data: Of arrests out of the hospital, 2 of 244 survive. Of unwitnessed arrests, 1 of 116 survive. Of asystole or EMD (electromechanical dissociation, a lethal heart arrhythmia), 1 of 237 survive. CPR is rarely effective for patients over 70. Of 503 arrests with CPR, 112 patients resuscitated, only 19 lived to discharge. When CPR was done on the patient for over 15 minutes, only 1 of 360 survived.

References: Various Authors, *JAMA*, 1988, articles on pp 2069, 2094, 2096, 2098.

Murphy, Donald J. et al, "Outcomes of CPR in the Elderly," *Annals of Internal Medicine*, 1989;111:199-205.

CPR is a procedure that is offered and done automatically for every patient even if it is not appropriate in a given case. Physicians and hospitals may fear that if they do not do CPR on all patients, they face losing a lawsuit. Not true. Caregivers are never required legally to do procedures that are useless, and indeed the reverse is true—they may find themselves sued for performing CPR without consent when the medical literature now clearly indicates the futility of the procedure in certain patients.

It has happened; after a no-code order, a patient was coded and stroked. He sued for two years of "wrongful life." The Ohio court said there was no law in Ohio giving the right to refuse treatment when not in a coma or terminally ill. The court got that reasoning from Ohio's living will law. The court said that life is not a harm and therefore dismissed the case.

The court also was concerned that allowing liability on the part of the hospital for CPR would discourage hospitals from doing CPR without authority on other patients.

Reference: *Hospital Ethics*, November–December 1991, p. 7. (See the wrongful life discussion in "A Time to Be Born.")

The law holds caregivers to the standard of practice of the community and the nation. The articles in JAMA and AIM will be evidence of what the standard of practice should be: No CPR unless it has a reasonable chance of success.

It is only a matter of time before Medicare and other insurers refuse payment for CPR ad libitum. If it is not clearly indicated by standards of practice, payment will be from the patient's funds or absorbed by the hospital. Probably only then will hospitals change the policy of automatic CPR on all patients. Patients not likely to benefit might have the procedure by requesting it be done and guaranteeing payment from their own funds.

A real problem is the hospice or other "no-code" patient outside the hospital, for whom EMS is called. Some people have gotten tags to wear as bracelets, and only half joking suggestions are made that one tattoo "DNR" on one's chest. The problem for the EMT is that she doesn't have time to be reading living wills and DNR orders, she's supposed to resuscitate first and discontinue later.

The states of Montana, New York, and Texas have put into statute provisions for community and nonhospital DNR orders. There are required forms, bracelets, and the obligatory nonliability for the EMT who honors the DNR in good faith.

Reference: Sachs, G., Miles, S., and Levin, R., "Limiting Resuscitation: Emergency Policy in the EMS," <u>Annals of Internal Medicine,</u> 1991;114:151–54.

DNR—THE ANSWER TO EVERYTHING?

With a present policy of automatic CPR for all, the DNR order becomes an issue. The order is more likely to be written for certain conditions, regardless of patient preferences. For patients with a five-year prognosis of survival, 52% of AIDS patients have DNR orders. Also with a five-year prognosis, patients with unresectable non small cell lung cancer have 47% DNR orders.

Patients with esophageal varices and cirrhosis also have only a five-year prognosis, but 16% of them have DNR orders. The five-year prognosis of death in patients with severe congestive heart failure with coronary artery disease prompted DNR orders in only 5%.

Reference: Wachter, R. M., et al, "Decisions about Resuscitation: Inequities Among Patients with Different Diseases but Similar Prognoses," *Annals of Internal Medicine,* 1989;111:525.

The American Medical Association says CPR doesn't need consent because it's an emergency. (Many practitioners will disagree that a code is always unanticipated). "No code" does not mean "no treatment", but after the DNR order, the aide will ask why she has to take the patient's blood pressure; "he's a no-code anyway".

The AMA says patients and family must be consulted before a DNR order is written. One case is reported of a suit for a DNR written without consulting a competent patient. The patient's estate counter-sued for this malpractice after the doctor sued the estate for the his bill. **Lesson:** don't sue for your bill if there's any possible problem.

Reference: AMA Council on Ethical and Judicial Affairs, "Guidelines for the Appropriate Use of DNR Orders," *JAMA*, 1991;265:1868–71.

FUTILITY IS THE ANSWER?

CPR is not necessary when it is futile. Theoretically, a DNR order does not need the patient's consent. The problem is, does the patient agree that the resuscitation will be futile? (See above discussion about value judgment of futility.)

In an emergency, we do CPR without consent. The patient doesn't have a say. If we say the CPR will be futile, we do not do CPR. We make the futility judgment, and decide no consent to withhold CPR is necessary. Again the patient doesn't have a say; this is one of the last areas of paternalism.

Reference: Scofield, Giles R. "Is Consent Useful When Resuscitation Isn't?" *Hastings Center Report*, November–December 1992, pp. 28–36.

DNR IN THE OR?

Many agencies routinely suspend DNR orders during surgery. Several reasons are given. The death is likely to be due to anesthesia or drugs administered, and is reversible. The OR and the anesthesiologist or anesthetist don't want the investigation that a death in the OR would bring. Traditionally, the primary physician's orders are superseded by the OR team during surgery.

A person who does not want resuscitation in a nonsurgery situation possibly would not want it during surgery either. This exception to the DNR order should be discussed with patient and family. They should be made aware of the hospital's policy and the possibility, likelihood, or certainty of resuscitation being performed if arrest happens during surgery. Funny, we don't call arrest "**death.**"

Reference: Walker, R. "DNR in the OR," *JAMA* 1991;266: 2407-11, and January 1992, *Medical Ethics Advisor*, 7-9.

Careful. At present, a living will is not the same as (and may not call for) a DNR order. And a DNR order may not mean that the patient wants to die. In future, we may see some rules that patients who have living wills, or who do not want resuscitation, will not be admitted to the hospital. Perhaps they will be keep out of ICU's where one of the goals is to save live with resuscitation and all available means.

THIS IS THE ANSWER

Should the policy of agencies be that no CPR be used on any patient over 70, or with sepsis, or with any form of cancer? The problem with present policy is that it applies to all. That would be the problem with a broad DNR policy as well. CPR, as with any other extraordinary invasive procedure, should be done only if ordered by the physician and consented to by the patient in advance. If that is the hospital policy (selectively ordered CPR) then no DNR order   ever need be discussed or written. Patients will assume they will not be resuscitated unless they request it. An order for CPR will be written and consented to, as orders for surgery are discussed and consented to.

If for some reason the patient cannot communicate, the same rules apply as in other invasive procedures. The physician will decide in an emergency, especially if an arrest happens immediately after admission or in the ER. If no emergency exists the physician will consult with the family or guardian before ordering CPR be done in the event of death.

CPR is an extraordinary measure to be instituted only when specifically ordered by the physician and consented to in advance by the patient.

Reference: Hall, Jacqulyn, "Call the Code," *The Aspec Review*, 1989; 2:15. Academy of Senior Professionals at Eckerd College

STUDY QUESTIONS

1.   What is the definition of "euthanasia?"

2.   What Nazi assumption allowed the killing of millions of people?

3.   What are the three pairs of conditions applied to euthanasia?

4.   What is the difference between "active" and "passive euthanasia?"

5. What is the difference between "voluntary" and "involuntary euthanasia?"

6. What is the difference between "direct" and "indirect euthanasia?"

7. What is the definition of "suicide?"

8. What is the definition of "assisted suicide?"

9. Do you agree or disagree with the statement and why? Euthanasia or assisted suicide is a relatively new ethical conflict.

10. What are some examples of attempts to pass laws allowing assisted suicide in the U.S.

11. What is the position of the Catholic Church on pain control and death?

12. What is your opinion on whether Nancy Cruzan's death was euthanasia and whether it was caused directly or indirectly, actively or passively, voluntarily or involuntarily?

13. What are some of the values present in an assisted suicide conflict?

14. Why do societies either make suicide illegal or discourage it?

15. What are some examples of the preoccupation about death?

16. What are the reasons some give that the practitioner should assist suicide?

17. What are the reasons some give that practitioners should not assist suicide?

18. Do you agree or disagree with this statement and why? Euthanasia is legal in Holland.

19. Why you think the Dutch guidelines for euthanasia should or should not be adopted in this country?

EUTHANASIA

I had a country mouse friend who was disappointed every time she heard that a program about this topic was coming on the radio. She'd get all interested and ready to hear about young people in China or something, and on would come this stuff about death and old people.

Whatever proportions [Nazi] crimes finally assumed, it became evident to all who investigated them that they had started from small beginnings. The beginnings at first were merely a subtle shift in emphasis in the basic attitude of the physicians.

It started with the acceptance of the attitude, basic in the euthanasia movement, that there is such a thing as life not worthy to be lived. This attitude in its early stages concerned itself merely with the severely and chronically sick. Gradually the sphere of those to be included in this category was enlarged to encompass the socially unproductive, the ideologically unwanted, the racially unwanted and finally all non-Germans.

But it is important to realize that the infinitely small wedged-in lever from which this entire trend of mind received its impetus was the attitude toward the nonrehabilitable sick:

Alexander, Leo, "Medical Science under Dictatorship," *NEJM*, (July 14, 1949), 241:2;39-47.

Nurses and their organizations cooperated fully with the Nazis in killing patients under that government. Few nursing texts acknowledge the terrible active role that nurses took in Nazi euthanasia.

Little wedge: On the first day of World War II, September 1, 1939, Hitler charged Karl Brandt, official head of the medical profession with this duty:

Reichsleiter Bouhler and Dr. Brandt, M.D., are charged with the responsibility of enlarging the authority of certain physicians to be designated by me in such a manner that persons who, according to human judgment, are incurably sick may, upon the most careful diagnosis of their medical condition, be accorded a mercy death.

("Biomedical Ethics and the Shadow of Nazism: A Conference on the Proper Use of the Nazi Analogy in Ethical Debate," April 8, 1976, Hastings Center.)

This is not 1939, and in this country we have many kinds of people. We are not inflicted with aspiration to an ideal state inhabited by a pure race. But we have to keep in mind any possible analogy to that time and that aspiration, as we struggle to make ethical decisions about dying people now.

Euthanasia comes from "eu" Greek for "well," and "thanasia" for "dying," "death," so the phrase means "well or good death." Usually the term is applied to a painless easy death for people suffering from incurable and painful illness. We practitioners don't need to hide from ourselves that we are talking about death, so we will use English instead of Greek here. What are the arguments?

Six kinds of good death are possible. As you will recognize from other concepts, there are often two opposites created in theories, for three conditions. We can have active or passive good death, direct or indirect, voluntary or involuntary. Some prefer to add a non voluntary, for people in a coma who cannot consent to nor refuse killing. Suicide comes in here, and assisted suicide.

Active euthanasia has the practitioner doing something actively to cause the death of the patient. Passive is withdrawing or withholding treatment that preserves life. As we have discussed above, these are not very helpful distinctions except in the most obvious cases, such as actively administering a lethal injection.

Direct good death is a result of an act intended to cause death, while indirect good death is the result of an act not intended to cause death in the first instance but which has that result. Such is the case of that last injection of morphine for the pain, which also then causes respiratory depression and death results.

Voluntary good death is obvious; the patient wants the death. Involuntary is the opposite; death is caused without the request of the patient.

Suicide is the patient killing herself. An active, voluntary, direct, unassisted death is suicide. Assisted suicide is the helping by someone (in our discussion a practitioner) with the killing.

At this time we have not agreed that involuntary death is legal or ethical. Capital punishment is an exception, and we haven't agreed on that. The death of PVS patients is involuntary; they have no volition. We do not all agree that such patients wanted death, that they volunteered.

Many have agreed that an indirect death, as a result of pain control, especially, is acceptable. Passive death, as a result of withdrawing treatments that harm and do not help, is accepted if voluntary. Many would agree that voluntary death is acceptable; some would not.

Culling out most of what is at least less disagreeable, we come to the main disagreement: Should voluntary, direct, active death be permitted? If unassisted, that is suicide. Should practitioners be permitted or sanctioned to assist such suicide?

HISTORY

As are so many ethical conflicts we have discussed, this is an old issue. Peoples in prehistory, if behavior of aboriginal people is any indication, dealt with the dying and their "care." The Greeks talked a lot about good death and suicide. Suicide is a concept that is closely related to assisted suicide and euthanasia. Plato in his ideal society would have permitted voluntary, direct medical killing of the incurably ill or disabled.

Aristotle thought that suicide and mercy killing violated the deal, the social contract, that individuals had with each other. And it was not virtuous. Hippocrates said, "I will neither give a deadly drug to anybody if asked for it, nor will I make a suggestion to this effect."

The Saints, Augustine (5th century) and Thomas Aquinas (13th) (not New Orleans) opposed suicide on religious grounds. They thought suffering, and life, are given by God. Utopians, as characterized in the writing of Sir Thomas More of the 1500s, thought suicide would be part of the "good life." Christians were generally against it.

Concepts of individualism, freedom, and reason started new debate about the subject in the 17th, 18th, and 19th centuries.

A Euthanasia Society was founded in Great Britain in 1936. Initiatives to legalize euthanasia were started in Ohio in 1906, Nebraska in 1937, and New York in 1939. All failed. The Nazi experience of killing and calling it euthanasia gave the whole movement a bad name with which it still clings.

In 1957, Roman Catholic Pope Pius XII distinguished "ordinary versus extraordinary" and sanctioned terminal patients' use of pain medication even if life is shortened.

We have already seen several cases under "Withholding and Withdrawing" in which involuntary, direct, passive death has been caused. The Cruzan case is primary. The argument can be made that her death was voluntary in that she would have wished it. One can argue that it was indirect since no lethal injection was administered. The primary objective in removing her gastrostomy tube was to cause death.

The indirect-direct distinction is as unhelpful here as the withholding-withdrawing, and some other distinctions without difference. The rabbit analogy arises. You don't feed your rabbit, but you don't intend for him to die. When he dies, did you cause his death directly or indirectly? Was he "allowed to die?"

Tort law has for centuries dealt with actions and intentions. If the person does an act (not feeding or watering a dog, for instance, is deemed and act) and the person knows the consequences which will follow the act, he is assumed in law to have intended the consequence.

Our unwillingness to face the reality of what we intend, to take responsibility for what we are doing, causes us to be extremely cruel in "letting nature take its course." (Of course if these patients don't feel pain, then perhaps there's no ethical problem).

When we kill animals at the pound, we don't lock them up and deny them food and water, we "put them out of their misery." It seems odd that we would do less for a person (admittedly, some people do not think this is a human).

The interests here are those of the individual, in life. That interest may be secondary to relief of pain (autonomy). The family's interest is in helping a loved one (beneficence). The practitioner's interest is in helping, (beneficence), in not harming (nonmaleficence). All of us together as the state or society have some interest in protecting people unable to protect themselves (beneficence).

The question about suicide arises. Is suicide in the best interest of people who don't want to live, for whatever reason? Can we prohibit suicide, or helping people kill themselves, when we don't know their psychic pain?

Societies prohibit suicide because we assume it is an irrational act. We assume life is better than death, and someone choosing death who doesn't have physical pain is irrational and needs help to live, not to die. That is our rationale for making assisted suicide illegal; suicide itself usually is not. Virtually all people who kill themselves are depressed; treatment for depression has become dramatically more effective in the last decade."

More politically interesting are the initiatives in Washington State which failed in 1991, but garnered 46% of the people's support. The initiative would make legal voluntary, active, direct death. The rationale that many offer is the fear, not of death, but of dying a lingering death, attached to machines, among strangers, in pain, without dignity.

Such an initiative was proposed and failed for California in 1992, passed in Oregon in 1994, and the Washington law outlawing Assisted Suicide was held unconstitutional in 1996. A Supreme Court review of the issue is likely.

Other signs of the concern: A best seller was the suicide manual of the Hemlock Society, authored by the founder. The society was founded by Derek Humphrey in 1980. In his book, <u>Final Exit</u>, he gives instructions for suicide and advocates that practitioners prescribe and administer fatal drugs if asked to do so.

Dr. Jack Kevorkian is a retired Michigan pathologist who has helped several people commit active, voluntary, direct death—suicide—in Michigan. He asserts that he assisted the people in suicide. Assisted suicide was not against the law of Michigan at the time (it is in other states). He was acquitted of violating a subsequent law against assisting suicide.

Dr. Kevorkian's license to practice has been revoked in all states, and he has been disciplined for practicing in a "negligent or incompetent manner" and using drugs for other than lawful <u>therapeutic</u> purposes." (See the "Professionals and Employees" section for licensure discussion.)

Dr. Kevorkian has written a book (surprise!) which advocates his long-standing argument that death row inmates to be executed be allowed to choose anesthesia and organ donation so their bodies are not wasted. He calls his apparatus for administering lethal drugs a Mercitron and suggests a new specialty of medicine, Obitiatry, for such patients.
Another suggestion for specialty is a combination of care for the dying, hospice and good death—"telostics," advocated in Crisp, R., "A Good Death: Who Best to Bring It?" *Bioethics*, 1987;1:74-79.

Another recent book details a woman's assistance in her terminally ill mother's death by self-administered prescription drugs, Betty Rollin's<u>Last Wish</u>. Is there any ethical question about profiting, through book sales, from the misery of people who find life so painful that death is preferable?

Or are these writers performing a valuable service for those people, and deserve to be highly rewarded? Or is there any moral question at all, there's just a market and these people produce a product that people want?

The medical community has debated the issue with several incidents. In one, a physician claimed to have put to death a terminally ill young woman with a lethal injection. He then wrote a letter about it which was printed in a major medical journal (involuntary, direct, active death).

Reference: Anonymous, "It's Over, Debbie," *JAMA*, 1988; 259:272.

NOTES

And another physician wrote of his role in writing a prescription for his patient's use in suicide, and distinguished three levels of physician participation:

1. Administering euthanasia: voluntary or involuntary; direct, active;
2. Assisting suicide by prescription: voluntary, direct, active; and
3. Refusing treatment or abstaining from treatment: voluntary or involuntary, direct or indirect, passive.

As a result of his article in a medical journal, the patient's identity was made known, her cadaver discovered stored at a local community college for dissection. A grand jury heard charges of assisted suicide and failed to indict him for trial. The law asked if he "intentionally causes or aids another to commit suicide."

Reference: Quill, T., "Death and Dignity: A Case of Individualized Decision Making," *NEJM* 1991;324:691–94.

Predictably, reaction to the article was heated and varied. The assault to medical ethics are seen as follows:

1. The issue diverts and hides the real need to better manage dying care, especially pain control.
2. The image of practitioner as healer would be irretrievably lost.
3. The trust of the patient in practitioner would suffer.

As discussed in the section above on futility, practitioners who have acquiesced in other patient demands will find it hard to take a high moral ground in this patient demand.

On the pro side, the patient needs relief from suffering. Allowing a good death relieves and prevents loss of control; ends fear of dying among strangers, on machines, without dignity. The individual has a right to his own body, his autonomy, his freedom; he can forego treatment, so why can't he ask the practitioner to help him die instead of suffering longer?

On the "con" side, consider the slippery slope to involuntary killing. This will happen secretly, because voluntary death will first be tolerated, then encouraged, then pressure brought to bear to end life. Grandma would feel subtle pressure to request the death, to leave her assets for others. Women would be especially susceptible to pressure, giving to the end.

Soon there would be pressure to have a surrogate decide on the good death for patients who can't voluntarily request it, or who don't have good families who request it for them like Nancy Cruzan's. If we allow competent people to get out of terrible lives, how can we discriminate against the incompetent, the helpless trapped in hopeless existences?

There would be subtle but real discrimination as surrogates decide who would want involuntary death. The poor, old, black, handicapped (mental and physical), alcoholic, drug addicted, AIDS, all would be seen as more miserable than others, would they not?

Reference: Singer, Peter and Siegler, Mark, "Euthanasia: A Critique," *NEJM*, 1990;322:1881–83.

The government's position is this: "Policies prohibiting direct killing may also conflict with the important value of patient self-determination.... The Commission finds this limitation on individual self-determination to be an acceptable cost of securing the general protection of human life afforded by the prohibition of direct killing."

Reference: President's Commission, details above.

THE DUTCH DO IT BETTER?

Holland now has legalized intentional death. Earlier, they had an agreement that the law against active good death will not be prosecuted (enforced) if certain conditions were met.

The conditions are as follows:

1.   Patient must be competent (not Quinlan, Cruzan, newborns handicapped, Alzheimers).

2.   Patient must request voluntarily, consistently, repeatedly over reasonable time and document these requests (not impulsive).

3. Patient must suffer intolerably, with no prospect of relief (no need to be terminal). Depression would not qualify, we have treatment; but a Dutch court exonerated a doctor who killed a patient merely depressed. But amyotrophic lateral sclerosis maybe (the disease the brilliant British physicist Stephen Hawking has survived with for 27 years).

4. Physician performs, with analysis by another doctor not involved in the original care.

Usually, death results after a barbiturate is given to put the patient to sleep, then curare is used to paralyze the breathing muscles.

The estimates vary widely as to how many deaths are caused in Holland yearly, from 2300 to 20,000. They believe a minimum 2% of all deaths are caused by physicians. The actual number is not known; despite the law's requirement, Dutch doctors don't put on the death certificate the required "unnatural causes." If this is listed, a formal inquiry must be held, so the doctors lie, though they have no liability if they comply with the list above.

Some 54% of Dutch doctors say they have performed intentional death, or assisted suicide. Assisted suicide is different from intentional death. Assisted suicide is prescribing drugs which patients later administer themselves. That prescribing is illegal in Holland. Only 186 intentional deaths were reported in Holland in 1988. Physicians admit, in an anonymous study, to assisting 386 suicides, causing 2318 deaths after request, and causing 1030 deaths without request (involuntary euthanasia).

Psychiatrists worry that many of the Dutch requesting death are depressed and could be helped with therapy if they were treated by other than general practitioners.

Still the problem remains: what about the patient who is terminally ill, unrelieved by medication? Or who wishes to have the struggle end, and who is not just suffering from depression. Shall we keep him alive, when our efforts have kept him alive to suffer?

Reference: Smith, Martin L., et al, "A Good Death: Is Euthanasia the Answer?" *Cleveland Clinic Journal of Medicine*, 1992;59:99–109.

Perhaps practitioners will recognize that their patients die, and they need care in dying as much and more than in getting "well." Perhaps practitioners will work to control their patient's pain, as Pope Pius XII sanctioned in 1957 and the American Nurses Association said in 1992.

Increasing titration of medication to achieve adequate symptom control, even at the expense of maintaining life or hastening death secondarily, is ethically justified. (Position Statement on Promotion of Comfort and Relief of Pain in Dying Patients. The American Nurse, *February 1992, p. 7.)*

But is Assisted Suicide Ethical for the Practitioner?

The national standard of ethics for nurses is that nurses do no assist patients to kill themselves, but already threat of Measure 16 has caused erosion of that standard in Oregon.

The American Nurses Association maintains that nurses may not ethically assist suicide (as they would be asked to do under Measure 16):

"Nurses, individually and collectively, have an obligation to provide comprehensive and compassionate end-of-life care which includes the promotion of comfort and the relief of pain, and at times, foregoing life-sustaining treatments. The American Nurses Association (ANA) believes that the nurse should not participate in assisted suicide. Such an act is in violation of the Code for Nurses With Interpretative Statements (Code for Nurses) and ethical traditions of the profession."

Position Statement on Assisted Suicide. American Nurses Association, Washington, D.C., 1994, p.1.

The National Oncology Nurses Society endorsed the ANA position in 1995, in their document, Endorsement of ANA Position Statement on Active Euthanasia and Assisted Suicide, Oncological Nurses Society, 1995. The National Association of Profile Nurses, and its Oregon Affiliate, Oregon Nurses for Life and Health, oppose assisted suicide in the strongest terms, believing it tantamount to euthanasia:
"The public must be assured that we will not participate in euthanasia or refer people to individuals and organizations supporting euthanasia,and that we consider euthanasia to be medical murder."

Valko, Nancy Guilfoy, National Nurses Group Supports Resistance to Euthanasia.

National Association of Prolife Nurses, Elysian, MN, 1994.

Though addressed to the prohibition against nurses' participation in executions, the following ecompasses the ethical standard of the ANA for causing death in patients:

"Regardless of the personal opinion of the nurse on the moral appropriateness of capital punishment, either generally or specifically, it is a breach of the ethical tradition of nursing, and its Code for Nurses, to participate in taking human life, even through a legally authorized civil or military execution."

Position Statement on Capital Punishment. American Nurses Association, Kansas City, MO: 1988

> Brief of Amicus Curia, National Association of Profile Nurses. Lee v. Oregon, Ninth Circuit of Appeals 95-3505 et seg (1996)

Reference: Kass, Leon R., "Neither for Love Nor Money: Why Doctors Must Not Kill," *The Public Interest*, No. 94, Winter 1989, pp. 25-46.

STUDY QUESTIONS AND ANSWERS

These are suggested answers. If you have something like these answers in your own words, consider yourself successful. If you have more (quality, not quantity) than these answers, consider yourself excellent.

1.   What is the error in the idea that to get old is to have failed?

- People who "fail" at surviving are dead
- The old are the successful people at surviving

2.   What is the definition of "end-of-life?"

   A euphemism for dying and death

3.   What is the definition of "longevity?"

- The length of life a person will achieve
- Not life expectancy, which is the average length of life of a mythical person born this year

4.   How is life expectancy computed? Give a phrase as a synonym!

- Add up the ages of all the people who died last year, and divide by the number of people who died
- A synonym is "average age of people who died last year"

5. What is one factor that affects life expectancy numbers?

   The age at death, especially the infant mortality rate (number of infants dying before one year of age)

6. Which is the correct statement: People are living to be older now. More people are living to be old now.

   Second statement

7. What is your own personal risk of heart attack if you are in a group whose risk (lass probability) of heart attack is 30%?

   Your own personal probability (called case probability) of heart attack is either 100% or 0%

8. What are the values encountered in ethical conflicts around the time to die?

   • Life
   • Autonomy
   • Beneficence
   • Nonmaleficence
   • Though it isn't in the text, that value always underlying—Money-work

9. What is a complicating factor in our relationships with patients that affects our work as practitioners?

   We are strangers more than in times past

10. What did you observe on your visit to a nursing home, and would you rather be there as a patient or dead?

    • Do this exercise for this class, but more for your own self to dispel some myths—or confirm some fears?

11. What is the definition of "insanity" given by the physician in the text?

    Refusal to consent

12. What is the greatest fear the competent have of becoming incompetent?

    Loss of control over everything

13. What is the difference between people who are "incompetent" and people who are "incapacitated?"

    - The words are different
    - The people are the same

14. Another two-word term for "competency" is _____.

    Decisional capacity

15. Is the determination of competence a legal process only?

    Competence is a legal determination too, but in dealing with patients practitioners make such determinations daily

16. What are the three components of decisional capacity?

    1. Patient can receive and evaluate information
    2. Patient can think about information and communicate the decision
    3. Patient knows the consequences of his decision.

17. Describe a patient who seems to have capacity but fails the third part of the test, the knowledge of consequences of his decision.

    You probably have seen cases like this; for example, a little old lady refuses surgery on her broken hip and yet believes she can go home and walk on it

18. Why is the practitioner's standard for decisional capacity or competence always a personal one at first?

    - We cannot get inside another's skin
    - So we must start with what our own reasoning and reactions and decisions would be
    - And measure the patient against that

19. A person who has been adjudged incompetent in a court proceeding is called the _____; the person who is appointed to make decisions for her is the _____.

    - Ward
    - Guardian

20. What is the definition of "advance directives."

    Written or spoken directives that competent people make for their care or treatment in the event that they become incompetent

21. What is the effect of advance directives if the patient is competent?

   - The advance directive is of no effect
   - It is only implemented when and if the patient becomes incompetent

22. What is the difference between a living will and a durable (springing) power of attorney?

   - A living will is an advance directive to anyone who may be a practitioner for the patient after she is incompetent, saying what treatment she wants or doesn't want
   - A durable power of attorney is an advance directive to one person, saying who the patient wants to make decisions for her after she is incompetent

23. Are spoken living wills of any use?

   - Living wills need not be written to be effective
   - Spoken statements to friends or family can be used to determine what the person's wishes for treatment were in the event she became incompetent
   - They were used in the Cruzan case

24. What relationship do we now have with patients which has in part caused the increased use of advance directives?

   We are strangers to our patients, so instead of knowing what they want because we know them, we must rely on formal directives

25. Why don't people write living wills or durable powers of attorney?

   - I don't know, so whatever you wrote may be better than my answer
   - Maybe they don't want to think about dying
   - Maybe they think their family will make the right decisions
   - Maybe they don't think they'll get sick
   - Maybe, just maybe, they want all the treatment you can provide for them; may be they don't want to die.

26. What should be the attitude of the practitioner toward advance directives that seem inappropriate in the circumstances?

    - As always, the practitioner must take responsibility for appropriate care, taking into account the patient's wishes as expressed in an advance directive
    - The advance directive cannot substitute for judgment

27. Why do most people seem not to want their advance directives followed rigidly?

    Because the future is a difficult thing to predict, and the patient does have trust in the practitioner and family to act for his beneficence— even if the practitioner is a stranger

28. Why do some people think a written advance directive is preferable to a spoken one?

    Because written evidence is easier to produce and prove in court.

29. What is the validity of a spoken advance directive, compared to a written one?

    - They are of equal validity
    - The written one is easier to prove in court, and perhaps in the hospital too

30. What are the ethics of ignoring the directives in a living will or durable (springing) power of attorney?

    - If the directives are appropriate in the judgment of the practitioner, then to ignore them is to violate the patient's autonomy
    - The problem is that the practitioner must evaluate their appropriateness, to use the judgment and beneficence expected and required of the practitioner
    - This in turn opens the danger of paternalism, of the practitioner doing good for the patient at the expense of the patient's autonomy

31. What is one ethical concern that has been raised about advance directives?

    - People are unable to project from a position of health, well-being, and competence what their wishes would be from a very different perspective

- The advance directive might be different from what they would want and different from what is in their best interest when they are later in different circumstances

32. What is the main requirement of the Danforth Amendment to the Medicare law (the Patient Self-Determination Act)?

    Patients must be told of their right to refuse treatment

33. What do you believe is the purpose of the law?

    - Whatever you believe is valid, but you should have mentioned one of the following:
    - The increase of knowledge of the patient about right to refuse treatment and about advance directives
    - The economic benefit if long-term or expensive care is refused by patients
    - And the belief that practitioners prolong lives out of greed

34. What is the meaning of the terms "withhold" and "withdraw," "active" and "passive," and "to treat" versus "to limit treatment?"

    - Withhold and withdraw are in theory the same, though they seem different in practice
    - Active and passive are not helpful distinctions regarding decisions about limiting treatment
    - The actual difference is between treating and limiting treatment
    - The idea of no treatment for ill people is difficult for the practitioner to conceptualize

35. What is the mental condition of the patients that most ethical conflicts are about?

    Incompetent

36. What are two of the myths about terminating life support that are false?

    Pick the two from the list in the text that are most prevalent at your institution and give examples of statements that real people have made

37. What value is highest in the American Thoracic Society's guidelines for terminating futile treatment?

    - The value of the practitioner's autonomy, her freedom to decide when a treatment is futile

- At that point the practitioner can withdraw treatment regardless of the patient or surrogate's wishes

38. What are the values in the futility issue—specifically, the Helga Wanglie case?

   - Patient autonomy
   - Practitioner autonomy (determination of what is futile treatment)
   - Beneficence and nonmaleficence not so much
   - Money-work--for the hospital, for the staff, for the insurance company in this case, but in general for whomever pays the bill

39. Could the doctors have handled this case differently?, or might they have wanted to go to court?

   - We cannot know their motives
   - There is no evidence that they engaged in an ethical conflict-solving process with Mr. Wanglie
   - They could have made the decision to discontinue the ventilator without going to court
   - Mr. Wanglie could not sue them if the court ordered the ventilator removed
   - This medical center is the home of Dr. Ronald Cranston, a well-known advocate of discontinuing life support for PUPs

40. What would an opposite decision have meant regarding futility of treatment?

   - Doctors could decide when treatment is futile without considering patient wishes
   - The value of practitioner autonomy would be more important than the value of patient autonomy
   - Doctors would have the authority to terminate life support without patient or family permission; they would have gotten authority without responsibility

41. What are examples of practitioner acquiescence to patient demands, which may make it harder for practitioners to assert their autonomy to decide when treatment is futile?

   Any treatment that practitioners give which does not have medical necessity erodes the authority of practitioners to later assert that they do not have to give treatment that is not medically necessary

42. What is the primary purpose of any "tool" or measurement of health or illness or quality of life?

    To obtain a number that makes a subjective evaluation seem or be objective

43. What is evidence that courts are not often involved in decisions to limit treatment?

    - 1.3 million people die yearly, 20 million since 1976, from decisions to limit treatment (usually with DNR orders)
    - Yet only 60 or so cases around this issue have been reported in the law

44. What is the difference in the use of the terms "substituted judgment" from "best interest?"

    - "Substituted judgment" is used when another substitutes his judgment for the patient; he judges what the patient would want
    - "Best interest" is used when the decision maker decides what is in the best interest of the patient (it's hard to see how best interest is different from just interest)
    - Since the judgment of the patient would be in his interest, the tests do not really differ
    - The result will be the same using either test

45. Why are family or people close to the patient named as decision makers?

    Because they know the patient well, they are better able to guess what she would judge for herself, and they will be affected

46. What are the three standards of evidence discussed and used in American law? List them from the most difficult to prove to the easiest, and give examples where each is used.

    - Beyond a reasonable doubt; criminal cases
    - Clear and convincing evidence; to prove patients like Nancy Cruzan wanted no treatment
    - Preponderance of the evidence; in civil cases like malpractice

47. Why is the Cruzan case so significant in American bioethics?

    - It's the first case of its kind (not the last-assisted suicide is coming) to be decided by the U.S. Supreme Court
    - It establishes for the first time a constitutional, not just state law, right to refuse treatment

48. What is one reason the courts might want to impose a standard of clear and convincing evidence before terminating treatment?

   • Because the decision to terminate is fatal, thus irreversible
   • Sometimes patients do recover
   • Or do they just want people to suffer?

49. What is another source of rights, remedy, or relief for persons who want treatment terminated, other than the U.S. Constitution's right to refuse treatment under the 14th Amendment liberty interest?

   The state constitution may have a specific written privacy right

50. What is the definition of "Persistent Vegetative State."

   • A relatively newly defined condition in which the patient has brain stem function, but no apparent "higher" brain function of thought, emotion, or voluntary motion
   • A synonym for Permanently Unconscious

51. What is the definition of "death?"

   • As a starting point—cessation of spontaneous respiration and heartbeat
   • That won't do, because we have had people maintained on ventilators some believed were "dead" (and we need their body parts)
   • Add, then, the cessation of all brain function as determined on 2 EEGs taken 24 hours apart (the definition in some state laws)
   • That won't do, we still have people lying in institutions not thinking, that some believe are "dead"
   • Go on to include diagnosis as being in a Persistent Vegetative State
   • That won't do; perhaps, we must include the absence of life in the absence of a clear consensus

52. What are the consequences of declaring PVS patients to be dead?

   • They will not be treated
   • They will be allowed to die by dehydration and be buried
   • Or their bodies might be used for organ retrieval

53. In which disease was the patient diagnosed as such declared to be dead.

   Leprosy

54. What is the difference between "artificial" and "natural" feeding?

- Start with artificial: IV's, total parental nutrition, nasogastric tube, gastrostomy, liquid formulas by bottle, "force feeding" with a spoon, spoons, cooked food.
- Natural: Apples, as in the garden of Eden; back to romanticism?

55. What is the year that closed chest massage at a fast rate was first reported?

1891

56. What are the conditions for which CPR was first considered effective?

- Young patients
- Witnessed arrests
- Drowning
- Anesthesia deaths

57. For which conditions is CPR done in the hospital or nursing home setting?

Any death

58. Which is presently the only condition under which CPR is not performed in most institutions?

When a DNR order is written

59. What is the ethical problem facing the Emergency Medical Technician on a call to a hospice patient?

She would like to honor patient autonomy, but her duty under the beneficence value is to resuscitate when called, and not to spend time with decisions about living wills

60. What discrimination is evident in DNR orders?

For the same five-year prognosis, some conditions (AIDS, lung cancer) are much more likely to have DNR orders than other conditions; such as coronary artery disease with congestive heart failure

61. What is the connection between futility and the DNR order?

- Theoretically, if the practitioner feels a treatment is futile, no treatment need be given. CPR is such a treatment

- However, as noted above, futility is a subjective judgment by the practitioner and always involves assessment of someone else's quality of life
- Discussion with patient and family at a minimum would be required for a finding of futility

62. What is your opinion of whether DNR orders should be suspended in the OR?

- Whatever you think, but include discussion about patient autonomy versus practitioner autonomy to decide treatment
- Some economic interest may be here, too, in the "OR record" of the surgeon and anesthesia team

63. What is CPR policy recommended in the text?

- The recommended policy is that CPR not be done without an order and consent, just as surgery is
- CPR would be done if the patient arrested on first admission before orders were written
- Since no code would be done without an order, no DNR order would ever be needed

64. What is the definition of "euthanasia."

- In Greek, good death
- As used in English discussions of euthanasia, intentionally causing death
- In some other definitions, "mercy killing"

65. What Nazi assumption allowed killing of millions of people?

That some lives were not worth living

66. What are the three pairs of conditions applied to euthanasia?

- Active-passive
- Voluntary-involuntary
- Direct–indirect

67. What is the difference between "active" and "passive euthanasia?"

While not a helpful distinction, active is (for instance) giving a lethal injection, while an example of passive is removing a ventilator

68. What is the difference between "voluntary" and "involuntary euthanasia?"

- "Voluntary death" occurs when the patient wishes it
- "Involuntary death" is death without the patient's wishing it

69. What is the difference between "direct" and "indirect euthanasia?"

- "Direct" is accomplished when you intend the patient's death
- "Indirect" is when you did not intend it, but it happened as a result of your actions

70. What is the definition of "suicide?"

- Active, direct, voluntary killing of oneself
- Or just killing oneself

71. What is the definition of "assisted suicide?"

- Assisting a suicide
- Suicide will always be a voluntary act by definition
- So assisting a patient to die who isn't volunteering cannot be assisting suicide
- It must be some kind of killing, whether mercy or not

72. Do you agree or disagree with the following statement and why? Euthanasia, and assisted suicide, are relatively new ethical conflicts.

- You should have disagreed
- Like most of the ethical conflicts you have studied, this is not new
- In your answer you should give an example from history about suicide
- You're right we are recently giving it more attention

74. What are some examples of attempts to pass laws allowing assisted suicide in the U.S.?

You should mention the Ohio, Nebraska, or New York attempts earlier this century and more recent law in Oregon and court decision finding the Washington Law unconstitutional

75. What is the position of the Catholic Church on pain control and death?

In 1957, the Pope gave sanction to the use of pain control, even if the medication hastened death secondarily

76. What is your opinion on whether Nancy Cruzan's death was euthanasia, was caused directly or indirectly, actively or passively, voluntarily or involuntarily.

   Whichever you answered is right, as long as you discuss all the concepts in terms of a permanently unconscious patient whose feedings and fluids were discontinued

77. What are some of the values present in an assisted suicide conflict?

   - Autonomy
   - Life
   - Beneficence
   - Nonmaleficence
   - And, of course, money-work

78. Why do societies either make suicide illegal or discourage it?

   - Because it is in opposition to our assumption that people act in their own best interest
   - So we assume they are irrational and need help to live, not die

79. What are some examples of the preoccupation about death?

   - Possible answers are the initiatives in Washington, California and Oregon to permit assisted suicide
   - A best seller about suicide
   - A doctor with a "suicide machine," and other books and articles in medical journals about the practitioner's role in suicide and death of patients
   - Possibly even the relatively recent interest in advance directives

80. What are the reasons some give that the practitioner should assist suicide?

   - The patient got into this painful death with the practitioner's assistance—the practitioner should not abandon him
   - The patient wants it
   - The practitioner has no business substituting his paternalistic judgment for the patient's autonomy
   - The knowledge that the practitioner will help allows the patient control, and avoids the fear of dying among strangers in pain

81. What are the reasons some give that practitioners should not assist suicide?

     •   The slippery slope goes from assisting voluntary suicide to involuntary killing
     •   If practitioners will assist with suicides, people will feel pressure to choose it, to spare their families concern and money
     •   Poor and the minorities in the society would be the easiest to kill, since their lives are seen as the worst

82. Do you agree or disagree with the following statement and why? Euthanasia is legal in Holland.

     It's not illegal, if done within guidelines

83. Why you think the Dutch process should or should not be adopted in this country?

     Whatever you believe is right, as long as you defend your belief with an explanation of what the Dutch procedure or experience is, and how it would translate into America

UNIT FIVE EXAM

HSM 510
Ethical Considerations in Health Care Delivery

SCANTRON FORM INSTRUCTIONS

Please follow these instructions for completing your Scantron form:

1. Use a #2 pencil **only.**

2. Enter the five-digit Test Number in the box marked **TEST No.** Shade in the corresponding boxes.

    The test number for this exam is: **51005**

3. Enter your Social Security Number in the box marked **SOCIAL SECURITY NUMBER.** Shade the corresponding boxes.

4. Enter your Course Code number in the box marked **COURSE CODE.** Shade in the corresponding boxes.

    The course code is: **510**

5. Print your name, address, and social security number on the lines provided.

6. Enter the estimated number of hours (to the nearest whole hour) you spent on this lesson (this is for our statistical purposes only). Fill in the appropriate boxes.

7. Be careful to darken the entire area within the boxes.

8. Do not make any marks outside the boxes. Completely erase all mistakes. **Do not use whiteout.**

9. Send the Scantron form to CCHS for grading. Your test results will be mailed to you.

If you have any questions regarding your exams or any other questions or comments, please write them on a **Request for Help** form and send it in to CCHS with the Scantron form. **DO NOT STAPLE** anything to the form. Be sure to write your name, SSN, phone number (optional), and Test Number on the **Request for Help** form. GOOD LUCK!!

UNIT FIVE EXAM

MULTIPLE CHOICE

Select the *best* answer to each of the following questions. Mark your responses on the Scantron form.

1. Lifespan is _____.

    a. life expectancy
    b. the length of life actually lived
    c. the average age at death last year
    d. the years of life you are expected to live

2. Identify one factor that does **not** affect life expectancy numbers.

    a. the quality of health care in the future
    b. the age of people dying last year
    c. infant mortality rates
    d. the number of people who died last year

3. Which is true?

    a. More individuals live to be old now than formerly
    b. Individuals live to be older now than formerly

4. If you are in a group whose risk, or class probability, of heart attack is 30%, what is your personal case probability of heart attack?

    a. 100%
    b. 30%
    c. either A or D will be correct eventually
    d. 0%

5. Which is the definition of "insanity" given by the physician in the text regarding consent.

    a. the patient is insane, he refused treatment
    b. the patient is sane, he refused treatment
    c. the patient is insane, he consented to treatment
    d. the patient is sane, he consented to treatment

6. Differentiate between people who are incompetent and people who are incapacitated.

   a. there is no difference
   b. incompetent people are unable to do things competently
   c. incapacitated people have lost their capacitors
   d. "incapacitated" sounds nicer

7. Define "competency."

   a. Ability to do complicated tasks.
   b. Having decisional capacity.
   c. Able to make good decisions.
   d. Making decisions the practitioner recommends.

8. Which is NOT a component of decisional capacity?

   a. able to think and decide
   b. able to understand information
   c. able to make a living will
   d. able to understand the consequences of a decision

9. The title of the person appointed by a court for an incompetent person is the _____ of the ward.

   a. attorney in fact
   b. surrogate decision maker
   c. health care director
   d. guardian

10. What is the effect of advance directives if the patient is competent?

    a. no effect
    b. effective
    c. revoked
    d. operative

11. A spoken advance directive, a living will, was used in which case?

    a. Busalacchi
    b. Cruzan
    c. O'Connor
    d. Quinlan

12. Why do some people think a written advance directive is preferable to a spoken one?

    a. signed by the maker
    b. written by a lawyer
    c. more easily proved in court
    d. uses legal language

13. State the main requirement of the Danforth Amendment to the Medicare law (or the Patient Self-Determination Act).

    a. educate the public about advance directives
    b. write policies for staff education
    c. inform staff of patient's rights
    d. inform patients of their rights

14. Which distinction is most helpful?

    a. withhold versus withdraw
    b. active versus passive
    c. limit treatment versus treat
    d. withhold versus refuse

15. Which is truth, not myth, about terminating life support?

    a. a court order is necessary to withdraw treatment
    b. patients have rights to refuse treatment
    c. withdrawing is legally more difficult than withholding treatment
    d. discontinuing treatment is murder

16. Which is an example of practitioner acquiescence to patient demands that will not make it harder for practitioners to assert their autonomy to decide when treatment is futile?

    a. appendectomy
    b. abortion
    c. cosmetic surgery
    d. sterilization

17. When a "tool" or measurement of health or illness or quality of life is made, the attempt is to make the measurement _____.

    a. subjective
    b. objective
    c. accurate
    d. infallible

18. Of the 20 million people who have died from decisions to limit treatment since the 1976 <u>Quinlan</u> case, about how many court cases on that issue have been recorded?

   a. 6000
   b. 600
   c. 60
   d. 6

19. Distinguish between the use of the term "substituted judgment" and "best interest."

   a. "substituted judgment" is subjective
   b. "best interest" is objective
   c. "best interest" is too many words
   d. the end result of the test is the same

20. Which is <u>not</u> one of the three standards of evidence discussed and used in American courts.

   a. preponderance of the evidence
   b. beyond a reasonable doubt
   c. clear and convincing beyond a reasonable certainty
   d. clear and convincing

21. Identify a source of rights, remedy, or relief for persons who want treatment terminated, other than the U.S. Constitution.

   a. state statutes
   b. state constitutions
   c. federal statutes
   d. federal regulations

22. Define "death."

   a. absence of life
   b. cessation of respiration and pulse only
   c. brain stem death
   d. persistent vegetative state

23. Identify a disease in which the patient diagnosed as such was declared to be dead.

   a. syphilis
   b. leprosy
   c. cancer
   d. plague

24. Which is most clearly artificial, not natural, feeding.

    a. cooked food
    b. with a spoon
    c. feeding tube
    d. bottle and nipple

25. Which is not one of the conditions under which CPR was considered effective in the first instance.

    a. terminal cancer
    b. drowning
    c. anesthesia collapse
    d. witnessed arrest

26. Describe the only condition under which CPR is not performed in most institutions.

    a. cancer diagnosed
    b. age over 80
    c. DNR ordered
    d. nursing home resident

27. Identify the Nazi assumption that allowed killing of millions of people.

    a. some lives were not worth living
    b. some people did not want to live
    c. some people did not fit with the ideal person
    d. some people were not really persons

28. Which is not one of the three pairs of conditions applied to euthanasia.

    a. direct or indirect
    b. killing or letting die
    c. passive or active
    d. voluntary or involuntary

29. Euthanasia and assisted suicide, are relatively new ethical conflicts.

    a. True
    b. False

30. Euthanasia is not illegal in Holland.

    a. True
    b. False

31. People who get old have failed to take care of themselves in some way.

    a. True
    b. False

32. The determination of competence is a legal process only.

    a. True
    b. False

33. The practitioner's standard for decisional capacity or competence is always a personal one at first because we have only our own reasoning as a guide; we must first measure the patient's against that.

    a. True.
    b. False.

34. Advance Directives as they are used in illness care, do not include _____.

    a. living wills.
    b. durable power of attorney for health care.
    c. health care surrogate document.
    d. last will and testament.

35. Spoken living wills are _____.

    a. valid.
    b. invalid.
    c. written.
    d. incompetent.

36. According to studies, most people do not want their advance directives followed rigidly.

    a. True.
    b. False.

CALIFORNIA COLLEGE FOR HEALTH SCIENCES
FINAL EXAM SCHEDULING CARD

FOR ASSOCIATE, BACHELORS, AND MASTERS COURSES

The Final Exam Scheduling Card must be submitted at least one month prior to the date that you wish to take the Final Exam.

All courses at California College for Health Sciences include at least one exam that requires the assistance of a proctor. Such an exam is sent directly to the proctor who administers the exam and returns the results to the College for scoring. The proctor is expected to verify that the student has completed the exam without the aid of study materials or outside assistance of any kind. It is up to you and your proctor to arrange a time and a place for the exam that is convenient for both of you.

You are responsible for identifying someone who is willing to serve as a proctor and for getting that person's qualifications submitted to the College for approval. The proctor should be a disinterested party who has no direct personal or professional involvement with you. Individuals who qualify as proctors include personnel such as: hospital administrators, Director of Personnel/Human Resources, librarians, counselors, Director of Education. If an approved proctor becomes unavailable, you must find a suitable replacement and submit a new Final Exam Scheduling Card. DO NOT submit the Final Exam Scheduling Card until all Unit Exams are successfully completed.

To prepare for the Final Exam, review your lessons, Unit Exams, and reading assignments. The testing staff is here to help you through final testing smoothly and without problems. If you have any questions, please call. Study hard and good luck!

Final Exam grades will NOT be released over the phone.
You can expect to have your exam results within three weeks of the completed
exam being mailed to **CCHS** by your proctor.

Please RUSH! This is my

Request for Help

The QUICKEST AND EASIEST way for you to get help in your CCHS program is to use this form. Your questions or comments may be on the course materials, your student account, or anything else related to your program. Mail or FAX this form, and your questions will be answered promptly.

Name: _____ **Date:** _____

Address: _____

City: _____ **State:** _____ **Zip:** _____

Course: _____ **Social Security #:** _____

Home Phone #: ( ) _____ **Work Phone #:** ( ) _____

☐ **YES! I would like CCHS to FAX the response to me at** ( ) _____

Instructions: Please type or write legibly and state your question clearly.

CCHS RESPONSE

If you need further assistance, please feel free to contact me. We appreciate your questions or comments, and we are pleased to be able to assist you.

Response prepared by: _____ Date: _____

Please RUSH! This is my
Request for Help

The QUICKEST AND EASIEST way for you to get help in your CCHS program is to use this form. Your questions or comments may be on the course materials, your student account, or anything else related to your program. Mail or FAX this form, and your questions will be answered promptly.

Name: _____ **Date:** _____

Address: _____

City: _____ **State:** _____ **Zip:** _____

Course: _____ **Social Security #:** _____

Home Phone #: (   ) _____ **Work Phone #:** (   ) _____

❏ **YES! I would like CCHS to FAX the response to me at** (   ) _____

Instructions: Please type or write legibly and state your question clearly.

CCHS RESPONSE

If you need further assistance, please feel free to contact me. We appreciate your questions or comments, and we are pleased to be able to assist you.

Response prepared by: _____ Date: _____

Please RUSH! This is my
Request for Help

The QUICKEST AND EASIEST way for you to get help in your CCHS program is to use this form. Your questions or comments may be on the course materials, your student account, or anything else related to your program. Mail or FAX this form, and your questions will be answered promptly.

Name: _____ **Date:** _____

Address: _____

City: _____ **State:** _____ **Zip:** _____

Course: _____ **Social Security #:** _____

Home Phone #: ( ) _____ **Work Phone #:** ( ) _____

☐ **YES! I would like CCHS to FAX the response to me at** ( ) _____

Instructions: Please type or write legibly and state your question clearly.

CCHS RESPONSE

If you need further assistance, please feel free to contact me. We appreciate your questions or comments, and we are pleased to be able to assist you.

Response prepared by: _____ Date: _____